NEURODEGENERATIVE DISEASES - LABORATORY AND CLINICAL RESEARCH

THE PRION PHENOMENA IN NEURODEGENERATIVE DISEASES

NEW FRONTIERS IN NEUROSCIENCE

NEURODEGENERATIVE DISEASES - LABORATORY AND CLINICAL RESEARCH

Additional books in this series can be found on Nova's website under the Series tab.

Additional e-books in this series can be found on Nova's website under the e-book tab.

NEURODEGENERATIVE DISEASES - LABORATORY AND CLINICAL RESEARCH

THE PRION PHENOMENA IN NEURODEGENERATIVE DISEASES

NEW FRONTIERS IN NEUROSCIENCE

GIUSEPPE LEGNAME
AND
GABRIELE GIACHIN
EDITORS

New York

Library of Congress Cataloging-in-Publication Data

ISBN: 978-1-63483-399-8
Library of Congress Control Number: 2015945228

Published by Nova Science Publishers, Inc. † New York

CONTENTS

Preface **vii**

About the Editors **ix**

List of Contributors **xi**

Chapter 1 Neuropathological Phenotypes in Human Prion Disorders **1**
Gianluigi Zanusso, Sergio Ferrari and Salvatore Monaco

Chapter 2 X-ray Fiber Diffraction from Prions: Of Mice and Beta-Solenoids **15**
Holger Wille

Chapter 3 Neurotoxicity in Prion Disease: Relationships with Other Neurodegenerative Diseases and Outlooks for Therapeutic Intervention **29**
Cathryn L. Ugalde, Victoria A. Lawson, David I. Finkelstein and Andrew F. Hill

Chapter 4 Glycosaminoglycans in Prion and Prion-like Diseases **67**
Tuane C. R. G. Vieira and Jerson L. Silva

Chapter 5 Complexity of Aggregation Pathway of α -synuclein **89**
Leonid Breydo and Vladimir N. Uversky

Chapter 6 Structural Characterization of α-synuclein Amyloids **111**
Wolfgang Hoyer, Hamed Shaykhalishahi, Santhosh Ayalur-Karunakaran and Henrike Heise

Chapter 7 Prion-Like Spreading of Aβ and tau Aggregates and their Relevance as Drivers of Pathology in Alzheimer's Disease **129**
Giuseppe Di Fede, Marcella Catania and Fabrizio Tagliavini

Chapter 8 Tau Strains and Their Propagation in Experimental Disease Models **157**
Kyle P. McHugh, Olga A. Morozova and David W. Colby

Chapter 9 Prion-Like Mechanisms in Amyotrophic Lateral Sclerosis **177**
Leslie I. Grad, Edward Pokrishevsky and Neil R. Cashman

Chapter 10	Prions in Yeast: Thinking Outside of the Brain *Polina Drozdova and Andrew Matveenko*	**209**
Chapter 11	Functional Prions: The Case Study of Aplysia *Eric R. Kandel*	**237**
Chapter 12	Concluding Remarks *Giuseppe Legname, Suzana Aulić and Gabriele Giachin*	**255**
Index		**263**

"Oh how I shall enjoy the journey back! Every station will be bringing me nearer to my soul's peace. O how I shall feel when I see the castle of Miramar among the trees and the long yellow quays of Trieste! Why is it I am destined to look so many times in my life with my eyes of longing on Trieste?"

James Joyce (1882-1941), Letter to Nora Barnacle, 27th October 1909.

PREFACE

Aberrant protein folding and self-assembly underlie over 30 untreatable human diseases called protein misfolding diseases or proteinopathies. These diseases range from tissue-specific to systemic and from genetic to sporadic. Some of the most devastating protein-related disorders are those that affect the central nervous system, such as Alzheimer's disease (AD), Parkinson's disease (PD), prion diseases and amyotrophic lateral sclerosis (ALS). In each disease, one or more proteins self-associate into toxic oligomers that disrupt cellular function and communication, and proceed to form insoluble amyloid aggregates characterized by fibrillar morphology and cross-β structure. Recent evidence argues that specific protein prions feature in the pathogenesis of several neurodegenerative diseases.

Prions are the causative agents of rare human and animal neurodegenerative diseases denoted transmissible spongiform encephalopathy (TSE). The most fascinating and unique feature of TSE is that it is caused almost exclusively by a proteinaceous and infectious particle termed prions, a concept introduced by S.B. Prusiner, who discovered this class of pathogens. In 1990s the mad-cow disease—a disease caused by prions acquired through foodborne transmission—provoked an unprecedented public scare due the concrete possibility that prions in animals could be transmitted to humans through the food chain and from human to human during surgical practices. For about two decades, prions were under deep scrutiny by scientists and public institutions everywhere. These investigations have led our community to a better risk management of prion diseases in humans and in animals, substantially limiting the possibility of new epidemics in the world.

Nowadays, prions have again been brought to the foreground after the discovery that a variety of neurodegenerative diseases—for instance, AD, PD and ALS—share features with prions, including protein misfolding and aggregation in the brain, as well as cell-to-cell transmission.

The increasing interest of the scientific community toward the prion phenomena in other neurodegenerative diseases, as well as the outstanding quality of the research papers published in the field, gave us the idea to publish this book. This happened during the PRION 2014 (May 27-30, 2014), the world's largest research congress on prion and protein misfolding diseases held in Trieste, Italy, in the middle of the old Europe. At that time, the forum for discussing the prion phenomena started to be particularly vibrant and accelerated the interest of the scientific community toward new investigations in this direction.

The Prion Phenomena in Neurodegenerative Diseases: New Frontiers in Neuroscience is a book project that benefits from the contribution of research groups who brought an extensive set of experiences and knowledge in different fields of neuroscience. The generous collaboration with these talented scientists has led to the collection of original chapters that cover the prion phenomena at structural, molecular, clinical and functional levels.

The chapters discuss in detail different diseases associated with protein misfolding and aggregation, providing an overview about the general mechanisms of cytotoxicity induced by amyloidogenic proteins and about the structural organization of these amyloidal protein aggregates. In particular, special emphasis is given on the correlation existing between the molecular and pathological features of human prion diseases (e.g., Creutzfeldt Jakob diseases) and other common age-related disorders, such as AD, PD and ALS. Finally, this book also covers the recent findings on physiological prions discovered in lower model organisms—such as in yeasts and in the sea slug *Aplysia californica*—as functional epigenetic factors.

This book represents an up-to-date review of different protein-misfolding diseases, serving as an invaluable tool for both specialized researchers working in the field of neurodegeneration and for a broad spectrum of academic readers that wish to learn more about the prion phenomena.

As editors of this book, we wish to express our sincere thank you to all the authors that contributed to this project: without their knowledge, enthusiastic participation and generosity in providing outstanding scientific material within their chapters, this book would not have been possible. Lastly, we would like to thank our publisher, Nova Science, for their great support and for patience in allowing us to assemble this multidisciplinary text.

The Editors

ABOUT THE EDITORS

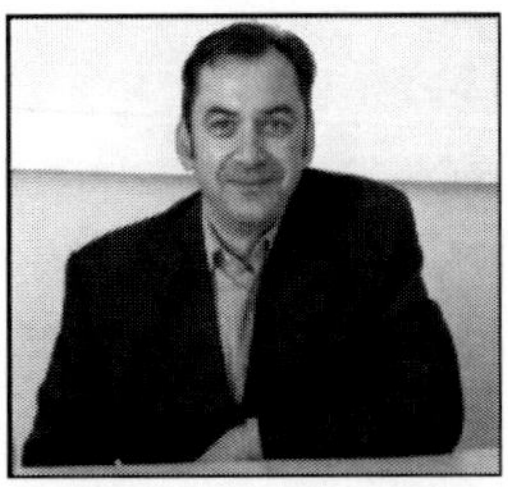

Professor Giuseppe Legname earned his Doctor of Philosophy at the University of Warwick, UK. After a long spell in industry in the field of immunotherapy, he moved to the National Institute for Medical Research (NIMR), Medical Research Council in London, UK as a Research Associate. In 1999 he became Assistant Adjunct Professor, and later Associate Adjunct Professor, at the Institute for Neurodegenerative Diseases (IND), University of California at San Francisco, USA, under the direction of 1997 Nobel Laureate Professor Stanley B. Prusiner. Since then he has been involved in basic research projects in the field of Prion Biology and Disease. In 2006 he joined the faculty of SISSA in Trieste as Associate Professor at the Department of Neuroscience. Currently he is the Coordinator of the PhD Program in Functional and Structural Genomics at SISSA and member-elect of the Academic Senate. He is a reviewer for several international journals and co-author of various patents. The main focus of his research program is the physiological function of the prion protein in mammals and the mechanisms of prion replication as well as the structural characterization of molecular determinants for prion infectivity.

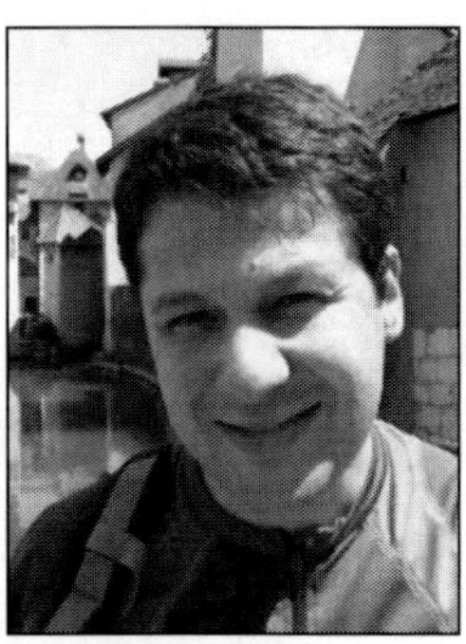

Dr. Gabriele Giachin is a structural biologist. After his M.Sc. in Agricultural Biotechnology at the University of Udine (Italy), he joined the group of Prof. Giuseppe Legname at SISSA (Trieste, Italy) where he earned his Ph.D. degree in Functional and Structural Genomics in 2012. During his Ph.D. he investigated the structural events leading to the conversion of the prion protein into pathological prions. He mainly used NMR approaches and at the Slovenian NMR centre (Prof. J. Plavec's group, Ljubljana, Slovenia) he obtained the NMR structures of different human prion protein mutants: these findings highlighted the role of the β_2-α_2 loop as hot spot for prion conversion. In his postdoctoral research at SISSA, he focused on the effect of mutations on copper coordination using cell biology and EXAFS techniques. He also investigated the role of Nanobodies as a drug able to halt prion propagation and with the J. Steyaert's group (Vrije Universiteit Brussel, Belgium) he solved the first X-ray crystal structure of the prion protein bound to a Nanobody. In October 2014 he joined the Structural Biology Group headed by Dr. Leonard Gordon at the European Synchrotron (ESRF, France) where he is working as a postdoctoral researcher with Dr. Montserrat Soler-Lopez, and studying by X-ray crystallography the structural features of novel Alzheimer disease-linked proteins, particularly the ECSIT proteins.

LIST OF CONTRIBUTORS

Suzana Aulić, MSc
Department of Neuroscience, Scuola Internazionale Superiore di Studi Avanzati (SISSA), Trieste, Italy

Dr. Santhosh Ayalur-Karunakaran, PhD
Heinrich Heine University Düsseldorf, Institute of Physical Biology, Universität, Düsseldorf, Germany

Leonid Breydo, PhD
Department of Molecular Medicine and bByrd Alzheimer's Research Institute, Morsani College of Medicine, University of South Florida, Tampa, Florida, United States

Neil R. Cashman, MD
Department of Medicine (Neurology), Djavad Mowafaghian Centre for Brain Health, University of British Columbia, Wesbrook Mall, Vancouver BC, Canada

Marcella Catania, PhD
Fondazione IRCSS "Carlo Besta" Neurological Institute, Division of Neurology V and Neuropathology, via Celoria, Milan, Italy

David W. Colby, PhD
Department of Chemical and Biomolecular Engineering, University of Delaware, Newark, Delaware, United States

Giuseppe Di Fede, PhD, MD
Fondazione IRCSS "Carlo Besta" Neurological Institute, Division of Neurology V and Neuropathology, via Celoria, Milan, Italy

Polina Drozdova, MSc
Dept. of Genetics and Biotechnology, Saint Petersburg State University, St. Petersburg, Russia

Sergio Ferrari, MD
Department of Neurological and Movement Sciences, University of Verona, Verona, Italy

David I. Finkelstein, PhD
Florey Institute for Neuroscience and Mental Health, Parkville, Victoria, Australia

Gabriele Giachin, PhD
Structural Biology Group, European Synchrotron Radiation Facility (ESRF), Grenoble, France

Leslie I. Grad, PhD
Department of Medicine (Neurology), Djavad Mowafaghian Centre for Brain Health, University of British Columbia, Wesbrook Mall, Vancouver BC, Canada

Prof. Dr. Henrike Heise, PhD
Heinrich Heine University Düsseldorf, Institute of Physical Biology, Universität, Germany

Andrew Francis Hill, PhD
Department of Biochemistry and Molecular Biology, Bio21 Molecular Science & Biotechnology Institute, The University of Melbourne, Parkville, Victoria, Australia

Dr. Wolfgang Hoyer, PhD
Heinrich Heine University Düsseldorf, Institute of Physical Biology, Universität, Düsseldorf, Germany

Eric R. Kandel, MD
Zuckerman Mind Brain Behavior Institute; Department of Neuroscience; Kavli Institute for Brain Science; Howard Hughes Medical Institute, College of Physicians and Surgeons of Columbia University, New York State Psychiatric Institute, Riverside Drive, New York, NY, United States

Victoria A. Lawson, PhD
Department of Pathology, The University of Melbourne, Parkville, Victoria, Australia

Giuseppe Legname, PhD
Department of Neuroscience, Scuola Internazionale Superiore di Studi Avanzati (SISSA), Trieste, Italy

Andrew Matveenko, MSc
Dept. of Genetics and Biotechnology, Saint Petersburg State University, St. Petersburg, Russia

Kyle P. McHugh, MSc
Department of Chemical and Biomolecular Engineering, University of Delaware, Newark, Delaware 19716, United States

Salvatore Monaco, MD
Department of Neurological and Movement Sciences, University of Verona, Verona, Italy

Olga A. Morozova, MSc
Department of Chemical and Biomolecular Engineering, University of Delaware, Newark, Delaware, United States

Edward Pokrishevsky, MSc
Department of Medicine (Neurology), Djavad Mowafaghian Centre for Brain Health, University of British Columbia, Wesbrook Mall, Vancouver BC, Canada

Dr. Hamed Shaykhalishahi, PhD
Heinrich Heine University Düsseldorf, Institute of Physical Biology, Universität Düsseldorf, Germany

Jerson L. Silva, Ph.D., MD
Centro Nacional de Ressonância Magnética Nuclear Jiri Jonas, Instituto de Bioquímica Médica Leopoldo De Meis, Instituto Nacional de Ciência e Tecnologia de Biologia Estrutural e Bioimagem, Universidade Federal do Rio de Janeiro, Rio de Janeiro, Brazil

Fabrizio Tagliavini, MD
Fondazione IRCSS "Carlo Besta" Neurological Institute, Division of Neurology V and Neuropathology, via Celoria, Milan, Italy

Cathryn L. Ugalde, BSc(hons)
Department of Biochemistry and Molecular Biology, Bio21 Molecular Science & Biotechnology Institute, The University of Melbourne, Parkville, Victoria, Australia

Vladimir N. Uversky, PhD, DSc
Department of Molecular Medicine and bByrd Alzheimer's Research Institute, Morsani College of Medicine, University of South Florida, Tampa, Florida

Tuane C. R. G. Vieira, PhD
Instituto Federal do Rio de Janeiro, Rio de Janeiro, Brazil

Holger Wille, PhD
Centre for Prions and Protein Folding Diseases and Department of Biochemistry, University of Alberta, Edmonton, Alberta, Canada

Gianluigi Zanusso, PhD, MD
Department of Neurological and Movement Sciences, University of Verona, Verona, Italy

In: The Prion Phenomena in Neurodegenerative Diseases
Editors: Giuseppe Legname and Gabriele Giachin
ISBN: 978-1-63483-399-8

Chapter 1

NEUROPATHOLOGICAL PHENOTYPES IN HUMAN PRION DISORDERS

Gianluigi Zanusso*, Sergio Ferrari and Salvatore Monaco

Department of Neurological and Movement Sciences,
University of Verona, Verona, Italy

ABSTRACT

Although novel diagnostic tests provide *intra vitam* detection of prions, neuropathology remains the gold standard for definite diagnosis in human prion disorders. In particular, the classification of prion affected subjects in specific groups, as well as the identification of novel phenotypes, is mainly based on the characteristics of spongiform changes distribution, astrogliosis and pattern of PrP^{Sc} deposition. Moreover, in sporadic Creutzfeldt-Jakob disease (sCJD), the implementation of neuropathology with molecular typing allowed to identify distinct disease phenotypes related to the glycotype of protease-resistant PrP^{Sc} and the polymorphism methionine/valine at codon 129, but also to identify atypical cases which differed from conventional cases. In addition, neuropathology allows the characterization of prion strains following experimental transmission to rodents. In this chapter, we show the spectrum of different pathological phenotypes observed in typical and atypical sCJD showing distinct pathological features. Finally, we show the neuropathological features and pattern of prion protein deposition distinctive of sCJD phenotypes and other human forms, such as Gerstman-Straussler-Scheincker.

INTRODUCTION

Prion diseases or transmissible spongiform encephalopathies (TSEs) are fatal neurodegenerative disorders of humans and animals. They occur as sporadic, genetic or acquired forms and include Creutzfeldt-Jakob disease (CJD), Gerstmann-Sträussler-Scheinker

* Corresponding Author address. Email: gianluigi.zanusso@univr.it.

(GSS), and fatal familial insomnia (FFI) in humans [1, 2, 3]. Genetic prion diseases are associated with different mutations in the prion protein gene (*PRNP*) which segregate with distinct clinical and pathological phenotypes [4, 5, 6]. Sporadic CJD (sCJD) is the most common form and thus it has been here extensively reviewed, including the clinical features associated with each molecular subtype, neuroimaging findings, cerebrospinal fluid markers. Definite diagnosis is still based on post mortem examination of brain relying on the detection of proteinase-K resistant PrP (PrP^{Sc}) and on specific neuropathological alterations [7]. Biochemical analysis is extremely useful, and consists of a rapid test which provides a series of basic information linked to PrP^{Sc} glycotyping, such as the distinction between sporadic CJD and variant, and between CJD and GSS, furthermore it identifies the occurrence of atypical glycotypes. Neuropathological examination is a final step for case definition, it is based on the recognition of the extent of spongiform changes, gliosis, neuronal loss. PrP^{Sc} pattern of deposition is also addressing the diagnosis and, although neuropathology is an old fashioned procedure, it allows a prion disease diagnosis nearly to 100% of cases [4].

SPORADIC CREUTZFELDT-JAKOB DISEASE

Sporadic Creutzfeldt-Jakob disease (sCJD) accounts for 85% of all CJD cases with annual worldwide incidence of 1-2 cases/million population [8]. The peak age of onset is between 65 and 75 years, albeit cases younger than 20 years and older than 90 years have been reported [9, 10]. sCJD diagnosis is based on clinical symptoms characterized by a rapidly progressive dementia accompanied to cerebellar signs, visual disturbances, pyramidal and extrapyramidal signs, myoclonus, ending in akinetic mutism. Supportive investigations include the detection of 14-3-3 protein in the cerebrospinal fluid (CSF), the evidence of hyperintense signals on T2, FLAIR or diffusion-weighted sequences (DWI) in basal ganglia or in cortical ribbon of cerebral cortex at magnetic resonance imaging (MRI), and the demonstration of typical complexes of periodic sharp and slow wave at electroencephalogram (EEG) [11, 12, 13]. On the basis of clinical signs and supportive tests, current diagnostic criteria classify sCJD cases as possible and probable, while definite diagnosis relies on neuropathology showing the typical spongiform changes and/or on detecting the disease-associated proteinase-K resistant prion protein or PrP^{Sc} in the brain tissue [14].

sCJD is characterized by an heterogeneous number of clinical variants including Heidenhain, classical, myoclonic, thalamic, cerebellar or ataxic, and panencephalopathic form [15, 16, 17, 18]. More recently, clinical variants were grouped within distinct molecular subtypes. Molecular classification was originally proposed by Parchi et al., and accounts for *PRNP* polymorphism methionine (M) valine (V) at codon 129 and for the glycotype (type 1 or type 2) of the protease-resistant component of PrP^{Sc} [5, 19, 20]. The combination between M129V genotypes and the two PrP^{Sc} glycotypes results in distinct pathological subtypes of sCJD (Figure 1 and Table 1).

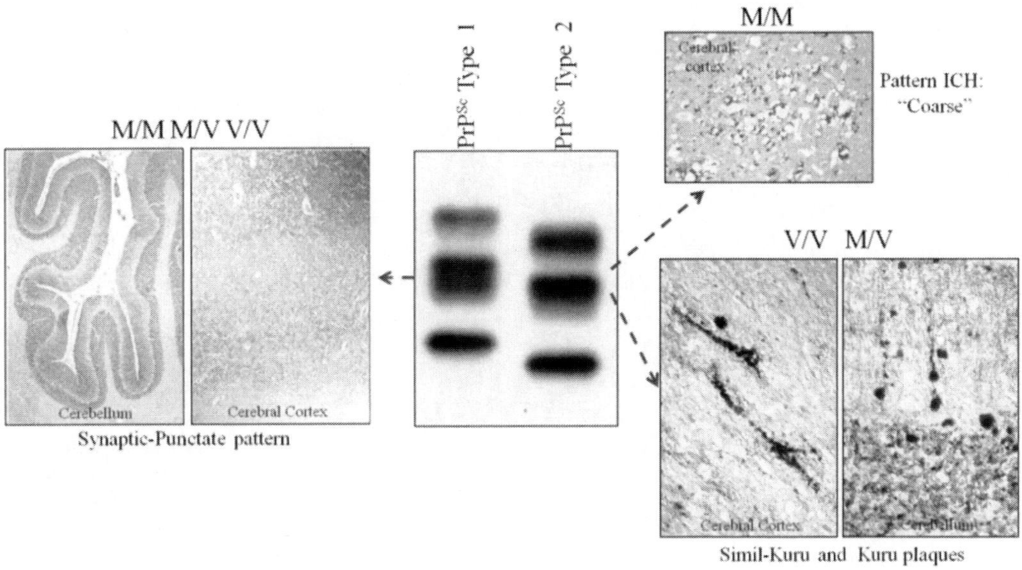

Figure 1. Molecular basis of pathological phenotypes in sCJD. PK-resistant PrPSc glycotypes, PrP^{Sc} type 1 and PrP^{Sc} type 2 in combination with polymorphisms M or V at codon 129 correlate to distinct pathological phenotypes. PrP^{Sc} Type 1 combined with 129 MM, MV or VV result in a synaptic punctate pattern of PrP^{Sc} deposition. Differently, PrP^{Sc} type 2 combined with a MM results in large vacuoles and coarse perivacuolar PrP^{Sc} deposition or if the host is MV or VV at codon 129 PrP^{Sc} pattern is characterized by large aggregates (VV) or amyloid plaques (MV).

Table 1. Demographic, clinical and neuropathological characterisitcs of sCJD molecular subtypes

Molecular subtypes	Clinical variants	Relative %	Mean duration (months)	Clinical features at onset	Diagnosic test			Neuropathology
					PSWCs	14-3-3	MRI	
MM1 or MV1	Myoclonic, heidenhain variant	70	3.9	Rapidly progressive dementia, myoclonus, visual signs	80%	90%	Striatum and cortical ribbon	Spongiosis with small vacuoles (<10mm) predominantly in neocortex, striatum, focal in cerebellar cortex, with sparing of hippocampus. Synaptic punctate pattern of PrP^{Sc} deposition in spongiotic areas.
VV2	Ataxic Variant	16	6.5	Ataxia	50%	100%	Striatum and cortical Ribbon	Spongiosis predominates in deep layers of neocortex, limbic cortex, hippocampus, striatum, thalamus and brainstem. Large and plaque-like aggregates of PrP^{Sc} in affected areas. Perineurial and intracellular staining in deep layers of cerebral cortex.
MV2	Kuru-Plaque variant amyotrophic	9	17.1	Ataxia, extrapyramidal signs	30%	50%	Cortical ribbon striatum and thalamus	Spongiosis anf PrP^{Sc} deposits similar to VV2 type, but presence of Kuru-type amyloid plaques, also identifiable in haematoxylin-eosin stain and PrP^{Sc} positive predominantly in molecular and granular layer of cerebellum.
MM2 Thalamic	Thalamic variant	2	15.6	Insomnia, ataxia	-	-	Thalamus	Athophy and slight spongiosis of medial thalamic and inferior olivary nuclei. Faint synaptic staining of PrP^{Sc}.
MM2 Cortical	Cognitive	2	15.7	Progressive dementia	-	50%	Cortical ribbon	Large vacuoles of confluent spongiosis predominatly in cerebral cortexes and striatum. Perivacuolar and “coarse” pattern of PrP^{Sc} deposits.
VV1	Not established	1	15.3	Progressive dementia	-	-	Cortical ribbon	Fine vacuoles of spongiosis in cerebral cortex and striatum, Fine and faint punctate pattern of PrP^{Sc} deposition.

Clinical and Pathological Features of Sporadic Creutzfeldt-Jakob Disease in Each Distinct Molecular Subtypes

MM1 and MV1 Subtype

This is the most common subtype of sCJD accounting for 60–70% of all cases is MM1. It corresponds to the clinical variant previously described as myoclonic or 'classic' and Heidenhain's variant. The mean age of disease onset of the symptoms is 68 years with a range of 17–99 years and a mean clinical duration of 4 months with a range of 1–18. Prodromal symptoms are usually psychiatric changes characterized by depression and anxiety followed by a rapidly progressive cognitive decline, gait ataxia or hallucinations. The EEG is typical in about 80% of all cases, 14-3-3 protein is positive and MRI shows a hyperintense signal in FLAIR and DWI in striatum and in the cortical ribbon [21]. Neuropathologically it is characterized predominantly by microspongiosis, astrogliosis and neuronal loss. Spongiform degeneration affects all the brain areas but in particular the occipital and frontal cortex, but is evident also in molecular layer of cerebellar cortex. PrP^{Sc} shows a punctate pattern of synaptic staining with an intensity extent related with spongiform changes (Figure 2, A-D). In this group, around 30% of cases show "mixed" pathological changes characterized by brain areas with typical spongiform changes and a synaptic pattern of PrP^{Sc} deposition together with areas showing large vacuoles with perivacuolar PrP^{Sc} deposits. These pathological features might be observed in the same patient in different brain areas or in the same brain area. These cases with a co-occurence of different pathological pattern have been classified as mixed type1/2 and conventionally named as 129 genotype and 1/2 (i.e., MM1/2) (Figure 2, G, H) [22, 23, 24].

MM2 Cortical Subtype

MM2 cortical occurs in 2–8% of cases. The mean age at onset is 60 years with a 44–70 year range, and the average disease duration is 16 months. A progressive dementing illness involving all cognitive domains is the main clinical feature, and thus the diagnosis of sCJD might be overlooked [25]. In the late course of the illness patients develop myoclonic jerks or epileptic seizures. The EEG characteristically shows non-specific slowing, albeit occasionally non-periodic paroxysmal discharges might be observed. 14-3-3 protein in CSF might be positive in 50% of cases depending on the degree of disease progression. MRI shows a hyperintense signal involving the whole cortical ribbon with a relative sparing of basal ganglia. The hallmarks of MM2 subtype are spongiform changes characterized by large vacuoles in the cerebral cortex, basal ganglia and thalamus which might be confluent. It is important to underline that in MM2 cerebellum is spared distinguishing those MM1/2 from pure MM2. PrP^{Sc} surrounds the vacuoles showing a "coarse" pattern of deposition (Figure 2, E, F).

MM2 Thalamic Subtype

MM2 thalamic subtype accounts for about 2% of all cases, corresponding to the thalamic variant of sCJD. Originally it was described by Gambetti in 1998 showing that it is clinically indistinguishable from that of fatal familial insomnia (FFI) and is named as sporadic fatal insomnia (sFI) [26, 27]. The mean age at onset is 50 years (range, 36–70 years) and the mean duration 24 months (range, 15–53 months). The clinical presentation commonly includes ataxia, visual signs and cognitive impairment. Most patients eventually show insomnia, dementia, and motor signs including ataxia, dysarthria, tremor, myoclonus and spasticity. The EEG shows non-specific slowing. The major pathological changes are centred in the thalamus especially the medial dorsal and anterior ventral nuclei, and consist in severe astrogliosis and neuronal loss but generally without spongiform degeneration. The inferior olivary nucleus also shows similar lesions. Other brain regions are less affected. Minimal focal spongiform degeneration affects anterior neocortical regions and the entorhinal cortex. PrP^{Sc} deposition is inconsistent or weak and localized in entorhinal cortex [28].

MV2 and VV2 Sutypes

In these subtypes, accounting for 15% in VV2 and 8% in MV2, the mean age at onset is around 60 years with a range of 41–81 years and the clinical duration is 6 months for VV2 but patients MV2 show a disease duration lasting till 72 months [29]. Depression and anxiety might be symptoms preceding neurological signs. While in VV2 the clinical presentation is always characterized by a subacute ataxia in the absence of dementia, in MV2 multiple neurological signs at onset are always found including ataxia, extrapyramidal features and cognitive deterioration. As disease progresses, dementia and subsequently myoclonus are observed in all patients. In a relatively rare number of cases of MV2 subjects, an involvement of motor neurons might be observed showing the clinical features of an amyotrophic variant. The EEG shows non-specific slowing in more than 90% patients and 14-3-3 protein might be negative in the early disease course becoming positive in the late stages of illness. MRI scans show a hyperintense signal in DWI and FLAIR sequences, on the whole cortical ribbon, basal ganglia and medial thalamus but sparing pulvinar. A blind study showed that the MRI distinction between MV2 and variant CJD is based on the preferential hyperintense signal in the striatum in MV2 and thalamus in vCJD. In particular, MV2 cases with amyotrophic variant shows hyperintensities in DWI at the level of the motor cortex, which is spared in all sCJD subtype [29, 30].

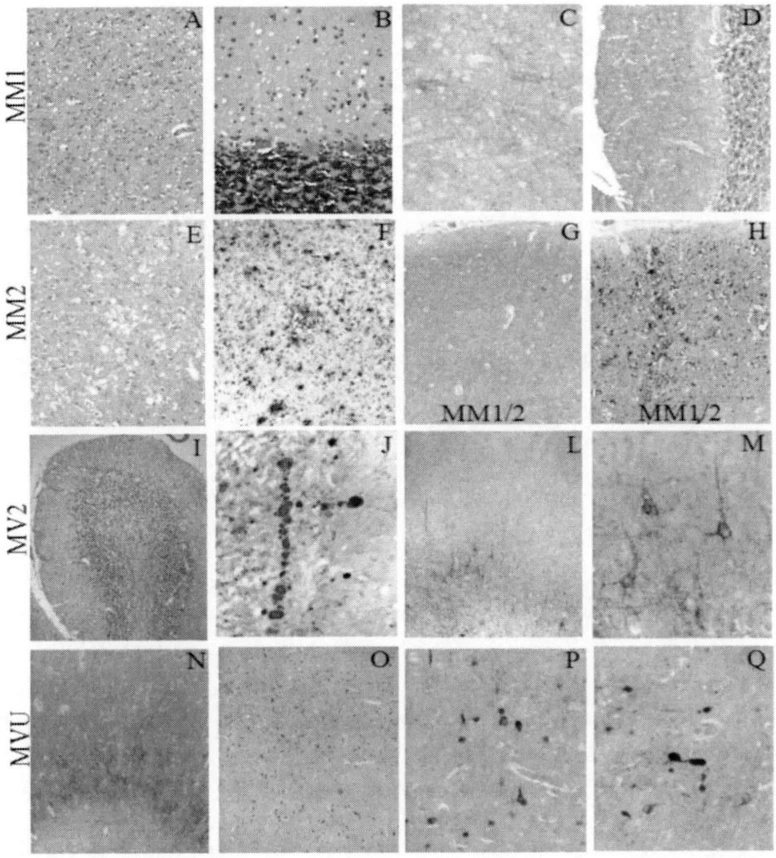

Figure 2. Histopathology and patterns of PrP^{Sc} immunoreactivity in CJD subtypes. In MM1 (A-D), spongiform changes with small vacuoles are observed in frontal cortex and molecular layer of cerebellum (A, B). Immunohistochemistry for PrP^{Sc} shows a homogeneous punctate pattern of deposition (C, D). In MM2 (E,F), spongiform changes are characterized by large vacuoles, often confluent resulting in cases with a long duration in status spongiosus, in contrast with the high involvement of cerebral cortexes, cerebellum is spared. PrP^{Sc} immunohistochemistry a perivacuolar while in the cerebellum PrP^{Sc} aggregates are very rarely observed in the molecular layer. In the same section of a frontal cortex from a patient with MM 1/2, the co-occurrence of a synaptic or coarse patterns of PrP^{Sc} deposition are observed (G,H); typical spongiosis is observed in the molecular layer of cerebellum in MV2 cases; Kuru plaques are shown in granule cell region of the cerebellum (I); immunohistochemistry shows a granular PrP^{Sc} deposition in deep layers of frontal cortex as well as a strong immunoreaction around neuronal somata and apical dendrites (L,M); In MVU subtype, PrP^{Sc} is mainly deposited in the deep layers of occipital cortex with a granular patter (N); a characteristics intracellular PrP^{Sc} deposition is observed in frontal cortex neurons (O, P) as well as positive axonal swellings in the thalamus (Q).

Neuropathologically, basal ganglia and cerebellum are highly affected while in frontal and occipital lobes the extent of pathology is related to disease duration. The late involvement of cerebral cortex represents the kinetics of disease spreading in both VV2 and MV2. Therefore, in cases with a relatively short duration brain biopsy might be non-diagnostic in cerebral cortex. Immunohistochemistry shows a PrP^{Sc} with a laminar distribution mainly deposited in deeper cortical layers under major aggregates or amyloid plaques, in VV2 and MV2 cases, respectively. Perineuronal and apical dendrites staining are also observed particularly in basal ganglia (Figure 2, M). Cerebellum is highly affected showing an intense immunostaining in the molecular and granular layer associated with the presence of numerous plaque-like VV2 or amyloid plaques in MV2 (Figure 2, I-M).

VV1 Subtype

VV1 subtype of sCJD occurs very rarely and it affects about 1% of all cases. Age at onset is 39 years and the mean duration is 15 months (range, 14–16 months). It is characterized by behavioural changes similar to what is observed in fronto-temporal dementia. EEG is usually slow but never typical. Positivity for 14-3-3 protein is unclear as well as the MRI pattern. In VV1 subtype, pathology affects cortico-striatal regions with severe spongiform changes. PrP^{Sc} immunostaining shows a faint synaptic pattern [31].

MVU Subtype

We originally described a 69-year-old woman with depression, behavioral disturbances and a severe rapidly evolving dementia. On the disease course she developed a social neglect, disorientation obsessive-compulsive behaviors, transient hallucinations evolving to akinetc mutism. MRI was negative. CSF showed a positive 14-3-3 protein and increased tau protein levels (1388 pg/ml). She died after 20 months from the onset. Differently from other sCJD, this cases showed a PrP^{Sc} glycotype lacking the diglycosylated isoform and PrP^{Sc} accumulated in neuronal perikarya and in axons (Figure 2, N-Q) [32]. 2D-PAGE analysis showed a pattern of PrP^{Sc} separation distinct from that observed in other sCJD subtypes and experimental transmission studies in TgHu mice revealed also a distinct pattern of propagation confirming that MVU subtype represents a novel prion strain (Galeno et al., unpublished observation).

Biochemical Typing Is a Criterion for Molecular Screening of sCJD Cases

In sporadic CJD (sCJD), the first step in sCJD definite diagnosis is based on PrP^{Sc} identification and glycotype characterization in brain tissue showing the different electrophoretic mobility of the unglycosylated form of PrP^{Sc}. Two distinct PrP^{Sc} glycotypes have been reported separating as three distinct bans representing the differently glycosylated isoforms of PrP^{Sc} migrating at 21 kDa and 19 kDa these glycotypes had been named respectively PrP^{Sc} type 1 and PrP^{Sc} type 2 [20, 33, 34]. However, we recently provided evidence that the molecular weights of PrP^{Sc} of type 1 and type 2 are 19 kDa and 17 kDa, respectively [35]. We described an additional PrP^{Sc} glycotype named type U lacking the diglycosylated isoform. However, a high percentage of sCJD shows a co-existence of both PrP^{Sc} types 1 and 2 correlating to distinct pathological phenotypes. This finding suggests that, rather than a pure type 1 or type 2 PrP^{Sc}, a variable mixture of PrP^{Sc} fragments are present in the brain generating confusion in molecular classification of a given sCJD case (Figure 3).

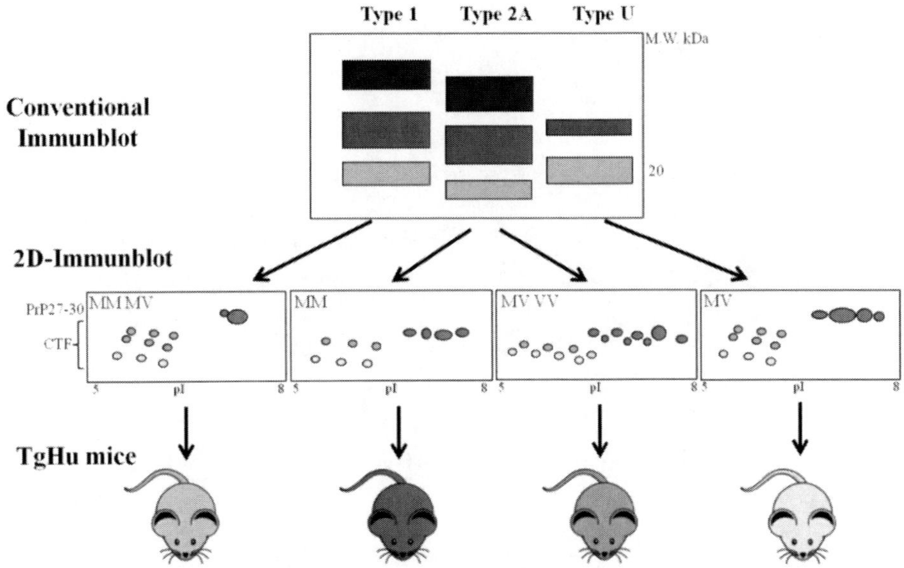

Figure 3. sCJD associated PrP^{Sc} glycotypes following 1D and 2D-PAGE analyses and transmission properties. The typical banding pattern of type 1 and type 2 PrP^{Sc} glycotypes is different from type U which lacks the highly glycosylated isoform, after SDS-PAGE analysis; following 2D-PAGE while PrP^{Sc} type 1 separates an homogeneous pattern regardless 129 polymorphisms, PrP^{Sc} type 2 shows two distinct patterns of separation in MM and in MV-VV subtypes; finally, PrP^{Sc} type U separates as an additional distinct pattern. After transmission in TgHu mice carrying all 129 genotypes, four distinct strains are defined: one associated with PrP^{Sc} type 1 MV and MM, one with PrP^{Sc} type 2 MM, one with PrP^{Sc} type 2 MV and VV and another with PrP^{Sc} type U, as observed following 2D separations [37].

Biochemical Characterization of PrP^{Sc} Using 2D-PAGE and Prion Strain Definition

Over the last years, we bypassed the conventional PrP^{Sc} typing adopting two-dimensional electrophoresis (2D-PAGE). Using this technique, we provided an extremely deep and informative characterization of PrP^{Sc} showing in sCJD three distinct groups of disease-associated PrP^{Sc} species are associated to type 1 PrP^{Sc}, MM and MV at codon 129 and other two associated with type 2 one in subjects MM and another in MV/VV (Figure 3). We claimed to have recognized by 2D-PAGE analysis the fingerprints of specific biochemical strain linked to distinct disease phenotypes [34, 36]. A subsequent study, confirmed our finding following transmission of brain samples from different sCJD subtypes (MM1/MV1, VV1, MM2c, MV2, VV2) into humanized transgenic mice resulting in four distinct sCJD strain of agent. Sporadic CJD MM1 and sCJD MV1 isolates showed identical transmission properties for all three genotypes of mice, MV2 and VV2 isolates had very similar transmission properties, and MM2 behave differently from other isolates [37]. Unfortunately, 2D-PAGE is demanding and rare laboratories were able to set up the technique and a large scale application was precluded.

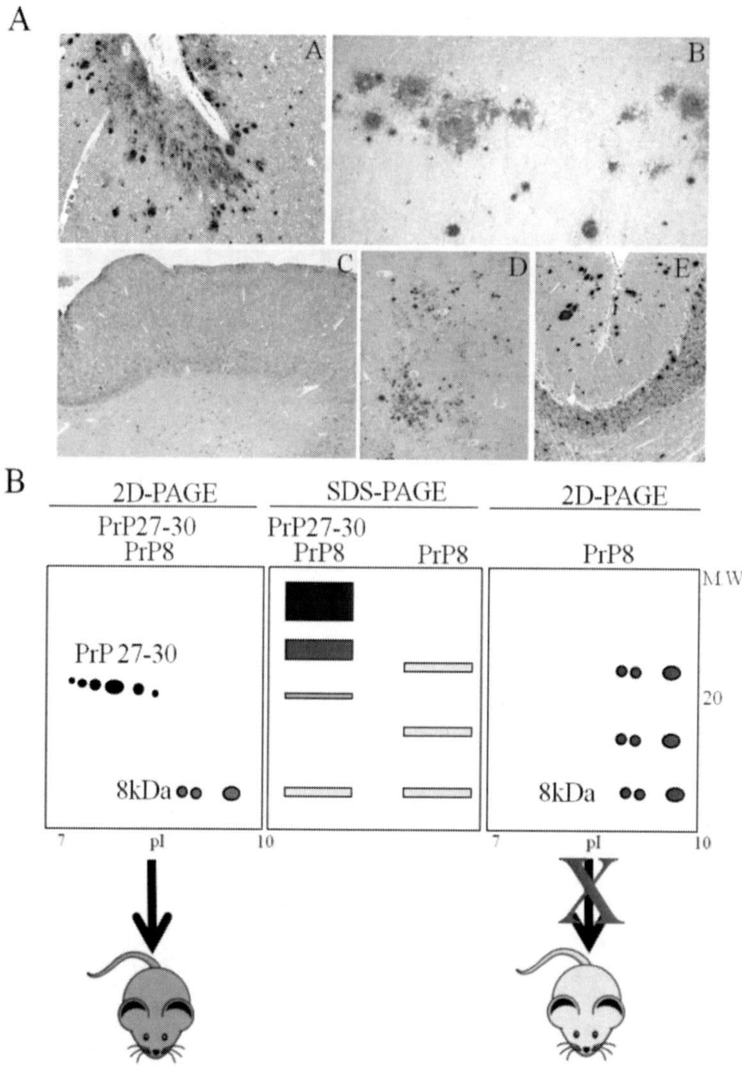

Figure 4. Immunohistochemistry showing PrP^{Sc} pattern associated with GSS P102L mutation. Panel A. Frontal cortex showing diffuse and multicentric amyloid PrP^{Sc} plaques in the outer layers of cerebral cortex and in the white matter (A, B); PrP^{Sc} deposition involving homogeneously the whole occipital cortex (C); multicentric PrP^{Sc} plaques (D); widespread deposition of amyloid palques in molecular and granular layers of cerebellum (E). Biochemical characterization and transmission properties of PrP^{Sc} associated with GSS P102L mutation. Panel B. Western blot analysis of proteinase K-resistant PrP^{Sc} in GSS P102L mutation shows the presence of two patterns one associated with three bands migrating at 29, 25 and 20 kDa, (PrP 27-30) in addition to variable amounts of an 8 kDa fragment and one lacking PrP 27-30.

In Vivo Diagnosis of sCJD

Biochemical and immunohistochemical examinations of brain tissue obtained by biopsy were considered definite methods for diagnosing CJD *in vivo*. This procedure allows to detect PrP^{Sc} and determine glycotype as well as to show typical neuropathologic changes. However, as carefully reported in previous paragraphs, in specific sCJD subtypes brain biopsy might provide a false negative result related to the kinetics of specific molecular subtypes. In the past, we also considered biopsy of the olfactory mucosa as a potential diagnostic tissue but this procedure was not further pursued because the information provided was sometimes inconclusive. Recently, a revolutionary diagnostic procedure such as RT-QuIC assay allows an *intra vitam* diagnosis of sCJD with a sensitivity and specificity nearly to 100%. This quantitative assay detects seeding activity in brain homogenate from sCJD in the order of femtograms. RT-QuIC was applied to cerebrospinal fluid samples from patients with and patients without sporadic Creutzfeldt–Jakob disease showing sensitivity in the order of 80 to 90% and a specificity of 100% [38, 39]. More recently, we provided evidence that a noninvasive procedure such as nasal-brushing, which allows a gentle collection of olfactory mucosa from a wide surface area of olfactory epithelium, improved RT-QuIC assay sensitivity to 100% [40, 41, 42, 43].

Gerstmann-Sträussler-Scheinker Syndrome (GSS)

Autosomal dominant inheritance of *PRNP* mutations may also lead to Gerstmann-Sträussler-Scheinker Syndrome (GSS). The peculiarity of GSS is that it shares the hallmarks of neurodegenerative disorders. It is characterized by a slowly progressive neurologic disease, extended over a period of 10 years with a wide spectrum of symptoms, including dementia, ataxia, paraparesis, extrapyramidal and pyramidal signs depending on a specific mutation and pathologically, it shows a widespread of PrP^{Sc} amyloid deposits accompanied with neurofibrillary tangles and dystrophic neurites. Furthermore, GSS are not transmissible and not spongiform changes are observed breaking the dogma of prion disorders with the exemption of P102L mutation. Several *PRNP* mutations have been shown to segregate with GSS: P102L, P105L, A117V, Y145X, Q160X, F198S, Q217R, Y218N, Y226X, Q227X and the most common mutation is P102L [44, 45, 46, 47, 48, 49]. This mutation has been largely studied phenotypic heterogeneity is also observed both within and between pedigrees with the same mutation, especially in P102L GSS cases. Accordingly, while in some P102L patients progressive gait disturbances, truncal ataxia, lower limb hyporeflexia and dysarthria are the presenting clinical features, followed over years by dementia and pyramidal signs, in other cases a rapid evolving dementia, indistinguishable from sporadic CJD (sCJD), is observed. Neuropathological examination in GSS P102L discloses marked variation in the degree and brain regional distribution of spongiform changes, which largely correlates with the biochemical detection of proteinase K (PK)-resistant PrP^{Sc} with a core fragment of 21 kDa (Figure 4). In P102L, biochemical analysis of P102L brain homogenates showed a group of subjects with both PrP 27-30 and an intermediate fragment of 8 kDa (spanning residues 80-150) and another group showing only 8 kDa PrP and lacking PrP 27-30 [50]. The presence of PrP 27-30 is associated with spongiform changes and transmissibility while cases with only 8 kDa fragments do not show spongiform changes and are not transmissible and show widespread amyloid PrP^{Sc} deposits and neurofibrillary tangles, as in non prion related neurodegenerative diseases (Figure 4).

REFERENCES

[1] Prusiner SB (1998) *Prions.* Proc Natl Acad Sci U S A 95: 13363-13383.
[2] Zanusso G, Monaco S (2005) Molecular mechanisms of human prion diseases. *Drug Discovery Today: Disease Mechanisms* 2: 511-518.
[3] Kraus A, Groveman BR, Caughey B (2013) Prions and the potential transmissibility of protein misfolding diseases. *Annu Rev Microbiol* 67: 543-564.
[4] Wadsworth JD, Hill AF, Beck JA, Collinge J (2003) Molecular and clinical classification of human prion disease. *Br Med Bull* 66: 241-254.
[5] Kovacs GG, Puopolo M, Ladogana A, Pocchiari M, Budka H, et al. (2005) Genetic prion disease: the EUROCJD experience. *Hum Genet* 118: 166-174.
[6] Mead S (2006) Prion disease genetics. *Eur J Hum Genet* 14: 273-281.
[7] Budka H, Aguzzi A, Brown P, Brucher JM, Bugiani O, et al. (1995) Neuropathological diagnostic criteria for Creutzfeldt-Jakob disease (CJD) and other human spongiform encephalopathies (prion diseases). *Brain Pathol* 5: 459-466.
[8] Ladogana A, Puopolo M, Croes EA, Budka H, Jarius C, et al. (2005) Mortality from Creutzfeldt-Jakob disease and related disorders in Europe, Australia, and Canada. *Neurology* 64: 1586-1591.
[9] Knight R (2006) Creutzfeldt-Jakob disease: a rare cause of dementia in elderly persons. *Clin Infect Dis* 43: 340-346.
[10] Buganza M, Ferrari S, Cecchini ME, Orrico D, Monaco S, et al. (2009) The oldest old Creutzfeldt-Jakob disease case. *J Neurol Neurosurg Psychiatry* 80: 1140-1142.
[11] Zanusso G (2006) Should MRI signs be included in the diagnostic criteria for sporadic Creutzfeldt-Jakob disease? *Nat Clin Pract Neurol* 2: 68-69.
[12] Vitali P, Maccagnano E, Caverzasi E, Henry RG, Haman A, et al. (2011) Diffusion-weighted MRI hyperintensity patterns differentiate CJD from other rapid dementias. *Neurology* 76: 1711-1719.
[13] Tagliapietra M, Zanusso G, Fiorini M, Bonetto N, Zarantonello G, et al. (2013) Accuracy of diagnostic criteria for sporadic creutzfeldt-jakob disease among rapidly progressive dementia. *J Alzheimers Dis* 34: 231-238.
[14] Zerr I, Kallenberg K, Summers DM, Romero C, Taratuto A, et al. (2009) Updated clinical diagnostic criteria for sporadic Creutzfeldt-Jakob disease. *Brain* 132: 2659-2668.
[15] Heidenhain A (1929) Klinische und anatomische Untersuchungen über eine eigenartige organische Erkrankung des Zentralnervensystems im Praesenium. *Zeitschrift für die gesamte Neurologie und Psychiatrie* 118: 49-114.
[16] Alema G, Bignami A (1959) [Subacute degenerative presenile polioencephalopathy with akinetic stupor and decorticate rigidity with myoclonus ("myoclonic" variety of the Jakob-Creutzfeld disease)]. *Riv Sper Freniatr Med Leg Alien Ment* 83(4)Suppl: 1485-1623.
[17] Nowacki P, Kulczycki J, Narolewska A, Grzelec H (2000) Amyotrophic form of Creutzfeldt-Jakob disease with rapid course in 82-year-old man. *Folia Neuropathol* 38: 161-163.
[18] Mittal M, Hammond N, Husmann K, Lele A, Pasnoor M (2010) Creutzfeldt-Jakob Disease Presenting as Bulbar Palsy. *Muscle & Nerve* 42: 833-835.

[19] Salvatore M, Genuardi M, Petraroli R, Masullo C, D'Alessandro M, et al. (1994) Polymorphisms of the prion protein gene in Italian patients with Creutzfeldt-Jakob disease. *Hum Genet* 94: 375-379.

[20] Parchi P, Giese A, Capellari S, Brown P, Schulz-Schaeffer W, et al. (1999) Classification of sporadic Creutzfeldt-Jakob disease based on molecular and phenotypic analysis of 300 subjects. *Ann Neurol* 46: 224-233.

[21] Zanusso G, Fiorini M, Ferrari S, Gajofatto A, Cagnin A, et al. (2011) Cerebrospinal fluid markers in sporadic Creutzfeldt-Jakob disease. *Int J Mol Sci* 12: 6281-6292.

[22] Puoti G, Giaccone G, Rossi G, Canciani B, Bugiani O, et al. (1999) Sporadic Creutzfeldt-Jakob disease: co-occurrence of different types of PrP(Sc) in the same brain. *Neurology* 53: 2173-2176.

[23] Uro-Coste E, Cassard H, Simon S, Lugan S, Bilheude JM, et al. (2008) Beyond PrP res type 1/type 2 dichotomy in Creutzfeldt-Jakob disease. *PLoS Pathog* 4: e1000029.

[24] Puoti G, Bizzi A, Forloni G, Safar JG, Tagliavini F, et al. (2012) Sporadic human prion diseases: molecular insights and diagnosis. *Lancet Neurol* 11: 618-628.

[25] Krasnianski A, Meissner B, Schulz-Schaeffer W, Kallenberg K, Bartl M, et al. (2006) Clinical features and diagnosis of the MM2 cortical subtype of sporadic Creutzfeldt-Jakob disease. *Arch Neurol* 63: 876-880.

[26] Parchi P, Capellari S, Chin S, Schwarz HB, Schecter NP, et al. (1999) A subtype of sporadic prion disease mimicking fatal familial insomnia. *Neurology* 52: 1757-1763.

[27] Mastrianni JA, Nixon R, Layzer R, Telling GC, Han D, et al. (1999) Prion protein conformation in a patient with sporadic fatal insomnia. *N Engl J Med* 340: 1630-1638.

[28] Scaravilli F, Cordery RJ, Kretzschmar H, Gambetti P, Brink B, et al. (2000) Sporadic fatal insomnia: a case study. *Ann Neurol* 48: 665-668.

[29] Heinemann U, Krasnianski A, Meissner B, Varges D, Kallenberg K, et al. (2007) Creutzfeldt-Jakob disease in Germany: a prospective 12-year surveillance. *Brain* 130: 1350-1359.

[30] Krasnianski A, Schulz-Schaeffer WJ, Kallenberg K, Meissner B, Collie DA, et al. (2006) Clinical findings and diagnostic tests in the MV2 subtype of sporadic CJD. *Brain* 129: 2288-2296.

[31] Meissner B, Westner IM, Kallenberg K, Krasnianski A, Bartl M, et al. (2005) Sporadic Creutzfeldt-Jakob disease: clinical and diagnostic characteristics of the rare VV1 type. *Neurology* 65: 1544-1550.

[32] Zanusso G, Polo A, Farinazzo A, Nonno R, Cardone F, et al. (2007) Novel prion protein conformation and glycotype in Creutzfeldt-Jakob disease. *Arch Neurol* 64: 595-599.

[33] Zanusso G, Farinazzo A, Fiorini M, Gelati M, Castagna A, et al. (2001) pH-dependent prion protein conformation in classical Creutzfeldt-Jakob disease. *J Biol Chem* 276: 40377-40380.

[34] Zanusso G, Farinazzo A, Prelli F, Fiorini M, Gelati M, et al. (2004) Identification of distinct N-terminal truncated forms of prion protein in different Creutzfeldt-Jakob disease subtypes. *J Biol Chem* 279: 38936-38942.

[35] Zanusso G, Fiorini M, Ferrari S, Meade-White K, Barbieri I, et al. (2014) Gerstmann-Straussler-Scheinker disease and "anchorless prion protein" mice share prion conformational properties diverging from sporadic Creutzfeldt-Jakob disease. *J Biol Chem* 289: 4870-4881.

[36] Zanusso G, Righetti PG, Ferrari S, Terrin L, Farinazzo A, et al. (2002) Two-dimensional mapping of three phenotype-associated isoforms of the prion protein in sporadic Creutzfeldt-Jakob disease. *Electrophoresis* 23: 347-355.

[37] Bishop MT, Will RG, Manson JC (2010) Defining sporadic Creutzfeldt-Jakob disease strains and their transmission properties. *Proc Natl Acad Sci U S A* 107: 12005-12010.

[38] Atarashi R, Satoh K, Sano K, Fuse T, Yamaguchi N, et al. (2011) Ultrasensitive human prion detection in cerebrospinal fluid by real-time quaking-induced conversion. *Nat Med* 17: 175-178.

[39] McGuire LI, Peden AH, Orru CD, Wilham JM, Appleford NE, et al. (2012) Real time quaking-induced conversion analysis of cerebrospinal fluid in sporadic Creutzfeldt-Jakob disease. *Ann Neurol* 72: 278-285.

[40] Orru CD, Bongianni M, Tonoli G, Ferrari S, Hughson AG, et al. (2014) A test for Creutzfeldt-Jakob disease using nasal brushings. *N Engl J Med* 371: 519-529.

[41] Orru CD, Groveman BR, Hughson AG, Zanusso G, Coulthart MB, et al. (2015) Rapid and sensitive RT-QuIC detection of human Creutzfeldt-Jakob disease using cerebrospinal fluid. *MBio* 6.

[42] Tabaton M, Monaco S, Cordone MP, Colucci M, Giaccone G, et al. (2004) Prion deposition in olfactory biopsy of sporadic Creutzfeldt-Jakob disease. *Ann Neurol* 55: 294-296.

[43] Zanusso G, Ferrari S, Cardone F, Zampieri P, Gelati M, et al. (2003) Detection of pathologic prion protein in the olfactory epithelium in sporadic Creutzfeldt-Jakob disease. *N Engl J Med* 348: 711-719.

[44] Hsiao K, Dlouhy SR, Farlow MR, Cass C, Da Costa M, et al. (1992) Mutant prion proteins in Gerstmann-Straussler-Scheinker disease with neurofibrillary tangles. *Nat Genet* 1: 68-71.

[45] Kitamoto T, Amano N, Terao Y, Nakazato Y, Isshiki T, et al. (1993) A new inherited prion disease (PrP-P105L mutation) showing spastic paraparesis. *Ann Neurol* 34: 808-813.

[46] Kitamoto T, Iizuka R, Tateishi J (1993) An amber mutation of prion protein in Gerstmann-Straussler syndrome with mutant PrP plaques. *Biochem Biophys Res Commun* 192: 525-531.

[47] Ghetti B, Piccardo P, Spillantini MG, Ichimiya Y, Porro M, et al. (1996) Vascular variant of prion protein cerebral amyloidosis with tau-positive neurofibrillary tangles: the phenotype of the stop codon 145 mutation in PRNP. *Proc Natl Acad Sci U S A* 93: 744-748.

[48] Piccardo P, Dlouhy SR, Lievens PM, Young K, Bird TD, et al. (1998) Phenotypic variability of Gerstmann-Straussler-Scheinker disease is associated with prion protein heterogeneity. *J Neuropathol Exp Neurol* 57: 979-988.

[49] Jansen C, Voet W, Head MW, Parchi P, Yull H, et al. (2011) A novel seven-octapeptide repeat insertion in the prion protein gene (PRNP) in a Dutch pedigree with Gerstmann-Straussler-Scheinker disease phenotype: comparison with similar cases from the literature. *Acta Neuropathol* 121: 59-68.

[50] Monaco S, Fiorini M, Farinazzo A, Ferrari S, Gelati M, et al. (2012) Allelic origin of protease-sensitive and protease-resistant prion protein isoforms in Gerstmann-Straussler-Scheinker disease with the P102L mutation. *PLoS One* 7: e32382.

In: The Prion Phenomena in Neurodegenerative Diseases ISBN: 978-1-63483-399-8
Editors: Giuseppe Legname and Gabriele Giachin

Chapter 2

X-RAY FIBER DIFFRACTION FROM PRIONS: OF MICE AND BETA-SOLENOIDS

Holger Wille*

Centre for Prions and Protein Folding Diseases and Department of Biochemistry, University of Alberta, Edmonton, Alberta, Canada

ABSTRACT

Only limited information is available about the structure of the infectious prion protein, PrP^{Sc}, and of its proteolytically truncated homolog, PrP 27-30. Their insolubility and propensity to aggregate have frustrated all attempts to determine their structures by conventional approaches such as X-ray crystallography and solution NMR spectroscopy. X-ray fiber diffraction, however, has been used to analyze the structures of PrP^{Sc} and PrP 27-30 amyloid fibrils purified from the brains of infected laboratory rodents. The structures of eight rodent-adapted natural isolates and seven "synthetic" prion strains that originated *in vitro* were analyzed. The diffraction patterns from all brain-derived prion strains exhibited the same repeating unit of 19.2 Å, represented by a series of meridional diffraction signals at 4.8, 6.4, and 9.6 Å. The underlying structure, which appears to form the general architecture for the infectious mammalian prion, was identified as a four-stranded ß-solenoid in a cross-ß arrangement. In contrast, recombinant prion protein that was fibrillized *in vitro* was found to posses a different structure altogether, with a repeating unit of 4.8 Å per molecule and a characteristic equatorial diffraction signal at ~ 10 Å, indicative of stacked ß-sheets. A variety of shortened prion protein constructs and peptides were found to adopt structures of a reduced complexity, often in a stacked ß-sheet configuration. Therefore, studies to investigate the structure of the infectious mammalian prion cannot rely on more convenient surrogates.

* Corresponding Author address. Email: wille@ualberta.ca.

INTRODUCTION

Prions are responsible for a variety of neurodegenerative diseases in humans, agriculturally important livestock, and wild cervids. These diseases, which are invariably fatal, include Creutzfeldt-Jakob disease (CJD) in humans, bovine spongiform encephalopathy (BSE) in cattle, chronic wasting diseases (CWD) in deer, elk, and moose, as well as sheep and goat scrapie [1]. The mammalian prion protein (PrP) was found to undergo a profound structural change in its conversion from the benign, cellular isoform (PrP^C) to the disease-causing, infectious conformer (PrP^{Sc}) [2, 3]. The structure of PrP^C is reasonably well known through studies of recombinantly expressed PrP (recPrP) by solution NMR spectroscopy and X-ray crystallography [4]. In contrast, the structure of PrP^{Sc} is poorly understood owing to its propensity to aggregate and its general insolubility [5]. Numerous analytical techniques such as Fourier-transform infrared (FTIR) and circular dichroism (CD) spectroscopies, electron microscopy and electron crystallography, as well as mass spectrometry in concert with limited proteolysis, surface reactivity, and H/D exchange studies have been used to investigate the structure of PrP^{Sc} [6]. The conclusions drawn from these diverse experimental approaches have been limited by the inherent difficulties of working with an aggregated and insoluble protein.

In this chapter, I am summarizing the results of a series of studies on the structure of PrP^{Sc} and its N-terminal truncated variant PrP 27-30, using X-ray fiber diffraction [7, 8]. These studies spanned well over a decade and involved fruitful collaborations with many scientists, particularly Gerald Stubbs and his team at Vanderbilt University were indispensable for the success of the experiments. These long-term efforts were rewarded by unique insights into the fold of the infectious conformer. X-ray fiber diffraction, as a technique, gained fame by providing the experimental data that led to the discovery of the structure of DNA [9, 10] and has also been used to determine the structure of complex assemblies such as intact tobacco mosaic virus (TMV) [11].

PrP^{Sc} and PrP 27-30 are prone to aggregate into a variety of different quaternary structures such as amorphous aggregates, two-dimensional crystals, and amyloid fibrils [12]. Prominent among those structures are the amyloid fibrils, from which, because of their regular and repeating structure, detailed structural information about their underlying molecular architecture can be extracted. X-ray fiber diffraction takes advantage of the repeating nature of the protein subunits that make up the amyloid fibrils, and thus provides unique insights into the molecular architecture of the infectious conformer in its native state.

In order to collect useful X-ray fiber diffraction data from our experiments with PrP^{Sc} and PrP 27-30 we tried a variety of sample preparation techniques, but discovered that an approach similar to the one that was used to determine the structure of DNA gave the best results. We prepared dried fibers from suspensions of both PrP^{Sc} and PrP 27-30 amyloid fibrils. The dried fibers were made in microchambers fashioned from standard microcuvettes that are commonly used for spectroscopy [13]. The microchambers allowed the humidity of the sample to be controlled using concentrated salt solutions as desiccants in a closed environment (Figure 1). The humidity control proved to be essential to maintain a biologically relevant conformation, as had been demonstrated through X-ray fiber diffraction analyses of both Sup35 amyloid fibrils [13, 14] and fungal HET-s prions [15]. In fully dried samples the structures had collapsed into degenerate stacked β-sheet amyloids, while the humidity controlled samples retained their native structure (a β-solenoid in case of the fungal HET-s prion [16]).

PrP^{Sc} and N-Terminally Truncated PrP 27-30

Samples of full-length PrP^{Sc} and PrP 27-30 were purified from the brains of Syrian hamsters, wild type mice, and transgenic mice (overexpressing PrP from other species) that were infected with prions from one of several rodent-adapted natural isolates. These prion strains showed a wide range of properties, for example the level to which the diseased brain contains pre-formed amyloid fibrils: RML prions in FVB mice are devoid of amyloid fibrils, [17, 18] while Sc237 prions in SHa have widespread amyloid plaques throughout their brain [19]. The purification of these diverse prion strains was based on the repeated precipitation with phosphotungstate anions (PTA), [20] which by itself induces amyloid formation *in vitro* with both PrP^{Sc} and PrP 27-30 [18]. The latter fact proved to be very useful for our X-ray fiber diffraction experiments and contributed to the overall quality and quantity of the purified PrP^{Sc} and PrP 27-30 amyloids [8].

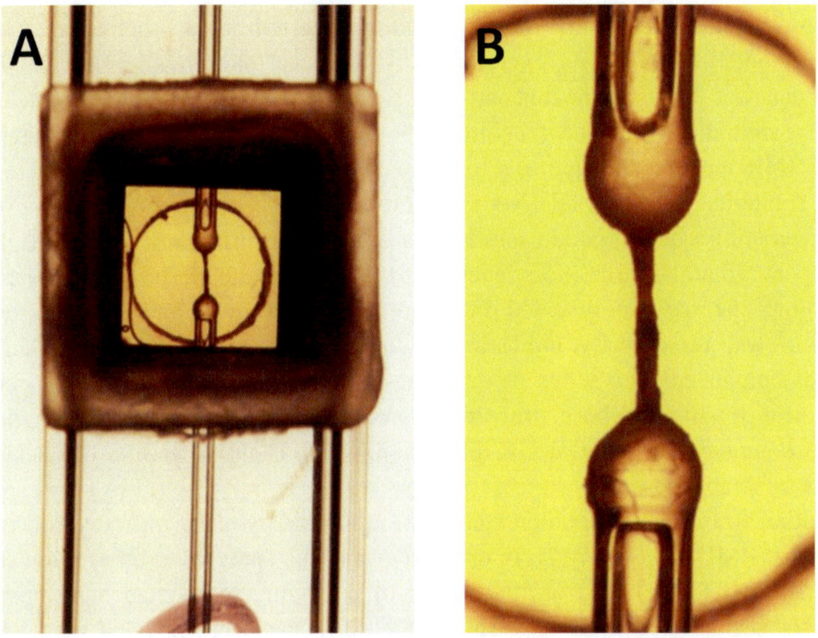

Figure 1. A dried fiber specimen of Syrian hamster (SHa) Sc237 PrP 27-30 in a humidity-controlled microchamber. (A) Low-power view of a microchamber with a single silicon-nitride window attached [13]. The silicon-nitride windows create a hermetic seal, while permitting the X-rays to reach the sample without undue scattering of the X-ray beam. Prior to the data collection at the synchrotron beamline, a lead-tape with a 5 mm pinhole to reduce unspecific X-ray scatter is attached (not shown). (B) High-power view of a dried SHa Sc237 PrP 27-30 fiber. The distance between the capped glass capillaries (top and bottom) is ~1.5 mm. While the fiber looks somewhat uneven, it did provide a fairly well-ordered diffraction pattern (comparable to Figure 2A).

The first X-ray fiber diffraction studies on PrP 27-30 were limited by the use of low intensity X-ray sources and the high degree of disorder in the prion samples [21]. In those diffraction patterns it was difficult to discern even the 4.8 Å diffraction on the meridian, which is a defining characteristic for the cross-β structure of amyloid [22]. Thus, no structural information was obtained at that time.

By using synchrotron-based X-ray sources (beamlines at the Stanford Synchrotron Radiation Laboratory (SSRL) and the Advanced Photon Source (APS)), which provide much higher intensity X-ray beams with a narrower collimation, we were able to collect diffraction patterns with unprecedented levels of information on the structure of prions. In addition, the use of PTA-purified prion preparations contributed significantly to the improved diffraction data [7]. The diffraction patterns from Syrian hamster PrP 27-30 revealed an axial repeating unit of 19.2 Å per molecule, represented by a series of meridional diffraction intensities at 4.8, 6.4, and 9.6 Å, respectively (Figure 2A, red arrows). This result indicated that the height of each molecule of PrP 27-30 is equivalent to four β-strands. The diffraction on the equator originated predominantly from lipid and detergent molecules (Figure 2A, black arrows), which co-purified with the prions or were added during the purification (as is the case with the detergent Sarkosyl). The absence of a strong ~10 Å equatorial diffraction, which is commonly seen with stacked β-sheet amyloids (compare Figure 2B), implied the presence of a β-helical or β-solenoidal structure instead [7].

Prior to our study, an X-ray fiber diffraction pattern from a β-helical or β-solenoidal amyloid had not been observed experimentally, and our interpretation of the PrP 27-30 diffraction data was the first time this particular fold had been suggested by this technique [7]. Fortuitously, around that time the structure of the fungal HET-s prion had been determined by solid-state NMR spectroscopy and was found to contain a two-rung β-solenoid [16, 23]. This structural similarity and the relative simplicity of expressing and refolding this non-pathogenic protein made it a good candidate for X-ray fiber diffraction studies. Right away it became apparent that the diffraction patterns of the β-solenoidal HET-s prion fibrils matched our prediction: The meridian revealed diffraction intensities at 4.8 and 9.6 Å (Figure 2C red horizontal arrows), respectively, indicating a two-stranded β-structure [24]. Furthermore, the equator was dominated by a series of intensities at 17 Å and 11 Å (Figure 2C red vertical arrows) typical of patterns whose structures approximate that of a solid cylinder such as a β-solenoid. A *dominant* ~10 Å equatorial diffraction, which is characteristic for stacked β-sheet amyloids, was notably absent.

The initial X-ray fiber diffraction studies were limited by using only two rodent-adapted scrapie strains: RML and Sc237 [7]. In order to extend the analyses to other prion strains, we purified PrP^{Sc} and PrP 27-30 from the brains of prion-infected Syrian hamsters, wildtype mice, and transgenic mice expressing sheep or elk PrP that were infected with a variety of rodent-adapted prion strains (Table 1). In detail, we examined four sheep or goat scrapie strains (Sc237, RML, 139H, and SSBP1), two transmissible mink encephalopathy (TME) strains (hyper and drowsy), and one isolate of bovine spongiform encephalopathy (301V) and chronic wasting disease each. Furthermore, we also included prions isolated from a transgenic mouse line expressing a P101L mutated version of PrP [25], which is analogous to the Gerstmann-Sträussler-Scheinker syndrome (GSS) mutation of P102L in human PrP [26].

With all of these prion strains we obtained nearly identical diffraction results (Table 1) indicating the presence of a four-rung β-helical or β-solenoid architecture, based on three orders of diffraction (9.6 Å, 6.4 Å, and 4.8 Å) of a 19.2-Å repeating unit in each case [8]. This also included the spontaneously arising prions from the P101L GSS mimic.

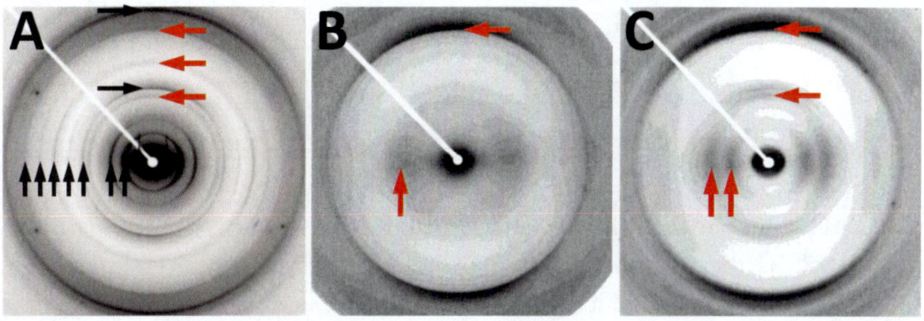

Figure 2. Comparison of X-ray fiber diffraction patterns from a rodent-adapted prion isolate, a recombinant PrP amyloid, and recombinant HET-s(218-289) amyloid. (A) Purified SHa Sc237 PrP 27-30 was used to produce a fairly well-ordered dried fiber (comparable to Figure 1B). The diffraction pattern contains signals originating from protein (red arrows) and lipid / detergent components (black arrows). Red arrows indicate meridional diffraction at close to 4.8, 6.4, and 9.6 Å (top to bottom), which correspond to the fourth, third, and second order diffraction of a 19.2 Å repeating unit. The lipid diffraction is dominated by meridional signals at 4.2 and 8.4 Å (black horizontal arrows), which stem from partially oriented lipids presumably associated with the glycosyl-phosphatidyl inositol (GPI) anchor of PrP. Lipid / detergent assemblies are responsible for a series of equatorial diffraction signals (black vertical arrows). The relatively high orders and sharpness of these intensities, as well as their spacings are characteristic of crystalline order [7]. (B) Diffraction pattern from recombinant murine PrP(89-230) amyloid that was fibrillized *in vitro*. The diffraction is dominated by meridional intensity at 4.8 Å (red horizontal arrow) and equatorial intensity close to 10 Å (red vertical arrow), typical of a stacked β-sheet amyloid [7, 24]. (C) Diffraction pattern from recombinant HET-s(218-289) amyloid fibrillized at pH 7. The structure of HET-s(218-289) amyloid had been determined by solid-state NMR spectroscopy to contain a two-rung β-solenoid structure [16, 23]. The meridional diffraction at 4.8 and 9.6 Å (red horizontal arrows, top to bottom) confirm the two-rung β-sheet conformation, while the equatorial diffraction at 11 and 17 Å (red vertical arrows, left to right) indicate the β-solenoid nature of this amyloid [24].

Table 1. X-ray fiber diffraction from rodent-adapted prion strains

Prion Strain	Disease of origin	Host species	β-sheet architecture
Sc237	Scrapie	Syrian hamster	4-rung β-solenoid[c]
139H	Scrapie	Syrian hamster	4-rung β-solenoid[c]
RML	Scrapie	mouse (FVB)	4-rung β-solenoid[a]
SSBP1	Scrapie	Tg14880 (sheep PrP)	4-rung β-solenoid[a]
301V	Bovine spongiform encephalopathy (BSE)	mouse (FVB)	4-rung β-solenoid[a]
Drowsy	Transmissible mink encephalopathy (TME)	mouse (FVB)	4-rung β-solenoid[b]
Hyper	Transmissible mink encephalopathy (TME)	Syrian hamster	4-rung β-solenoid[a]
Elk CWD	Chronic wasting disease (CWD)	Tg12584 (elk PrP)	4-rung β-solenoid[a]
GSS mutation (P102L)	Gerstmann-Sträussler-Scheinker syndrome (GSS)	Tg464 (mouse PrP: P101L)	4-rung β-solenoid[a]

Structure observed with [a] PrP^{Sc}, [b] PrP 27-30, and [c] PrP^{Sc} and PrP 27-30 preparations.

Data adapted from [8].

The general architecture for the structure of rodent-adapted prion isolates is shown in a cartoon depicting a four-rung β-helix or β-solenoid (Figure 3). At present, there is little evidence for structural elements beyond a β-helix or β-solenoid [6]. Therefore, the cartoon is limited to β-sheets in a roughly β-helical or β-solenoidal arrangement, no loops or other structural elements were included.

PrP Peptides and Recombinant PrP Amyloid

The difficulties that arise from working with infectious samples requiring biosafety level 2 conditions, such as the mammalian prions, limit the experimental techniques that can be employed. Furthermore, these difficulties also limit the researchers who can investigate these samples to those who have access to the appropriate facilities. To overcome this problem, synthetic peptides or short, recombinantly-expressed constructs of PrP are often used as surrogates for infectious specimens. While these models provide important insights into the behavior and folding properties of these surrogates, their relevance for the conformation of the biologically active, infectious prion is uncertain. This problem extends even to full-length recombinant PrP (recPrP(23-230)) and recombinant PrP(89-230) (recPrP(89-230)), which are often used to approximate PrP^{Sc} and PrP 27-30, respectively.

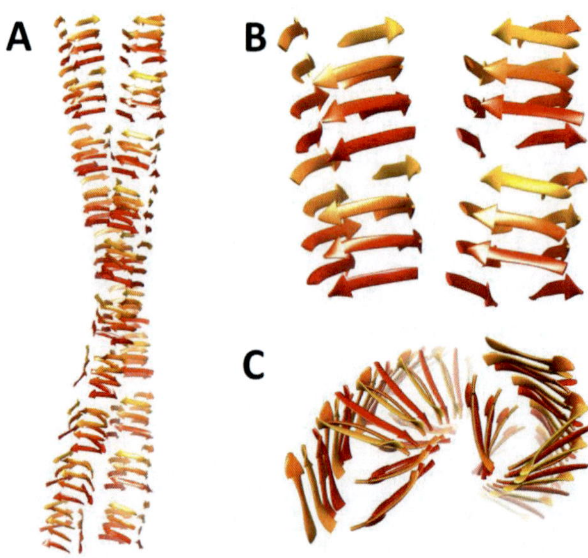

Figure 3. Cartoon graphic to illustrate the underlying structure that may give rise to the diffraction results obtained from brain-derived prion preparations. (A) Cartoon of two intertwined protein fibrils (protofilaments) consisting of individual molecules containing a four-rung parallel β-helix. (B) Detailed view of the top two molecules of the fibrils. In each case only the β-strands are depicted, loop and coil structures that would connect the individual β-strands are not shown. The four-rung β-helix has a height of 19.2 Å (= 4 x 4.8 Å). (C) View from the top of the fibrils illustrating two putative protofilaments.

In vitro generated amyloid from recPrP(23-230) and recPrP(89-230) conforms to the three hallmarks (compare [27]) that are required to use the term amyloid: 1) thin, unbranched protein fibrils, 2) which can be stained with Thioflavin T or Congo red dye, and which 3) display the typical cross-β diffraction [22, 28]. Nevertheless, the X-ray fiber diffraction data clearly reveal that the *in vitro* generated amyloid preparations (Figure 2B) are structurally distinct from those of brain-derived prions (Figure 2A). The former are dominated by a very strong meridional diffraction at 4.8 Å and a strong equatorial diffraction at ~10 Å (Figure 2B), which are the characteristics of a stacked β-sheet structure [7, 29, 30].

In the next round of experiments we used X-ray fiber diffraction to explore the amyloidogenicity of different PrP peptides and constructs, and to assess to what degree they would be able to recapitulate the structural features of brain-derived prions. We fibrillized the respective substrates under a variety of conditions, which resulted in structural variations of the generated amyloid and complicated the interpretation to some degree [31]. In all cases, we were unable to produce amyloid with structural properties identical to those of brain-derived prions (Table 2). Nevertheless, in some cases the diffraction data indicated the presence of a β-helix or β-solenoid (PrP(89-143,P101L) and PrP(89-177)), but those peptides were restricted to only two rungs of β-structure by the length of the corresponding peptide. Therefore, these shorter versions of PrP are unable to accommodate a four-rung β-structure by design.

Table 2. X-ray fiber diffraction from PrP peptides and recombinant PrP amyloid

PrP construct	Size (amino acids) & species	Source	β-sheet architecture
PrP(106-126) [c]	21, human	synthetic peptide	stacked β-sheet
PrP(89-143,P101L) [c]	55, mouse	synthetic peptide	stacked β-sheet or 2-rung β-solenoid [a]
PrP(89-177) [c]	89, mouse, bank vole	recombinant protein	stacked β-sheet or 2-rung β-solenoid [a]
PrP(90-231) [b]	142, Syrian hamster	recombinant protein	stacked β-sheet
PrP(89-230) [b]	142, mouse	recombinant protein	stacked β-sheet
PrP(23-230) [d]	208, mouse	recombinant protein	stacked β-sheet

[a] Different structures observed under different conditions.
Data adapted from [b] [7]; [c] [31]; and [d] [8].

The PrP(23-144) peptide, which is based on the human Y145Stop mutation [32], was found to adopt a one-rung β-solenoid conformation [33]. While this study did not contain enough detail to determine the full structure of PrP(23-144) amyloid, it provided a good comparison to our data on the PrP(89-143,P101L) peptide [31]. In our hands the PrP(89-143,P101L) peptide was structurally pleiomorphic and capable of adopting both a stacked β-sheet and a two-rung β-solenoid (Table 2), which constitutes an acceptable agreement with the earlier investigation.

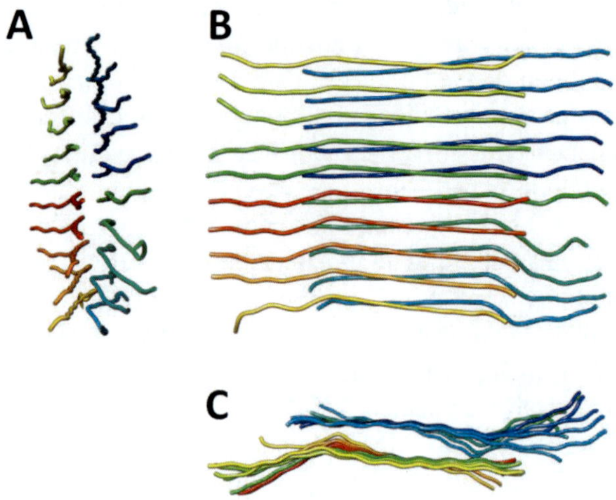

Figure 4. Graphic to illustrate the structure of a stacked β-sheet amyloid. The graphic is based on the PrP(106-126) peptide structure in its fibrillar state as determined by solid-state NMR spectroscopy [34]. (A, B) Two orthogonal side views of the stacked β-sheet amyloid structure of PrP(106-126). Each stack of molecules represents an independent β-sheet, formed through an in-register, parallel β-stacking of individual peptide molecules. The spacing between individual peptide strands in the β-sheet structure is 4.8 Å, which gives rise to a strong meridional diffraction signal at 4.8 Å. The β-sheet core of the amyloid structure is formed by the side-by-side association of two separate β-sheets (the overlapping region in B). (C) Top view of the fibril illustrating the ~10 Å spacing between neighboring β-sheets. This spacing is responsible for the 8-12 Å equatorial diffraction commonly seen with stacked β-sheet amyloid structures (compare Figure 2B). The PDB for this structure was kindly made available by Dr. Simon Sharpe (University of Toronto).

The structure of PrP(106-126) amyloid was determined by solid-state NMR spectroscopy [34], and is used here (Figure 4) to illustrate the general architecture of a stacked β-sheet amyloid. It is interesting to note that our X-ray fiber diffraction data from this peptide confirmed the general stacked β-sheet architecture, but that in our samples the peptide clearly formed a β-hairpin resulting in a molecular height of 9.6 Å [31]. Given the strength of the corresponding experimental data, this discrepancy cannot be attributed to experimental error, but instead re-emphasizes the structural pleiotropy of the prion protein and its truncated variants. This pleiotropy of the prion protein may also be a contributing factor to its ability to adopt distinct conformations such as those of PrP^{C} and PrP^{Sc}.

Synthetic Prions

While recombinant PrP (recPrP) amyloid clearly differs structurally from brain-derived, infectious prions (Figure 2), various preparations of recPrP amyloid have given rise to "synthetic" prion strains upon inoculation into indicator animals [35, 36, 37, 38, 39, 40]. This apparent discrepancy between structure and (mal-)function was resolved by studying the structure of synthetic prions after repeated passage through transgenic mice (Table 3).

Table 3. X-ray fiber diffraction from rodent-passaged synthetic prion strains

Synthetic prion Strain	Original inoculum	Host species	β-sheet architecture
MoSP1	seeded recPrP amyloid	Tg9949 (mouse PrP)	4-rung β-solenoid [b]
MoSP2	unseeded recPrP amyloid	Tg9949 (mouse PrP)	4-rung β-solenoid [b]
MoSP5	seeded recPrP amyloid	Tg4053 (mouse PrP)	4-rung β-solenoid [a]
MoSP6	seeded recPrP amyloid	Tg4053 (mouse PrP)	4-rung β-solenoid [b]
MoSP7	seeded recPrP amyloid	Tg4053 (mouse PrP)	4-rung β-solenoid [b]
'rPrP-res'	PMCA with lipids & RNA	Tg4053 (mouse PrP)	4-rung β-solenoid [b]
SSLOW	unseeded recPrP amyloid	Tg7 (Syrian hamster PrP)	4-rung β-solenoid [b]

Structure observed with [a] PrP^{Sc} and [b] PrP 27-30.
Data adapted from [7, 8].

PrP^{Sc} and PrP 27-30 from different synthetic prion strains were purified from the brains of infected transgenic mice in an equivalent manner to the rodent-adapted natural isolates mentioned earlier (Table 1). The X-ray fiber diffraction data from all of the synthetic prion strains displayed the same three orders of meridional diffraction at 9.6 Å, 6.4 Å, and 4.8 Å, indicative of a 19.2 Å repeating unit as was seen earlier with rodent-adapted natural isolates [7, 8]. Furthermore, these samples also lacked a strong equatorial diffraction at ~10 Å indicative of a β-helical or β-solenoidal architecture. This finding places the synthetic prion strains into the same structural class as the natural prion isolates, supporting the interpretation that there may be only one infectious fold for the mammalian prion protein.

While the X-ray fiber diffraction data resolved the apparent structural discrepancy between synthetic prions and natural isolates, it raised another question: How can recPrP amyloids cause a prion infection, if it is has a different structure? One possible answer lies in the heterogeneity of the recPrP amyloid preparations that was observed with both the X-ray fiber diffraction experiments (Figure 2B) as well as negative stain electron microscopy (data not shown) [7, 8]. Thus, the bulk recPrP amyloid preparations with their predominantly stacked β-sheet conformation may have hidden a minor fraction of protein in the infectious β-helix or β-solenoid fold. This structural heterogeneity could easily explain the relatively low titers that were observed in most, if not all, initial transmissions [35, 36, 37, 38, 39, 40].

An alternative explanation suggested that inoculated recPrP amyloid may be subjected to deformed templating (heterogeneous seeding) *in vivo*, which may then give rise to the infectious β-helix or β-solenoid conformer [41, 42]. While the first option is difficult to exclude (and they are not necessarily mutually exclusive), the current experimental data favor the deformed templating hypothesis as the more influential alternative [41].

CONCLUSION

The data presented in this chapter indicate that all infectious mammalian prions share a common four-rung β-helix or β-solenoid architecture. These results are not in contradiction to prior efforts by other investigators to assign distinct structural features to the different prion strains (for example [20, 43, 44, 45]). Our findings merely indicate that this structural diversity is based on a common four-rung β-helix or β-solenoid core. Thus the observed strain differences have to originate from more subtle structural differences.

The complex interplay between different levels of structure (secondary, tertiary, and quaternary structure), which define PrP^{Sc}, could explain the structural differences. For example, Aβ amyloid fibrils grown under quiescent or agitated conditions *in vitro,* showed clear differences in morphology and molecular architecture [46]. Electron paramagnetic resonance (EPR) spectroscopy demonstrated that morphological variations such as these could be based on relatively subtle differences in side-chain interactions between individual β-strands [47].

Moreover, the β-helix or β-solenoid fold has shown to provide sufficient variations to accommodate a wide range of molecular models for the structure of PrP^{Sc} [48, 49, 50, 51, 52, 53]. In all likelihood, none of the previously published models for the structure of PrP^{Sc} offer a realistic picture for the actual structure of the infectious prion [6]. Nevertheless, the β-helix or β-solenoid fold with its left- and right-handed variants represents a substantial territory of "fold-space," in which the structure of the infectious prion with all its strain variations can easily be accommodated. Together with the differences that can arise from subtle side-chain interactions alone [47], these alternatives provide enough structural variation to allow for distinct self-propagating prion folds, that is, strains.

ACKNOWLEDGMENTS

I would like to give special thanks to Gerald Stubbs for his advice and support in all matters X-ray fiber diffraction and his critical reading of the manuscript. Furthermore, I want to acknowledge Lillian Falese, Diane Latawiec, Ana Serban, Jan Stöhr, David W. Colby, Gültekin Tamgüney, Julian Ollesch, Alexander Borovinskiy, Amy Kendall, Michele McDonald, Wen Bian, and William Wan for their help in purifying the many prion samples and in collecting and analyzing the diffraction patterns. I am also indebted to Fred E. Cohen and Stanley B. Prusiner for their steadfast support for this project. Special thanks also belong to the beamline scientists at the Stanford Synchrotron Radiation Laboratory (SSRL) and the Advanced Photon Source (APS) for their support for the many data collection. Lastly, the experimental portions of this project were supported by grants from the National Institutes of Health (USA), the Fairchild Foundation, and the G. Harold and Leila Y. Mathers Foundation (to S.B.P., F.E.C., and G.S.). The writing of this chapter was backed by the Alberta Prion Research Institute (APRI) and the Helmholtz-Alberta Initiative on Neurodegenerative Disease Research (HAI-NDR).

REFERENCES

[1] Colby DW, Prusiner SB (2011) Prions. *Cold Spring Harb Perspect Biol* 3: a006833.

[2] Caughey BW, Dong A, Bhat KS, Ernst D, Hayes SF, et al. (1991) Secondary structure analysis of the scrapie-associated protein PrP 27-30 in water by infrared spectroscopy. *Biochemistry* 30: 7672-7680.

[3] Pan KM, Baldwin M, Nguyen J, Gasset M, Serban A, et al. (1993) Conversion of alpha-helices into beta-sheets features in the formation of the scrapie prion proteins. Proc Natl Acad Sci U S A 90: 10962-10966.

[4] Surewicz WK, Apostol MI (2011) Prion protein and its conformational conversion: a structural perspective. *Top Curr Chem 3*05: 135-167.

[5] Wille H, Prusiner SB (1999) Ultrastructural studies on scrapie prion protein crystals obtained from reverse micellar solutions. *Biophys J* 76: 1048-1062.

[6] Requena JR, Wille H (2014) The structure of the infectious prion protein: experimental data and molecular models. *Prion* 8: 60-66.

[7] Wille H, Bian W, McDonald M, Kendall A, Colby DW, et al. (2009) Natural and synthetic prion structure from X-ray fiber diffraction. *Proc Natl Acad Sci U S A* 106: 16990-16995.

[8] Wille H, Stöhr J, Bian W, Falese L, Tamgüney G, et al. (2015) *Manuscript in preparation.*

[9] Franklin RE, Gosling RG (1953) Molecular configuration in sodium thymonucleate. *Nature* 171: 740-741.

[10] Watson JD, Crick FH (1953) Molecular structure of nucleic acids; a structure for deoxyribose nucleic acid. *Nature* 171: 737-738.

[11] Namba K, Stubbs G (1986) Structure of tobacco mosaic virus at 3.6 A resolution: implications for assembly. *Science* 231: 1401-1406.

[12] Wille H, Shanmugam M, Murugesu M, Ollesch J, Stubbs G, et al. (2009) Surface charge of polyoxometalates modulates polymerization of the scrapie prion protein. *Proc Natl Acad Sci U S A* 106: 3740-3745.

[13] McDonald M, Kendall A, Tanaka M, Weissman JS, Stubbs G (2008) Enclosed chambers for humidity control and sample containment in fiber diffraction. *Journal of Applied Crystallography* 41: 206-209.

[14] Kishimoto A, Hasegawa K, Suzuki H, Taguchi H, Namba K, et al. (2004) beta-Helix is a likely core structure of yeast prion Sup35 amyloid fibers. *Biochemical and Biophysical Research Communications* 315: 739-745.

[15] Wan W, Stubbs G (2014) Fiber diffraction of the prion-forming domain HET-s(218-289) shows dehydration-induced deformation of a complex amyloid structure. *Biochemistry* 53: 2366-2370.

[16] Van Melckebeke H, Wasmer C, Lange A, Ab E, Loquet A, et al. (2010) Atomic-resolution three-dimensional structure of HET-s(218-289) amyloid fibrils by solid-state NMR spectroscopy. *J Am Chem Soc* 132: 13765-13775.

[17] Godsave SF, Wille H, Pierson J, Prusiner SB, Peters PJ (2013) Plasma membrane invaginations containing clusters of full-length PrPSc are an early form of prion-associated neuropathology in vivo. *Neurobiol Aging* 34: 1621-1631.

[18] Levine DJ, Stohr J, Falese LE, Ollesch J, Wille H, et al. (2015) Mechanism of Scrapie Prion Precipitation with Phosphotungstate Anions. *ACS Chem Biol* 10: 1269-1277.

[19] DeArmond SJ, McKinley MP, Barry RA, Braunfeld MB, McColloch JR, et al. (1985) Identification of prion amyloid filaments in scrapie-infected brain. *Cell* 41: 221-235.

[20] Safar J, Wille H, Itri V, Groth D, Serban H, et al. (1998) Eight prion strains have PrP(Sc) molecules with different conformations. *Nat Med* 4: 1157-1165.

[21] Nguyen JT, Inouye H, Baldwin MA, Fletterick RJ, Cohen FE, et al. (1995) X-ray diffraction of scrapie prion rods and PrP peptides. *J Mol Biol* 252: 412-422.

[22] Eanes ED, Glenner GG (1968) X-ray diffraction studies on amyloid filaments. *J Histochem Cytochem* 16: 673-677.

[23] Wasmer C, Lange A, Van Melckebeke H, Siemer AB, Riek R, et al. (2008) Amyloid fibrils of the HET-s(218-289) prion form a beta solenoid with a triangular hydrophobic core. *Science* 319: 1523-1526.

[24] Wan W, Wille H, Stohr J, Baxa U, Prusiner SB, et al. (2012) Degradation of fungal prion HET-s(218-289) induces formation of a generic amyloid fold. *Biophys J* 102: 2339-2344.

[25] Nazor KE, Kuhn F, Seward T, Green M, Zwald D, et al. (2005) Immunodetection of disease-associated mutant PrP, which accelerates disease in GSS transgenic mice. *EMBO J* 24: 2472-2480.

[26] Hsiao K, Baker HF, Crow TJ, Poulter M, Owen F, et al. (1989) Linkage of a prion protein missense variant to Gerstmann-Straussler syndrome. *Nature* 338: 342-345.

[27] Eisenberg D, Jucker M (2012) The amyloid state of proteins in human diseases. *Cell* 148: 1188-1203.

[28] Astbury WT, Dickinson S, Bailey K (1935) The X-ray interpretation of denaturation and the structure of the seed globulins. *Biochem J* 29: 2351-2360 2351.

[29] Jahn TR, Makin OS, Morris KL, Marshall KE, Tian P, et al. (2010) The common architecture of cross-beta amyloid. *J Mol Biol* 395: 717-727.

[30] Sunde M, Serpell LC, Bartlam M, Fraser PE, Pepys MB, et al. (1997) Common core structure of amyloid fibrils by synchrotron X-ray diffraction. *J Mol Biol* 273: 729-739.

[31] Wan W, Wille H, Stohr J, Kendall A, Bian W, et al. (2015) Structural Studies of Truncated Forms of the Prion Protein PrP. *Biophys J* 108: 1548-1554.

[32] Ghetti B, Piccardo P, Spillantini MG, Ichimiya Y, Porro M, et al. (1996) Vascular variant of prion protein cerebral amyloidosis with tau-positive neurofibrillary tangles: the phenotype of the stop codon 145 mutation in PRNP. *Proc Natl Acad Sci U S A 93*: 744-748.

[33] Skora L, Zweckstetter M (2012) Determination of amyloid core structure using chemical shifts. *Protein Science* 21: 1948-1953.

[34] Walsh P, Simonetti K, Sharpe S (2009) Core structure of amyloid fibrils formed by residues 106-126 of the human prion protein. *Structure* 17: 417-426.

[35] Colby DW, Giles K, Legname G, Wille H, Baskakov IV, et al. (2009) Design and construction of diverse mammalian prion strains. *Proc Natl Acad Sci U S A* 106: 20417-20422.

[36] Colby DW, Wain R, Baskakov IV, Legname G, Palmer CG, et al. (2010) Protease-sensitive synthetic prions. *PLoS Pathog* 6: e1000736.

[37] Deleault NR, Piro JR, Walsh DJ, Wang F, Ma J, et al. (2012) Isolation of phosphatidylethanolamine as a solitary cofactor for prion formation in the absence of nucleic acids. *Proc Natl Acad Sci U S A* 109: 8546-8551.

[38] Legname G, Baskakov IV, Nguyen HO, Riesner D, Cohen FE, et al. (2004) Synthetic mammalian prions. *Science* 305: 673-676.

[39] Makarava N, Kovacs GG, Bocharova O, Savtchenko R, Alexeeva I, et al. (2010) Recombinant prion protein induces a new transmissible prion disease in wild-type animals. *Acta Neuropathol* 119: 177-187.

[40] Wang F, Wang X, Yuan CG, Ma J (2010) Generating a prion with bacterially expressed recombinant prion protein. *Science* 327: 1132-1135.

[41] Makarava N, Kovacs GG, Savtchenko R, Alexeeva I, Budka H, et al. (2011) Genesis of mammalian prions: from non-infectious amyloid fibrils to a transmissible prion disease. *PLoS Pathog* 7: e1002419.

[42] Wan W, Bian W, McDonald M, Kijac A, Wemmer DE, et al. (2013) Heterogeneous seeding of a prion structure by a generic amyloid form of the fungal prion-forming domain HET-s(218-289). *J Biol Chem* 288: 29604-29612.

[43] Bessen RA, Marsh RF (1994) Distinct PrP properties suggest the molecular basis of strain variation in transmissible mink encephalopathy. *J Virol* 68: 7859-7868.

[44] Telling GC, Parchi P, DeArmond SJ, Cortelli P, Montagna P, et al. (1996) Evidence for the conformation of the pathologic isoform of the prion protein enciphering and propagating prion diversity. *Science* 274: 2079-2082.

[45] Peretz D, Scott MR, Groth D, Williamson RA, Burton DR, et al. (2001) Strain-specified relative conformational stability of the scrapie prion protein. *Protein Science* 10: 854-863.

[46] Petkova AT, Leapman RD, Guo Z, Yau WM, Mattson MP, et al. (2005) Self-propagating, molecular-level polymorphism in Alzheimer's beta-amyloid fibrils. *Science* 307: 262-265.

[47] Agopian A, Guo Z (2012) Structural origin of polymorphism of Alzheimer's amyloid beta-fibrils. *Biochem* J 447: 43-50.

[48] Wille H, Michelitsch MD, Guenebaut V, Supattapone S, Serban A, et al. (2002) Structural studies of the scrapie prion protein by electron crystallography. *Proc Natl Acad Sci U S A* 99: 3563-3568.

[49] Govaerts C, Wille H, Prusiner SB, Cohen FE (2004) Evidence for assembly of prions with left-handed beta-helices into trimers. *Proc Natl Acad Sci U S A* 101: 8342-8347.

[50] Stork M, Giese A, Kretzschmar HA, Tavan P (2005) Molecular dynamics simulations indicate a possible role of parallel beta-helices in seeded aggregation of poly-Gln. *Biophys J* 88: 2442-2451.

[51] Yang S, Levine H, Onuchic JN, Cox DL (2005) Structure of infectious prions: stabilization by domain swapping. *FASEB J* 19: 1778-1782.

[52] Kunes KC, Clark SC, Cox DL, Singh RR (2008) Left handed beta helix models for mammalian prion fibrils. *Prion* 2: 81-90.

[53] Shirai T, Saito M, Kobayashi A, Asano M, Hizume M, et al. (2014) Evaluating prion models based on comprehensive mutation data of mouse PrP. *Structure* 22: 560-571.

In: The Prion Phenomena in Neurodegenerative Diseases ISBN: 978-1-63483-399-8
Editors: Giuseppe Legname and Gabriele Giachin

Chapter 3

NEUROTOXICITY IN PRION DISEASE: RELATIONSHIPS WITH OTHER NEURODEGENERATIVE DISEASES AND OUTLOOKS FOR THERAPEUTIC INTERVENTION

Cathryn L. Ugalde[1,2,3], Victoria A. Lawson[2], David I. Finkelstein[3] and Andrew F. Hill[1,*]

[1]Department of Biochemistry and Molecular Biology, Bio21 Molecular Science & Biotechnology Institute, The University of Melbourne, Parkville, Victoria, Australia
[2]Department of Pathology, The University of Melbourne, Parkville, Victoria, Australia
[3] Florey Institute for Neuroscience and Mental Health, Parkville, Victoria, Australia

ABSTRACT

Prion diseases, or transmissible spongiform encephalopathies, are a group of infectious, invariably lethal neurodegenerative diseases. Traditional prion disease is pathologically characterized by the deposition of PrP^{Sc}; an aberrant, misfolded isoform of the normal cellular prion protein, PrP^{C}, in the central nervous system, widespread neuronal loss and reactive gliosis. Given its presence in the brain in disease, PrP^{Sc} was historically presumed to be the neurotoxic species. Current knowledge suggests toxicity instead precedes the accumulation of protein characteristic of disease, however the precise biochemical and molecular features of its development remains elusive. Amyloid-forming proteins associated with other neurodegenerative diseases, particularly α-synuclein and amyloid-β in Parkinson's disease and Alzheimer's disease respectively, share many similar characteristics with PrP, suggesting common mechanisms of neurotoxicity may exist amongst relatable diseases. Unifying current knowledge of prion-disease associated toxicity and relatable neurodegenerative diseases will be crucial to dissect the mechanisms of neurotoxicity and aid the development of appropriate strategies for early diagnosis and treatment of these currently untreatable, devastating diseases.

[*] Corresponding Author address. Email: Andrew.Hill@latrobe.edu.au.

INTRODUCTION

Prion diseases, or transmissible spongiform encephalopathies (TSEs), are a group of infectious, lethal neurodegenerative diseases that affect both humans and animals. A common feature of these diseases is the conformational misfolding of the normal cellular prion protein, PrP^C, into its disease associated isoform PrP^{Sc}. It is believed PrP^{Sc} either solely [1] or partially [2, 3] constitutes 'prions'; *proteinacious infectious particles* that are the transmissible, causative agent for prion disease [4]. In humans, disease can be caused by mutations in the PrP^C encoding gene, *PRNP*, causing familial Creutzfeldt-Jakob disease (CJD), fatal familial insomnia (FFI) or Gerstmann-Sträussler-Scheinker (GSS) syndrome as a result of misfolding of the cellular protein. Prion disease can also be contracted following exposure to infectious prions and include variant CJD (vCJD), kuru and iatrogenic CJD, or acquired by an as-yet unknown origin (sporadic CJD). Non-human prion diseases include scrapie in sheep and goats, bovine spongiform encephalopathy (BSE) and chronic wasting disease (CWD) in deer and elk, among others.

The conversion of PrP^C to PrP^{Sc} sees the molecule undergo significant structural alterations whereby it changes from a predominantly α-helical structure into a β-sheet rich conformation [5, 6] that is more susceptible to amyloid formation [7]. Through these changes PrP^{Sc} can adopt resistance to proteases such as Proteinase K (PK); a feature which is often exploited for its detection. Additionally, although PrP^C is encoded by the host genome, PrP^{Sc} harbours unique phenotypic characteristics, referred to as prion strains. Different isolated scrapie prion strains can be characterized by their variable incubation periods and distribution of disease-associated neuropathology in inbred mice [8]. These strains are not a result of differences in primary sequence given that their characteristics are conserved throughout serial passages in inbred mice with identical *PRNP* and can be re-isolated in mice following passage in intermediate species with different *PRNP* expression [9]. Unlike conventional pathogens where genomic alterations underlie strain variability, it is unknown how a polypeptide chain could encipher multiple disease phenotypes.

Established prion disease is characterized by accumulation of aggregated PrP^{Sc}, vacuolation and astrogliosis in the brain and associated neuropathological spongiform change. Given its capacity to transmit disease, and its presence in the brain, PrP^{Sc} was generally considered to be the neurotoxic agent. However it is now appreciated the generation of toxicity is much more complex. The deposition of PrP^{Sc} can occur in virtually all peripheral compartments that express PrP^C, particularly the secondary lymphoid organs, spleen and skeletal muscle [10], where PrP^{Sc} resides with no gross detrimental effects. Why prions preferentially cause toxicity to neurons remains unknown and an intense area of research.

Dissociation between aggregated PrP^{Sc} and neurotoxicity is typified by the observation that the abundance of PrP^{Sc} in the brain does not always correlate with the degree of neuronal cell death. Human post mortem studies reveal a large degree of variability in PrP^{Sc} load, where in some cases neurodegeneration occurs despite minimal PrP^{Sc} deposition [11, 12]. This feature extends to prion-infected animals, which represent *bona fide* models of human prion disease. Transgenic mice expressing human familial prion disease-associated mutations exhibit lower levels of PrP^{Sc} than wild-type counterparts at terminal stages of disease [13] or PrP^{Sc} deposition is entirely absent [14]. The prion protein contains a glycosylphosphatidylinositol (GPI) anchor sequence at its C-terminal end and hence is typically found anchored to the cellular membrane. Prion infected mice expressing truncated PrP lacking a GPI anchor tolerate abundant PrP^{Sc} deposition for extended periods of time prior to the development of clinical disease [15, 16]. Collectively these studies question whether PrP^{Sc} itself is the toxic agent and suggest it may instead represent an unrelated endpoint to disease pathogenesis.

Given that PrP knockout mice show no overt neurodegenerative phenotype [17], even when elicited postnatally [18], it is unlikely a loss of function of PrP^C following prion conversion contributes greatly to neuronal cell death. However neurotoxicity is intimately linked to prion replication, in view of the finding that only cells that express PrP^C are susceptible to the effects of PrP^{Sc}. PrP knockout mice are resistant to any toxic effects of PrP^{Sc} [19, 20]. This resistance occurs even in the presence of continual prion replication, as PrP^C knockout mice hosting grafted PrP^C-expressing neuronal tissue only develop neurodegeneration and spongiosis in the PrP-expressing grafted region following inoculation with infectious prions, whilst PrP^{Sc} deposition is rampant in both grafted and non-grafted brain regions [21]. In addition, viral mediated ablation of neuronal PrP expression in mice with established prion infection halts the development of clinical symptoms and reverses neurodegeneration [22, 23]. This occurs despite continual PrP^{Sc} production in glial cells, and as such these mice remain healthy whilst harbouring titres of PrP^{Sc} in the brain equivalent to end-stage titres in conventional mice [22]. These findings demonstrate that the expression of PrP^C by an infected cell is a critical requirement for the development of neurotoxicity.

The capacity by which PrP^C and/or PrP^{Sc} contribute to neurotoxicity in prion disease is not known. It is possible that the upstream neurotoxic agent in prion disease is: (i) PrP^{Sc} that is rate limited by PrP^C, (ii) PrP^C that is either mislocalised or has adopted a toxic gain-of-function, or (iii) another agent or variant of PrP entirely. The high degree of heterogeneity in the clinical presentation of prion disease suggests the generation of toxicity may not be a mutually exclusive entity; rather multiple overlapping pathways of toxicity may exist to explain all forms of disease. This chapter describes the key propositions of the toxic agent in prion disease, and how these studies are helping identify therapeutic targets for prion disease-induced neurodegeneration.

THE GENERATION OF A CANDIDATE TOXIC PRP SPECIES; PRP^L

Although prion disease can affect a wide range of animals, transmission between species is accompanied by a 'transmission barrier' whereby the incubation period is distinctly longer, or does not cause clinical disease, when infecting prions are from a different species. This lag-phase decreases following subsequent passages as it becomes adapted in the host species [24]. Subclinical infection has been shown in mice inoculated with hamster prions which sees early passage infections still replicate PrP^{Sc} to rates as high as seen in end-stage disease, yet to do exhibit any signs of clinical disease [25]. Numerous other studies report the existence of similar subclinical states where wild-type mice are unburdened by high PrP^{Sc} titres in the brain [26-29]. These studies suggest dissociation between what is transmissible in prion disease (propagating PrP^{Sc}) and the toxic agent. An explanation for this phenomenon is that the neurotoxic agent is a conformation of PrP distinct from that of PrP^C and PrP^{Sc}. Referred to as PrP* [30, 31] or PrP^L, denoting the *lethal* conformer of PrP [32, 33], it is generated either as an intermediate or by product of the conversion of PrP^C to PrP^{Sc} (Figure 1). According to this hypothesis, subclinical infection would occur when differences in primary sequences of host and infectious PrP^{Sc} translate to a slow conversion rate of PrP^C to PrP^{Sc}, which would mean either maturation of the toxic intermediate PrP^L to PrP^{Sc} occurs faster than its conversion, or the slow catalytic ability of PrP^{Sc} to form PrP^L from PrP^C as a toxic by product. In subsequent passages however, when infectious PrP^{Sc} is host-adapted, PrP^L generation is increased and disease, with associated clinical phenotype, develops as normal.

Kinetic studies further support an uncoupling of infectivity and toxicity. Rises in infectious PrP^{Sc} titres during disease does not linearly correlate with the development of clinical symptoms or neurodegeneration [4, 34-36]. This observation was described further in large cohort studies showing prion propagation could be separated into two phases: an initial phase where infectivity exponentially increases, which is followed by a second phase, distinguished by a plateau in the rising PrP^{Sc} titres [35, 36]. This plateau is independent of PrP^C concentration, given that transgenic mice expressing various levels of PrP^C are reported to have equivalent PrP^{Sc} titres upon the saturation of infectivity [35, 36]. This is in contrast to toxicity, whose generation is reliant on PrP^C expression. A study investigating prion kinetics in mice with variable PrP expression found mice with higher levels of PrP have a symptomatic period that is shorter as a proportion of the overall disease course compared to lower PrP-expressing counterparts [37]. In agreement to this, large cohort studies show the duration of the aforementioned plateau period is inversely correlated with PrP^C expression and determines the time until clinical onset [35, 36]. These studies strongly show infectivity and toxicity are two different processes with unique characteristics. A logical explanation for this uncoupling is differential PrP^L abundance between the infectious and toxic phases.

A caveat to the PrP^L hypothesis is that the morphology of the molecule is completely unknown and, given that no PrP isoforms aside from PrP^C and PrP^{Sc} have ever been reported to occur *in vivo*, its existence remains purely hypothetical. Still it is increasingly apparent that not all PrP^{Sc} molecules are identical; rather infectious PrP^{Sc} encompasses a heterogeneous mix of PrP^{Sc} quasi-species [38] and as such various sized PrP oligomers or variants are thought to exist. The identification of disease associated PK-sensitive PrP^{Sc} [39] is one such example and indeed is an attractive candidate for PrP^L. The expression of PK-sensitive PrP^{Sc} increases exponentially from the plateau in infectivity through until terminal disease [36] and certain mutations in PrP bias towards the generation of these species, which translates into reduced survival rates when inoculated into mice [40]. However a definition of what constitutes PK-sensitive PrP^{Sc} is lacking and as such various treatment regimes have been used to separate out PK-sensitive PrP^{Sc} from PrP^C and whether or not they isolate the same population is yet to be established. Other quantitative measures rely on indirect measurements by subtractive calculations of PK-resistant PrP^{Sc} from total PrP, which in order for correctness assumes total PrP levels remain unchanged during disease progression. Consensus for this facet of disease is lacking and while some have reported mRNA levels of *PRNP* remain unchanged during disease progression [41, 42], others report a decrease in PrP^C concentration (which would lead to an underestimation of PK-resistant PrP^{Sc} during infection) [43], or more detrimentally, an increase in *PRNP* mRNA and/or total PrP levels throughout disease until terminal stages [44-46]. Hence whether or not PK-sensitive PrP^{Sc}, or indeed any other putative PrP^L population which is distinct from PrP^{Sc}, is directly involved in the generation of neurotoxicity remains to be conclusively established.

TOXIC OLIGOMERS

The deposition of misfolded protein in the brain is not a unique feature of prion disease and occurs in many other neurodegenerative diseases. This includes amyloid-β (Aβ) in Alzheimer's disease (AD) and α-synuclein (αsyn) in synucleinopathies (the most common of which is Parkinson's disease; PD). Similar to prion disease, the presence of aggregated misfolded Aβ and αsyn is intimately linked with the development of neurodegeneration in their respective diseases. In these diseases, the aggregated protein deposits are predominately composed of mature amyloid fibrils however smaller intermediate conformations of misfolded protein also exist including oligomers and protofibrils. Numerous data suggest instead of large insoluble aggregates, soluble prefibrillar species of Aβ and αsyn may be the toxic entity in disease. This may have an equivalent in prion disease and as such review of relatable neurodegenerative diseases could shed light on prion disease-associated neurotoxicity.

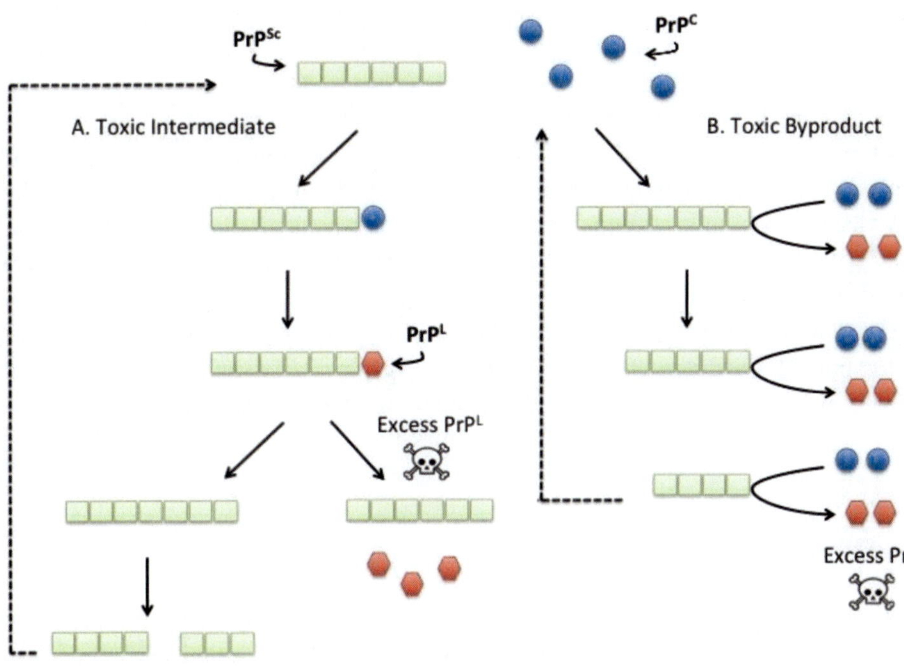

Figure 1. The hypothetical generation of PrP^L. PrP^L may be generated as a toxic intermediate in the conversion of PrP^C to PrP^{Sc} (A) or as a toxic byproduct of prion conversion (B). Adapted from [33].

Aβ oligomers

In AD, the relationship between neurodegeneration and amyloid burden is tenuous. The two do not correlate well in diseased human brain [47, 48], and in certain transgenic models expressing mutant amyloid precursor protein (APP; the precursor to Aβ) to model AD, lethality occurs in the absence of amyloid formation [49]. Instead, the degree of neurodegeneration correlates with the pool of soluble Aβ species [50, 51]. Animal studies reveal soluble Aβ oligomers impair rodent spatial memory [52] and cause dendritic spine retraction [53, 54]. They also block hippocampal long-term potentiation (LTP) and activate long-term depression (LTD) [55, 56], which are electrophysiological correlates of learning and memory. The notion of Aβ oligomer-induced toxicity is further supported by the observations that mutations which lead to particularly aggressive forms of AD, such as the 'Arctic' mutation in the APP gene (E693G), preferentially produces larger quantities of protofibrils *in vitro* [57] and apolipoprotein E (specifically the E4 allelic variant), the most relevant risk factor for AD, has been shown to alter Aβ oligomerization [58]. Collectively these studies give overwhelming evidence for a role of Aβ oligomers in mediating toxicity in AD.

The mechanisms underpinning these toxic effects have also been studied, where oligomer-induced alterations to LTP and LDP are caused by the N-Methyl D-Aspartate (NMDA) and metabotropic glutamate-5 (mGlu5) receptors respectively [54, 56]. The modulation of these receptors, however, is complex and interestingly seems to involve PrP^C, which has been shown to be a receptor for Aβ oligomers [59] and cause Aβ-induced synaptotoxicity likely by forming a complex with mGlu5 [60]. Accordingly, antibodies targeting PrP negate these Aβ-induced synaptotoxic effects [61].

Although dimeric forms of Aβ are considered the smallest toxic entity [56], other forms may also be relevant, such as the non-fibrillar 56-kDa Aβ oligomeric form, termed Aβ*56. Presumed to be composed of Aβ trimers because Aβ*56 dissociates into trimers before monomers [52], Aβ*56 induces cognitive dysfunction independent of amyloid deposition and neuronal loss when injected into rats [52]. In humans Aβ*56 is found in the brain and cerebral spinal fluid (CSF) where it correlates with several postsynaptic proteins in healthy control cognitively intact individuals [62, 63], thus Aβ*56 may play a role in early cognitive deficits in AD, prior to any overt symptoms of neuronal loss. However given that Aβ*56 cannot in itself induce AD, its contribution to the development of cognitive decline seen in progressed AD is not known.

αsyn Oligomers

Early αsyn aggregates have also been associated with toxicity in synucleinopathies; a broad term for diseases manifesting misfolded αsyn and includes PD, multiple system atrophy (MSA), dementia with Lewy Bodies (DLB) and AD. These diseases vary greatly in terms of their distribution of intracellular misfolded αsyn deposits (termed Lewy Bodies, LB) and pattern of selective neuronal susceptibility and hence it is considered they may represent distinct diseases.

Like PrP^{Sc} and Aβ, αsyn deposition in human brain does not correlate well with the degree of neurodegeneration [64-66]. This observation extends to animal models, where in transgenic fly and rodent models of PD, neurodegeneration can occur in the absence of any fibrillar αsyn deposits [67, 68]. Instead numerous data implicate αsyn oligomers as toxic in synucleinopathies. Small prefibrillar species are directly linked to neurodegeneration in DLB brain, where its aggregation at presynaptic terminals correlates with decreases in presynaptic markers and dendritic spine loss [69]. *In vitro* studies have demonstrated that subtypes of synthetic wild-type αsyn oligomers are extremely toxic to cultured cells [70]. Expression of wild-type αsyn induces disease in animals [68, 71-73] and mutations in αsyn that increase its propensity to oligomerize and decrease the formation of fibrils have been shown to be more toxic than wild-type αsyn when expressed in primary neuronal cultures and invertebrate models of PD (*C. elegans* and *Drosphilia melanogaster*) [74]. In addition, the expression of mutant αsyn that preferentially forms oligomers in rodents is associated with higher rates of toxicity compared to those mutations which form mature fibrils [75].

In vitro studies into the mechanisms of αsyn-induced toxicity suggest the most toxic species are small annular oligomers, 40-45 nm in diameter [70]. The discovery of these annular αsyn species from human MSA brain [76] confirms this species is relevant *in vivo*. Proposed mechanisms of αsyn oligomeric toxicity include pore formation [70, 77], Golgi fragmentation and trafficking malfunction [78] and mitochondrial impairment [79]. The finding that the mitochondria are the target for oligomers fits with a plethora of data implicating mitochondria dysfunction in synucleinopathies. Deficits in mitochondria complex I activity are found in PD brain tissue [80-82] and chemicals which induce mitochondrial dysfunction are capable of manifesting PD in humans and animals independent of αsyn accumulation [83-85]. Furthermore several genes associated with familial PD, including *LRRK2*, *Parkin*, *PINK1* and *DJ-1* have been shown to directly modulate mitochondria functioning [86]. Hence mitochondria dysfunction may be a central mechanism of toxicity that unifies the various subsets of synucleinopathies.

PrP Oligomers

Unlike Aβ and αsyn, the role of PrP oligomers in causing neurotoxicity is hampered by the fact these species are yet to be identified *in vivo*. Nonetheless, it is likely that amyloid-forming proteins form conserved prefibrillar oligomeric structures prior to the generation of mature fibrils. This is supported by the finding that synthetic antibodies are capable of recognizing oligomeric species irrespective of primary sequence from various amyloid-forming sources including Aβ, PrP, αsyn and islet amyloid polypeptide (IAPP; involved in type II diabetes) [87]. As such, it is possible small soluble PrP oligomers are the toxic agent in prion disease. Similarly, given that small aggregates, by virtue of size, have a higher proportion of exposed resides on their surfaces compared to larger aggregates [88] they are likely to exhibit a higher relative toxicity than larger aggregates. Indeed, it has been proposed the formation of amyloid plaques in neurodegenerative diseases is a mechanism employed by the cell to sequester the smaller, more toxic species away from vital cellular compartments where they can cause severe damage.

Studies using synthetic PrP have shown promising results where PrP species characteristic of oligomers have increased toxicity *in vitro* [89-91] and *in vivo* [91] compared to larger mature fibrils. It is believed monomeric PrP folds into an α-helical conformation prior to its dimerization and extension into oligomers [92], which may be the toxic species. Synthetically produced monomeric α-helical PrP is highly toxic to murine neuronal, but not fibroblast cell cultures and are toxic in a dose-dependent manner when injected into mouse brain [93]. In these studies there are contrasting reports on whether this observed toxicity is PrP^C dependent, which would have implications on the mechanisms of action. If PrP oligomer-induced toxicity is a PrP^C dependent process, the oligomeric species may simply appear highly toxic due to its small size containing an increased number of nucleation sites compared to mature fibrils and hence these species catalyse the production of other toxic species more rapidly. The identification of small non-fibrillar PrP^{Sc} aggregates of 14-28 PrP molecules as the most infectious size of PrP^{Sc} [94] supports this view, however this does not easily accommodate the kinetic studies showing an uncoupling of infectivity and toxicity [35, 36]. In the studies reporting toxicity independent of PrP^C expression, a mechanism of action unique to PrP-oligomers may exist. *In vitro* and biophysical studies report the ubiquitin/proteasome system (UPS) may be a target for PrP-oligomers, given that small aggregates of oligomeric β-sheet rich PrP can directly bind and inhibit the 20S subunit of the proteasome [95, 96]. However whether or not this interaction occurs *in vivo* remains to be established.

Despite the accumulating data implicating oligomers as the toxic entity in a number of neurodegenerative diseases, a common neurotoxic mechanism of action has yet to be identified. This may be due, in part, to variations in normal processes of the proteins, compartmental location and/or different sizes or conformations of the putative toxic species. The latter factor is particularly relevant given that, by definition, the term 'oligomer' refers to essentially any conformer of protein greater than a monomer and thus represents a wide range of various sized conformations. Oligomeric species exist in an equilibrium with each other, and as such identifying one species as toxic over another would be challenging; for example, the reported putative toxic Aβ dimers have been shown to rapidly aggregate into metastable protofibrils [97] which may be more toxic in nature. A further important consideration is that the fibrillization pathway taken by an amyloid-forming protein is highly specific to its environment and susceptible to artificial manipulation. The popular laboratory solvent SDS is capable of inducing artificial aggregation of Aβ [98] and αsyn [99], which in the case of αsyn follows an atypical pathway of fibrillization [99]. Thus the *in vitro* production of oligomers or preparations of tissue are pertinent considerations when deciphering the toxic oligomer. Although compelling, further elucidation of the mechanism of oligomer toxicity, including *in vivo* evidence of PrP oligomers is needed to confirm it as a viable neurotoxic agent in prion disease.

ALTERED PrP^C SIGNALLING

Changes to the *status quo* of PrP^C functioning and/or signalling are also thought to underlie toxicity in prion disease. Evidence for this is demonstrated by the lethal toxicity of structural PrP mutants where expressions of transgenic PrP mutations containing large amino-proximal deletions in PrP (such as residues 32-121 and 32-134) on a PrP knockout background are highly toxic in mice, with ataxia and cerebellar granule cell degeneration presenting and death occurring by 3-4 months of age [100]. This observed toxicity is thought to be a consequence of the deletion of the hydrophobic region of the PrP molecule given that total ablation of the hydrophobic region is extremely toxic whilst mutations covering only half the region are innocuous [101]. The hydrophobic region spans residues 112-133 and is situated in the 'hinge' region of the PrP molecule, where it separates the structured globular domain of PrP (amino acid residues: 124-230) from the unstructured flexible tail (amino acid residues: 23-123). It contains a palindromic region and glycine rich region and is almost perfectly conserved amongst mammals [102]. The hydrophobic region is implicated in the conversion process of PrP^{C} to PrP^{Sc} where it undergoes significant structural rearrangement: amino acid substitutions in this region significantly alter the infectivity of PrP^{Sc} [103] and antibodies targeting this region bind PrP^{C} but not PrP^{Sc} [104]. Further insights come from the toxicity observed in transgenic mice expressing Doppel (Dpl); a homolog of PrP which shows structural conformation to the globular domain but lack any alignment to the flexible tail [105]. The neurotoxicity of Dpl and the PrP deletion mutations may be overcome by co-expression with PrP^{C}. These findings suggest these toxic mutants may act by altering the normal function of PrP^{C}. Several mechanisms have been postulated to describe how altered PrP^{C} functioning may contribute to toxicity in prion disease.

One possibility is that PrP^{C} has neuroprotective properties that are abrogated by its conversion to PrP^{Sc}. Subtle phenotypic changes are observed in PrP knockout mice, which have higher levels of apoptotic cell death following ischemic or traumatic brain damage [106-109]. Primary neuronal cultures from PrP knockout mice are highly sensitive to apoptosis following serum withdrawal, which can be rescued by the expression of PrP^{C} or the anti-apoptotic molecule Bcl-2 [110] and human neurons are resistant to the pro-apoptotic stimuli Bax, when Bax is co-expressed with wild-type PrP^{C} [111]. The ability of PrP to rescue cells from apoptosis or PrP knockout mice from brain injury is ablated when PrP lacks the octapeptide repeat region of the flexible tail [111-113]. The octapeptide repeat region is a tandem repeat region of 4-5 glycine-rich octapeptides, spanning residues 59-89. Polymorphisms lacking one octapeptide repeat region occurs in approximately 1% of the population [114] whereas supernumerary insertions of various lengths in this region are linked to familial forms of prion disease [115-118]. In rodent animal models deleting or blocking the function of this region with antibodies slows disease progression [119, 120]. However given that the octapeptide repeat region is dispensable for the protective action of PrP^{C} towards both Dpl and toxic PrP mutants [100,121], a neuroprotective role for PrP^{C} is not considered associated with its ability to suppress toxicity of these molecules.

Another major proposal is that PrP^{C} itself acts as a receptor for PrP^{Sc}, and their interaction triggers the activation of a neurotoxic cascade by PrP^{C}. This hypothesis is supported by reports that antibodies targeting certain regions of the PrP molecule can cause rapid neurodegeneration in brain tissue [122, 123]. One study used a comprehensive panel of monoclonal antibodies targeting various regions of the PrP molecule to show those targeting the globular domain, particularly alpha helices 1 and 3 (such as POM1), are toxic in nanomolar concentrations to organotypic brain slices prepared from PrP overexpressing mice [123]. As with prion disease, the toxicity mediated by POM1 is PrP^{C} dependent (Figure 2A-B). These antibodies do not act by distorting the conformation of PrP, and given that various small antibody fragments could achieve equivalent toxicity, including small recombinant single chain Fv fragments, its toxicity is not due to cross-linking of PrP^{C} or complement [123]. Additionally the toxic signalling pathways elicited by these antibodies overlaps with those triggered by prions: POM1 treated and prion infected brain slices both induce the expression of reactive oxygen species (ROS) and calpains, and are protected by ROS scavengers and calpain-specific inhibitors [123-125]. Both activate components of the PERK signalling pathway [125]. Similarities are also found at the transcriptional level, with 80% of genes found down-regulated being conserved between the models [125]. Further support for PrP^{C} being the upstream neurotoxic agent was demonstrated in studies showing the toxicity of POM1 is mediated by the flexible tail of PrP^{C}. Organotypic brain slices prepared from transgenic mice expressing PrP that lack a flexible tail, PrP(Δ32-93), are resistant to the toxic effects of POM1, which also occurs when wild-type PrP overexpressing brain slices are co-treated with POM1 and antibodies, such as POM2, that target the octapeptide repeat region of the flexible tail [123] (Figure 2C-D). The binding of POM2 to PrP is likely to disrupt any putative native conformation of the octapeptide repeat region [126]. Similarly, prion infected organotypic brain slice cultures treated with POM2 are protected from neuronal loss [125]. These studies reveal PrP^C is capable of adopting a toxic gain-of-function, which is triggered by the flexible tail following stimulus in the globular domain, possibly following attachment to the cellular membrane (Figure 2E). This mechanism may also explain the toxicity of the PrP deletion mutants where PrP(Δ94-134) transgenic mice have a small, but significant, increase in median survival time when injected with POM2 compared to non-injected counterparts [123].

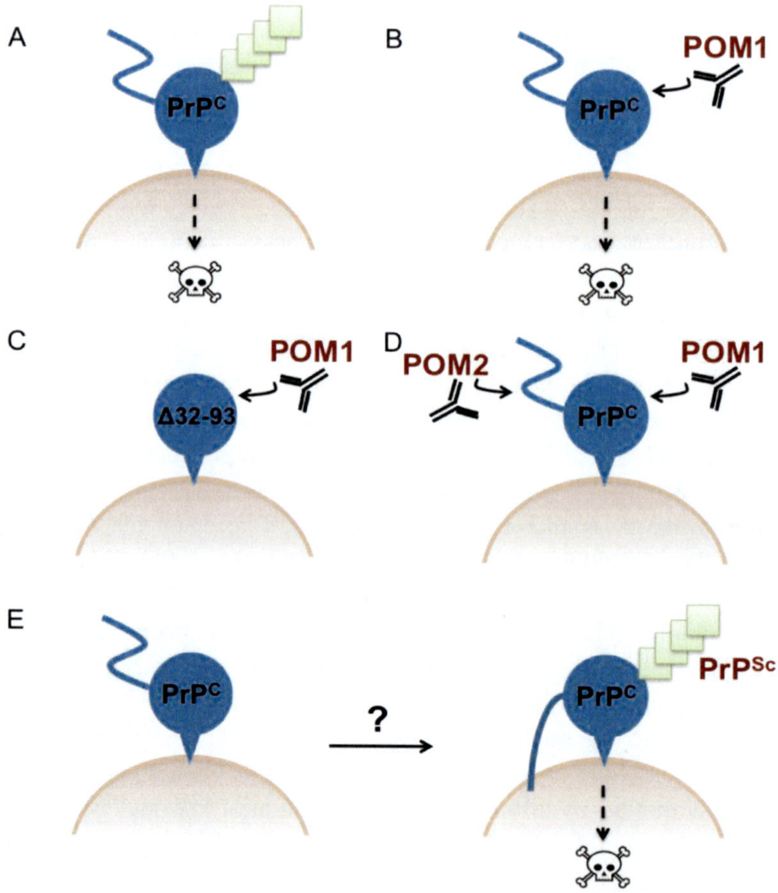

Figure 2. The flexible tail of PrP modulates toxicity in brain slices [123]. The expression of PrP^C is essential for toxicity in prion disease *in vivo* (A). A similar phenotype can be triggered in wild-type PrP overexpressing brain slices by antibodies, such as POM1, which target the globular domain of PrP (B). POM1 mediated toxicity requires a functioning flexible tail: transgenic mice expressing amino-truncated PrP, PrP(Δ32-93), are resistant to the effects of POM1 (C) as are wild type PrP overexpressing brain slices co-treated with POM1 and antibodies targeting the flexible tail, such as POM2 (D). This may mean toxicity is triggered by the flexible tail, possibly by alteration to the native conformation causing attachment to the cell membrane (E).

The capacity of the flexible tail to mediate a toxic signal fails to explain the toxicity of Dpl, or the observation that the toxic effects of Dpl or PrP mutants are abrogated by co-expression with PrP^{C}. Further insight may come from the finding that mice expressing anchorless PrP succumb to a variant of prion disease characterised by a long incubation period and atypical neuropathology where extensive PrP^{Sc} accumulation occurs but show no sign of spongiform change [15]. Given the overtly differential disease course and pathology in anchorless PrP transgenic mice compared to wild-type PrP counterparts, it is possible different mechanisms of neurodegeneration exist in these mice whereby the generation of 'acute' toxicity, *per se*, requires PrP^{C} to be attached to the cellular membrane. This further supports the idea that numerous pathways may contribute to prion disease-associated neuronal death, which may depend on the spatial and temporal status of PrP^{C}.

ALTERATIONS TO ENDOPLASMIC RETICULUM FUNCTION

Alterations to the homeostatic functioning of the endoplasmic reticulum (ER) may also contribute to prion-disease induced toxicity. The ER is essential for the co-translational or post-translational modification of various secretory and transmembrane proteins. Once targeted to the ER, these nascent proteins are modified and folded by chaperones and folding factors in order to form their proper tertiary structure, after which they are either targeted to the membrane or released from the cell via the secretory pathway. This process is strictly regulated by quality control mechanisms and disruption of this system leads to a state referred to as 'ER stress'. ER stress can be triggered by various stress stimuli, such as accumulation of misfolded protein, amino acid deprivation and viral replication [127]. Numerous studies, detailed below, suggest alterations to the normal processing of PrP within the ER and/or the activation of pathways associated with ER stress can contribute to toxicity in prion disease.

Mislocalization of PrP

Aside from PrP that is attached to the cellular membrane via a GPI anchor, several other variants of PrP exist. Random errors in processing can lead to the hydrophobic region of PrP adopting a transmembrane conformation with its COOH-terminus or NH_2-terminus facing the inside of the lumen of the ER, resulting in ^{ctm}PrP or ^{ntm}PrP respectively [128-130]. While under normal conditions these topological conformers make up a small per cent of the overall pool of PrP and are innocuous, even slight over expression of ^{ctm}PrP, or PrP mutations that preferentially produce it, lead to a non-transmissible neurodegenerative phenotype in mice that arises independently of PrP^{Sc} accumulation [128, 131]. In addition, PrP may be mislocalized to the cytosol if the degradative capacity of the proteasome is impaired [132, 133], or by stress triggering retrograde transport of PrP from the ER to the cytosol during ER associated degradation (ERAD) [134, 135]: a controlled process to remove unwanted or terminally misfolded protein by targeting them to the cytosol for proteasomal degradation. Increased expression of cytosolic PrP (cytPrP) in both neuronal and non-neuronal cells produces PrP^{Sc}-like self-perpetuating, amorphous aggregates that are highly toxic [136-138] and transgenic mice expressing mutant PrP lacking both its C and N terminus, which leads to accumulation of PrP in the cytosol, develop neurological illness characterized by substantial loss of granule cerebellar neurons and gliosis [137]. It has been reported both ^{ctm}PrP and cytPrP may cause toxicity by binding to and disrupting the actions of Mahogunin (MGRN1), a cytosolic E4 ligase [139]. In accordance to this, MGRN1 knockout mice exhibit pathological commonalities with prion disease such as spongiform degeneration [140]. However follow up studies have so far failed to find a role of MGRN1 in prion disease, as neither the up-regulation nor ablation of MGRN1 alters the pathology or course of disease [141, 142].

The mechanisms of ^{ctm}PrP or cytPrP production have been investigated. As a general rule increasing the hydrophobicity of PrP increases the production of transmembrane PrP variants [128, 143], which may explain toxicity in certain familial forms of prion disease. Alternatively, PrP^{Sc}-induced chronic ER stress has been proposed to trigger cytPrP accumulation via the activation of a pre-emptive quality control (pQC) system that acts to halt translocation of protein and increase retrotranslocation and degradation in the cytosol. If persistently activated, pQC may increase the level of cytPrP beyond the degradative capacity of the proteasome, resulting in accumulation of toxic PrP in the cytosol. In support of this, transgenic mice expressing a PrP variant that has low translocation potential (thus modelling a state of chronic activation of pQC) develop a mild neurodegenerative phenotype similar, in some aspects, with prion disease pathology [144]. In addition, it is feasible that proteasome inhibition caused by PrP oligomers [95, 96] may also lead to the accumulation of cytPrP, and hence provide a mechanism of action for oligomeric-PrP toxicity. However a role for ^{ctm}PrP or cytPrP in prion disease-associated neurotoxicity is questioned by the observation that *in vivo* models are only able to recapitulate certain aspects of disease. Several studies report the expression of cytPrP is non-toxic, perhaps even protective, in cell culture and animal models [145, 146]; hence any effects elicited by these variants in prion disease are not considered to be the sole contributors to toxicity.

The Unfolded Protein Response

A common feature of ER stress is protein misfolding in the ER, which in order to prevent perturbations in normal cellular activities, leads to the activation of the unfolded protein response (UPR). The UPR is a self-protective mechanism which aims to restore normal ER homeostasis by activating chaperones and enzymes associated with the folding pathway, activating ERAD and suppressing global protein synthesis. Conversely, under conditions of chronic or irreversible stress, the UPR can trigger apoptotic cell death, thus it represents a complex regulatory system that can signal both pro- and anti-cell survival signals. There are three signalling transduction components of the UPR: protein kinase RNA (PKR)-like ER kinase (PERK), inositol-requiring enzyme 1 (IRE1), and activating transcription factor 6 (ATF6) [127]. They are all activated by the heat-shock protein Grp78/BiP, which is reported to be constitutively bound to its signalling molecule in an 'inactive' state and dissociates to 'activate' its signalling molecule following the detection of rising levels of misfolded protein [147, 148]. Following activation, PERK oligomerizes and trans-autophosphorylates the cytosolic portion of its receptor complex, which leads to the activation and phosphorylation of its target protein, the alpha subunit of eukaryotic translation factor-2 (eIF2α). Phosphorylated eIF2α (p-eIF2α) triggers a suppression of global protein synthesis and induces the activation of activating transcription factor 4 (ATF4) that enters the nucleus to modulate target UPR genes. In particular, ATF4 regulates the functions of CHOP, which is believed to activate apoptotic pathways, and GADD34, which serves to provide a negative feedback loop by dephosphorylating eIF2α. IRE1 also activates via oligomerization and trans-autophosphorylation, which leads to cleavage and subsequent splicing of mRNA that encodes the transcription factor, x-box binding protein 1 (XBP1). Two splice variants of XBP1 are translated with opposing actions: one that activates UPR target genes, the other which represses them. Activation of the anchored transcription factor, ATF6, results in its translocation to the Golgi apparatus via a CREB/ATF bZIP transcription factor domain, where it is cleaved by proteases to yield a cytosolic fragment known ATF6f ('f' for fragment). ATF6f is capable of entering the nucleus where it also activates UPR target gene expression (Figure 3).

Grp78/BiP is found elevated in human CJD brain [149] and its expression is elevated in cells following exposure to PrP^{Sc} [149] or the toxic PrP fragment PrP(106-126) [150]. Downstream components of PERK signalling p-eIF2α and ATF4 are elevated in prion diseased organotypic brain slice cultures [125]. In prion infected mice, the rising levels of misfolded PrP^{Sc} correlates with increases in components of PERK signalling; phosphorylated PERK (p-PERK) and p-eIF2α, as well as decreases in synaptic proteins, leading to neuronal death [46]. In this model the overexpression of GADD35 or the knockdown of PrP was able to suppress PrP^{Sc}-induced toxicity, whereas treatment with salubrinal, a compound that inhibits the dephosphorylation of p-eIF2α, exacerbated neurodegenerative symptoms and enhanced disease progression [46]. In agreement to these findings, treatment with compounds targeting PERK, or downstream of eIF2α, GSK2606414 and ISRIB respectively, impede the development of clinical symptoms and neuropathology in prion diseased mice [151, 152]. Collectively these studies suggest PERK-mediated signalling greatly contributes to prion disease-induced neurotoxicity.

What causes the activation of PERK signalling in prion disease is unknown. The observation that toxic globular domain-directed antibodies activate components of the PERK signalling pathway [125] argues against PrP^{Sc} accumulation activating PERK signalling in prion disease. Given that some report PrP mRNA levels increase during prion infection [46] it is possible increased synthesis of native PrP activates the UPR. This is supported by studies showing the overexpression of protein production may trigger UPR markers [153]. However given that others report PrP mRNA levels to be unchanged throughout disease progression [41, 42], further elucidation is necessary to determine the activator/s of UPR signalling in prion disease. In addition, the mechanism of cell death by eIF2α may be multifaceted. Aside from a suppression of protein synthesis, cleaved caspase-12 (mouse homologue to human caspase-4) also correlates with neuronal cell loss in mouse models of prion disease [46, 149], which may indicate the activation of apoptosis. However neither ablation of caspase-12 [154], nor modulation of apoptotic mediators by Bax deletion or Bcl-2 overexpression [155] alters disease progression. Studies examining the effect of PERK signalling on gene expression by knocking down various components of the signalling pathway reveal nearly half of PERK-dependent targets are ATF4 independent [156], hence it cannot be excluded that other unknown downstream effectors also contribute to eIF2α-mediated neuronal cell death in prion disease.

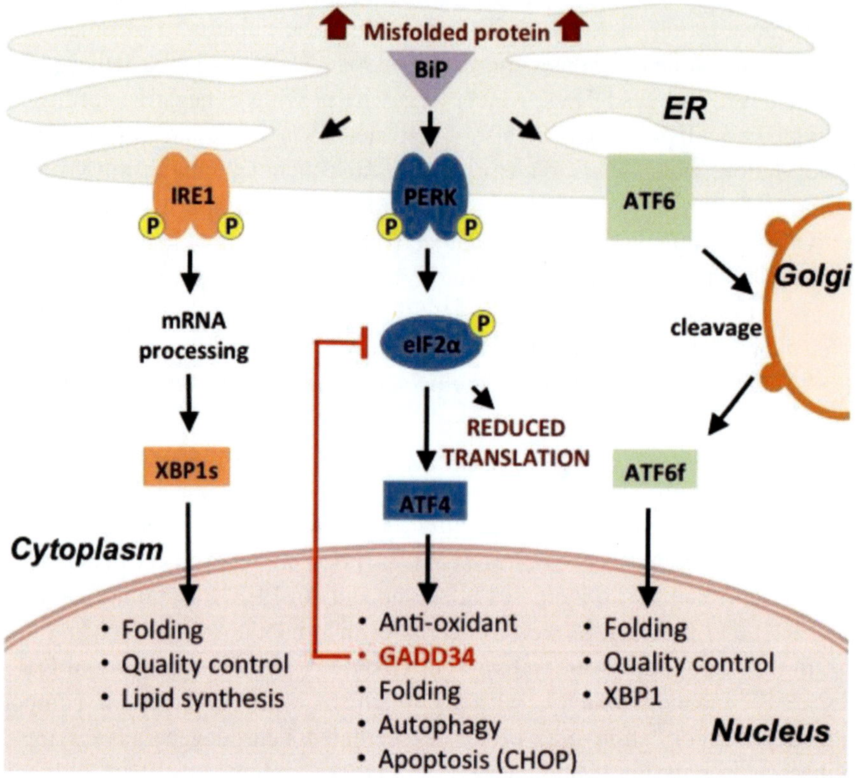

Figure 3. The unfolded protein response (UPR). Rising levels of misfolded protein triggers the activation of three signalling components of the UPR in the endoplasmic reticulum (ER). Activation of IRE1 occurs following trans-autophosphorylation of the receptor complex that in turn cleaves mRNA encoding XBP1. PERK also trans-autophosphorylates following activation, which in turn phosphorylates and activates its target eIF2α. The main outputs for p-eIF2α are a reduction in total protein synthesis and activation of transcription factor ATF4. Activated ATF6 transits to the Golgi apparatus where it is cleaved, releasing ATF6 fragment (ATF6f). XBP1s, AT4 and ATF6f are all capable of entering the nucleus to activate target UPR genes associated with various pro- and anti-survival signals. In particular, ATF4 can induce the expression of GADD34 that generates a negative feedback loop by targeting eIF2α for dephosphorylation.

PERK-mediated neurotoxicity may have an equivalent in relatable neurodegenerative diseases. Selective neuronal loss of dopaminergic neurons of the substantia nigra is a key feature of PD, and in this region p-PERK and p-eIF2α are found elevated in diseased brain compared to control brain, where p-PERK immunoreactivity co-localizes with areas of high αsyn expression [157]. Numerous studies support a role of αsyn in directly activating the PERK pathway. The accumulation of αsyn in dopaminergic cells leads to increases in both Grp78/BiP and ATF4 [158]. Manganese-induced ER stress causes αsyn to oligomerize and activate the PERK pathway in organotypic brain slice cultures [159] and ablation of αsyn in this model leads to a reduction in PERK-mediated signalling, while the levels of p-IRE1 and Xbp1 mRNA splicing remained unchanged [160]. It has also been proposed monomeric αsyn within the ER activates PERK signalling by binding directly to Grp78/BiP [158]. Importantly, cells expressing the PD-associated familial αsyn mutation, A53T, harbour elevated levels of p-eIF2α, Grp78/BiP and CHOP and increased cell death relative to wild-type cells, which in contrast to prion disease models, is partially reversed by treatment with salubrinal or inhibition of caspase-12 [161]. This suggests the PERK pathway may have contrasting effects in prion and PD. In support of this, A53T transgenic mice exhibit an attenuation in αsyn-mediated cell death following treatment with salubrinal [162].

In AD, Grp78/BiP, p-PERK and p-eIF2α are all found elevated in diseased brain [163,164] and mice overexpressing the human apoE4 allele [165]. In transgenic mice expressing the lethal APP/PS1 mutation to model AD, the observed decrease in synaptic proteins was found to be concomitant with increased p-eIF2α levels. Strikingly, the conditional deletion of PERK was able to rescue synaptic protein synthesis which improved behavioural spatial memory and suppressed the potentiation of LTP [166], hence giving strong evidence PERK signalling is involved in neurodegeneration in AD. The contributions of p-eIF2α to these effects may be multifaceted given that, in contrast to the reduced translation of protein synthesis elicited by p-eIF2α, it has also been shown to directly increase the translation of BACE1 [167-171]; a critical protease in the cleavage of APP to produce Aβ. Treating primary neurons with salubrinal results in a significant increase of BACE1 expression [167]. In agreement to these findings, reductions in PERK-dependent eIF2α phosphorylation suppress any elevation in BACE1 [172]. Another critical protein present in AD and other neurodegenerative diseases, hyperphosphorylated tau, is also associated with PERK activation. Increased levels of p-PERK and p-IRE1 associate with p-tau in the hippocampus of frontotemporal dementia cases that exhibit tau pathology [173] and genome-wide association studies reveal *EIF2AK3*, the gene that encodes PERK, as a risk factor for certain tauopathies [174]. In a mouse model of tauopathy, tau accumulation triggers activation of the UPR by blocking ERAD, which is reversible following depletion of tau [175]. Activation of the UPR may also contribute to tau pathology by upregulating glycogen synthase kinase 3β (GSK-3β); a kinase implicated in the phosphorylation of tau. In AD neurons, p-PERK is found in proximity to GSK-3β [163] and *in vitro* studies show activation of various components of the UPR induces the activity of GSK-3β [176, 177].

The UPR is reported to also be involved in animal models of amyotrophic lateral sclerosis (ALS). Mutations in Cu/Zn superoxide dismutase (SOD1) are linked to familial ALS and various transgenic mouse lines harbouring SOD1 mutations show elevations in virtually all components of the UPR including Grp78/BiP, PERK, IRE1 and ATF6 [178, 179]. A role of PERK signalling in ALS-induced toxicity is supported in other animal models of ALS, which overexpress proteins present in the toxic stress granules, such as TDP-43. When expressed in *Drosophila* and mammalian neuronal cell cultures, the toxic TDP-43 leads to increased p-eIF2α levels and its toxicity is ablated following treatment with GSK2606414 [180]. Other studies show reducing ATF4 expression in mutant SOD1 models delays disease progression, in part, associated with reductions in the pro-apoptotic molecules CHOP and Bim [181], suggesting PERK-mediated mechanisms aside from reduced protein translation may contribute to ALS disease-associated toxicity. However, in contrast to this, disease is accelerated in mutant SOD1 mice when only one allele of the gene encoding PERK is expressed [182] and zebrafish and *C. elegans* models of TDP-43 toxicity show reduced neurodegeneration following induction of p-eIF2α by various pharmalogical compounds, including salubrinal [183].

Collectively these studies give strong evidence that PERK-mediated signalling is implicated in toxicity in various neurodegenerative diseases; however it seems to have contrasting roles whereby it can act in either a protective or harmful capacity. The observed contrasting effect of salubrinal between prion disease and PD and ALS is one such example of this and highlights the complex nature of UPR signalling. Additionally although strong evidence suggests the UPR is involved in neurodegeneration in mice infected with prions [46], it may not be involved in familial forms of disease, given that transgenic mouse and cell models of familial prion disease report no alterations to UPR signalling [184]. Therefore further investigations are needed into establish the role the UPR plays in neurotoxicity in prion disease and relatable neurodegenerative diseases.

Therapeutic Strategies for Prion Disease-Associated Neurotoxicity

It has been over three decades since the first compounds were tested therapeutically in humans to treat prion disease. Since then, a large number of compounds have been found that exhibit prion-alleviating properties, with several compounds being trialled in humans (Table 1). The unsuccessful results from human studies are in part due to the difficulties in translation from *in vitro* systems to the human condition. This was exemplified by the promising *in vitro* results for the antimalarial and antipsychotic compounds quinacrine and chlorpromazine. Both compounds were found to inhibit PrP^{Sc} conversion in cultured cells [185-187] and given their safe efficacy in humans and ability to cross the blood brain barrier (BBB), quinacrine was quickly trialled in humans to treat prion disease despite a lack of *in vivo* evidence or known mechanism of action. Quinacrine was unsuccessful in improving disease parameters either individually [188-190], or in a combined treatment strategy with chlorpromazine [191, 192] (Table 1). After human use was started reports emerged showing quinacrine failed to extend survival in prion-infected mice [193-195] and its treatment is capable of generating drug-resistant prions [195] and can amplify prion replication in certain prion diseases [196]. These failed therapeutic attempts demonstrate that a reduction in PrP^{Sc} conversion *in vitro* is unlikely to be an appropriate readout of efficacy for the human condition.

One of the most promising compounds trialled in humans to date has been the polyanion, pentosan polysulfate (PPS). PPS interferes with prion replication and is efficacious in animal models to both peripheral [197-200] and CNS prions [194]. However human trials have had variable results [201-206] (Table 1) and a major limitation to its use *in vivo* is its inability to cross the BBB, which requires the compound to be administered intraventrically. More recent promising small compounds are able to transverse the BBB. Compound-B (cpd-B) extends survival of mouse-adapted scrapie infected mice by 2.3% when treatment is administered orally from the day of intracerebral inoculation with prions [207]. Due to the potential of cpd-B to generate toxic metabolites [208], less-toxic analogues have been generated with similar anti-prion effects, however they do not appear effective against human prion strains [209]. The compound IND24 significantly extends the lifespan of mice infected with mouse-adapted scrapie prion strains, however IND24 was ineffective to human prion strains, and has the capacity to generate drug resistant prions [210]. Luminescent Conjugated Polymers (LCPs) show high affinity to binding amyloid and certain compounds are capable of crossing the BBB [211]. Various LCPs have been shown to reduce PrP^{Sc} infectivity in infected brain homogenate and prion-infected organotypic brain slice cultures, potentially via hyperstabilizing PrP^{Sc} deposits [212]. The efficacy of prion-alleviating LCPs has yet to be reported using human prion strains and *in vivo* systems.

Table 1. Human trials performed for therapeutic intervention of prion disease

Compound	Effect of compound in animal models	Human study design	Outcome	Comments
Amantadine	No effect on survival [213,214]	Observational [215, 216]	No effect on patient survival	Anti-viral compound trialled when disease believed to be of viral origin
Flupirtine		RCT-DB [217]	No effect on patient survival	No justification given for its use in humans
Quinacrine	No effect on survival or PrP^{Sc} accumulation [193-195,218]	Observational [188-190]	Variable effect on survival	Treatment in humans started before animal testing
		RCT-DB [189]	No effect on patient survival	
Combined Chlorpromazine and Quinacrine		Case report [191, 192]	No effect on patient survival	
Doxycycline	Increase survival to peripheral and CNS prions [219]	Observational [220, 221]	Increase patient survival	
		RCT-DB [222]	No effect on patient survival	
		Preventative (EU clinical trial register: 2010-022233-28)	Currently underway in FFI presymptomatic carriers	
Intraventricular infusion of PPS	Increase survival to peripheral and CNS prions [194,197-200]	Observational [201, 202]	Variable effects on survival	Surgical complications common and toxicity observed in some human trials
		Case report [203-206]	Possible increase patient survival	

RCT-DB: Randomized double-blind placebo-controlled clinical trial; CNS: central nervous system; FFI: Fatal Familial Insomnia; PPS: Pentosan Polysulfate.

Targeting the neurotoxic agent would likely be an advantageous therapeutic strategy and given the plethora of data suggesting aggregated PrP^{Sc} is not the toxic agent, compounds acting to reduce PrP^{Sc} load may be ineffective. For example, PPS does not interfere with the toxicity of the globular domain-directed antibody POM1 [125] and therefore if PrP^{C} is the upstream neurotoxic agent, PPS will likely be of little therapeutic benefit. Compounds that act on potential neurotoxic pathways in prion disease show great promise. The small compound anle138b is efficacious to various strains of prions in mouse models of prion disease and acts by inhibiting the formation of PrP^{Sc} oligomers [223]. Strikingly, anle138b also inhibits the aggregation of αsyn *in vitro* and shows efficacy in mouse models of PD by reducing oligomer formation [223]. The capacity of anle138b to bind to a structure-dependent epitope suggests it may be effective in treating other neurodegenerative diseases associated with oligomer-induced toxicity. Targeting downstream components of the neurotoxic cascade have also showed promise as novel therapeutics for prion disease. The PERK-inhibitor compound GSK2606414 suppresses the manifestations of behavioural deficits and prion-disease associated neuropathology in mice when daily treatment was commenced in parallel with the first signs of synapse loss in diseased mice [151]. GSK2606414 easily crosses the BBB so can be administered orally, and has a high specificity for PERK [151, 224], making it an attractive therapeutic compound. Unfortunately the long-term survival of these mice has not been assessed due to excessive weight loss following treatment requiring the trial to be aborted [151]. This may reflect adverse side effects associated with targeting a major signal transduction pathway. Abnormal UPR signalling occurs in numerous conditions associated with ER stress including neurodegenerative disease, cancer, metabolic disease, inflammatory disease and cardiovascular disease [225] and thus represents a major stress pathway. Total suppression of PERK-mediated eIF2α phosphorylation leaves cells susceptible to death from ER stress [156, 226, 227] and PERK knockout mice exhibit exocrine pancreatic dysfunction and abnormalities associated with glucose and insulin metabolism [228]. In agreement to these findings, mice harbouring homozygous mutations in eIF2α at the serine residue which undergoes phosphorylation (Ser51Ala) succumb to death within 24 hours due to deficits in gluconeogenesis [227] and small chemical chaperones improves insulin signalling in type 2 diabetic mice by promoting protein folding and reducing ER stress [229]. This aligns with observations of mice treated with GSK2606414 that exhibit mild insulin resistance [151]. Recently another compound, ISRIB, which acts downstream of eIF2α, has been shown to be therapeutic to mouse models of prion disease. This compound penetrates the BBB and is less toxic than GSK2606414 [152]. Similar to GSK2606414, its efficacy was investigated in prion-infected mice when treatment commenced at the first signs of synapse loss. Daily intraperitoneal injection of ISRIB increased survival of prion-infected mice from 84±3 in vehicle treated controls to 96±4 days in ISRIB treated animals, however again the trial was aborted due to excessive weight loss [152]. Therefore although these preliminary reports are promising, further elucidation into the long term and off-target effects of GSK2606414 and ISRIB are important future directions.

The ability to rescue mice with established prion disease by ablating the expression of PrP^C [22], suggests targeting PrP^C may also be a viable therapeutic strategy. In cultured cells and cell-free systems, monoclonal antibodies that target PrP^C abolish prion replication [230-235]. Their effectiveness extends to *in vivo* animal models where two antibodies ICSM35 and ICSM18, that recognise residues 93-105 and 143-153 respectively, have been shown to completely ameliorate prion propagation of peripheral prions in infected mice when treatment starts before PrP^{Sc} reaches the brain [236]. This striking result is the only therapeutic strategy to date shown to clinically cure disease. ICSM18 and ICSM35 are non-toxic to mice [237] and appear to act by stabilising the conformation of PrP^C [238]. A humanized version of ICSM18 has been produced which is non-toxic at intravenous doses of up to 200 mg/kg in cynomolgus macaques [61], giving evidence for its safe use in human trials. Given its large size, the efficacy of PrP-directed antibodies decreases once prions reach the CNS and as such, its ability to cross the BBB is considered a large therapeutic challenge. However the observation that intraperitoneal injection of the PrP antibody 6D11 (amino acid specificity: 93-109) in APP/PS1 transgenic mice results in a reduction in behavioural deficits, gives proof-of-principle evidence that peripherally administered antibodies can reach the CNS [239]. In agreement to this, studies investigating Aβ-directed antibodies as a therapeutic for AD, showed small amounts of peripherally-administered antibodies were found in the brain [240, 241]. Additionally it has been reported the BBB is impaired in prion disease [242, 243] and as such the transverse of antibodies across the BBB may not be a major obstacle when treating progressed disease.

Despite the plethora of data showing PrP-targeted antibodies as therapeutic, concern is raised by reports showing that under certain conditions PrP antibodies can be neurotoxic [122, 123]. The antibodies D13 and P, which align to hydrophobic region PrP resides 95-105, have been reported to be toxic to wild-type mice, with widespread neuronal loss observed 24 hours post hippocampal injection [122]. However replication of this experiment could not be achieved by others [237]. Similarly 6D11 cures cells of prion infection and prolongs the incubation period of disease *in vivo* [244]. Antibodies targeting alpha helix 1 (amino acid residues: 145-155) and 3 (amino acid residues: 200-219) of the globular domain of PrP are highly toxic to PrP overexpressing organotypic brain slices [123, 125], however the alpha-helix 1 region aligns to the binding region of the non-toxic, therapeutic ICSM18 [236, 237]. Additionally, the antibody W226, which targets regions between 145-153 of the prion protein and has a 59% homology to ICSM18, is able to prevent prion replication in cultured cells, however exerts no protection to mice from peripheral prion infection [245]. The reason for the contrasting effects of these antibodies has not been elucidated. It may be a matter of dose threshold: either of the concentration of the antibody or expression of available PrP^C to bind. Additional factors may include the species specificity, binding affinity, mode-of-action, or the differences in epitope recognition of the antibody. Nonetheless the observations that under certain conditions PrP-directed antibodies have the capacity to be toxic should be addressed prior to its use in humans.

Aside from monoclonal antibodies, the search for other small compounds that bind PrP^C may prove rewarding. Although chlorpromazine is not effective at reducing PrP^{Sc} titres in animal models [218], a recent study suggests it acts by binding to the hydrophobic pocket of PrP^C and stabilises the protein [246]. If true, this advantageous mode-of-action supports further testing into its *in vivo* efficacy. An alternate approach to therapeutically target PrP^C is to alter its expression. This has been achieved by employing RNAi, where a study using lentiviral mediated shRNA against PrP^C in prion infected mice showed a single treatment of shRNA injected into each hippocampus when the first signs of neuropathological change occurred prevented the onset of behavioural deficits and reduced spongiform degeneration and neuronal loss [247]. These neuropathological changes were observed in sites surrounding the injection site and despite the small region of brain exposed to the RNAi, the mean survival of shRNA treated mice was 23.5% higher than untreated animals [247]. This demonstrates that even small reductions in PrP^C expression are likely to be therapeutic in prion disease. Using RNAi as a therapy also has great potential to treat familial forms of disease by generating allele-specific siRNA. Although studies on this are yet to be described for prion disease, preliminary studies have been performed for familial forms of other neurodegenerative diseases including AD [248], PD [249] ALS [250] and Huntington's disease [251] with promising results. Additionally the CRISPR/Cas-9 system has been utilized to correct a mutation associated with cystic fibrosis in patient-derived cultured intestinal cells, which when assayed in organoid culture, showed a rescue of disease-associated defects [252]. These encouraging studies for treating single-gene hereditary defects support the potential for tailored patient-specific therapy, which is considered the gold-standard for future therapeutic strategy.

Targeting regulators of PrP expression may also prove beneficial. The laminin receptor has been shown to bind to prions [253, 254] and its knockdown using RNAi significantly decreases PrP^{Sc} accumulation in cultured cells [255] and extends the preclinical incubation period in prion infected mice [256]. Alternatively, the transcription factors SP1 and metal transcription factor-1 regulate *PRNP* gene expression *in vitro* [257], however their role in prion disease is yet to be established. Targeting miRNA is another option, in view of the finding that miRNA profiles are deregulated in brain tissue of terminally ill prion infected animals [258, 259] and exosomes released from prion-infected cultured cells [260]. In these studies there is a degree of concordance between miRNA signatures, suggesting targeting prion disease-specific miRNA may be a viable option to treat disease.

Limitations to the use of RNAi as therapies are that they do not readily cross the BBB and have the potential to trigger off-target effects and/or toxicity due to over-loading the RNAi pathway. Various alterations to naked RNAi may improve these parameters, such as designing siRNA duplexes to decrease off-target effects, or fusing it to neuron specific markers such as rabies virus glycoprotein (RVG) to aid its delivery to the CNS. Alternatively, other methods of knockdown may reduce toxicity; miRNA appear generally better tolerated than siRNA or shRNA [261] and recently synthetic miRNA sequences have been used to target *PRNP* mRNA to produce PrP^C knockdown in cultured cells [262]. Additionally many studies have investigated using siRNA delivery vectors [263]. In particular, the naturally occurring RNA carriers exosomes show great potential in allowing the safe transport of siRNA over large distances where intravenous injections of exosomes fused to RVG are targeted to the CNS where they deliver siRNA cargo specifically to neurons [264]. This system has been successfully utilized to reduce levels of BACE1 in mouse brain by over 60% in the striatum, cortex and midbrain of wild-type mice [264]. In another study, exosomes were efficiently targeted to the brain via the intranasal route [265], suggesting a non-invasive mode of administration for RNAi molecules.

Conclusion

Prion disease and other neurodegenerative diseases associated with misfolded proteins are complex in origin and pathogenesis. In prion disease, it is becoming increasingly apparent that confounding factors such as prion strain, aetiology and mode-of-infection all impact the generation of disease. This notion is pertinent to the generation of neurotoxicity, where many processes and pathways are likely to be involved that converge on the point of toxicity. For example, the recent observation that PERK signalling is upregulated in POM1-induced toxicity in organotypic brain slice cultures [125] unifies several key hypotheses. It is also reasonable to assume that different PrP subtypes exist, which possess different molecular and biophysical characteristics, some of which are more toxic in nature than others. Therefore it will be important to address whether any conformation of PrP preferentially binds to PrP^C. Additionally, given that PrP^C anchorless mice still succumb to toxicity [15], further understanding of the locality of PrP^C and other PrP subtypes in the generation of neurotoxicity remain important avenues of research.

Future development of therapeutic strategies needs to encompass the evolving knowledge of neurotoxic mechanisms. Compounds targeting critical components of toxic pathways show great promise, as does gene-targeted therapies. The latter strategy may not only act to resolve sporadic disease but also correct mutations associated with familial forms of disease prior to the onset of symptoms. Given that the effectiveness of a compound increases the earlier the treatment regime starts, early diagnosis is also critical for future effective therapies. Currently a correct diagnosis is typically not made until clinical symptoms present, which is an advanced disease phenotype whereby prions have penetrated the CNS and large-scale neuronal loss has already occurred. Indeed, a retrospective medical review reports the mean time between onset of clinical symptoms and diagnosis is 7.9 months, or approximately 2/3 of the way through their disease course [266]. Therefore the discovery of biomarkers for early detection of disease should be considered a vital component for effective treatment. The search for biomarkers for neurodegenerative disease has resulted in the identification of various proteins in the brain and CSF of patients that correlate with AD, however these results have been largely inconsistent [267]. Recently miRNA has been used as a diagnostic tool in AD, where a panel of 16 exosome-specific miRNAs was able to predict disease with high sensitivity and specificity (87% and 77% respectively) [268] from patient serum, supporting the idea that miRNA profiles may be used to identify individuals at-risk of developing neurodegenerative disease well before any neurotoxicity occurs.

ACKNOWLEDGMENTS

C.L.U wishes to thank Dr. L.J. Vella for critical proofreading of the manuscript.

REFERENCES

[1] Legname G, Baskakov IV, Nguyen HOB, Riesner D, Cohen FE, et al. (2004) Synthetic mammalian prions. *Science* 305: 673-676.
[2] Weissmann C (1991) A unified theory of prion propagation. *Nature* 352: 679-683.
[3] Couzin J (2004) Biomedicine. An end to the prion debate? Don't count on it. *Science* 305: 589-589.
[4] Prusiner SB (1982) Novel proteinaceous infectious particles cause scrapie. *Science* 216: 136-144.
[5] Borchelt DR, Scott M, Taraboulos A, Stahl N, Prusiner SB (1990) Scrapie and cellular prion proteins differ in their kinetic of synthesis and topology in cultured-cells. *Journal of Cell Biology* 110: 743-752.
[6] Pan KM, Baldwin M, Nguyen J, Gasset M, Serban A, et al. (1993) Conversion of alpha-helices into beta-sheets features in the formation of the scrapie prion proteins. *Proceedings of the National Academy of Sciences of the United States of America* 90: 10962-10966.
[7] Merz PA, Somerville RA, Wisniewski HM, Iqbal K (1981) Abnormal fibrils from scrapie-infected brain. *Acta Neuropathologica* 54: 63-74.

[8] Fraser H, Dickinso.Ag (1973) Scrapie in mice - agent-strain differences in distribution and intensity of grey matter vacuolation. *Journal of Comparative Pathology* 83: 29-40.
[9] Bruce M, Chree A, McConnell I, Foster J, Pearson G, et al. (1994) Transmission of bovine spongiform encephalopathy and scrapie to mice: strain variation and the species barrier. *Philos Trans R Soc Lond B Biol Sci* 343: 405-411.
[10] Aguzzi A, Calella AM (2009) Prions: Protein aggregation and infectious diseases. *Physiological Reviews* 89: 1105-1152.
[11] Medori R, Tritschler HJ, Leblanc A, Villare F, Manetto V, et al. (1992) Fatal familial insomnia, a prion disease with a mutation at codon-178 of the prion protein gene. *New England Journal of Medicine* 326: 444-449.
[12] Collinge J, Owen F, Poulter M, Leach M, Crow TJ, et al. (1990) Prion dementia without characteristic pathology. *Lancet* 336: 7-9.
[13] Manson JC, Jamieson E, Baybutt H, Tuzi NL, Barron R, et al. (1999) A single amino acid alteration (101L) introduced into murine PrP dramatically alters incubation time of transmissible spongiform encephalopathy. *Embo Journal* 18: 6855-6864.
[14] Hsiao KK, Scott M, Foster D, Groth DF, Dearmond SJ, et al. (1990) Spontaneous neurodegeneration in transgenic mice with mutant prion protein. *Science* 250: 1587-1590.
[15] Chesebro B, Race B, Meade-White K, LaCasse R, Race R, et al. (2010) Fatal transmissible amyloid encephalopathy: A new type of prion disease associated with lack of prion protein membrane anchoring. *Plos Pathogens* 6.
[16] Chesebro B, Trifilo M, Race R, Meade-White K, Teng C, et al. (2005) Anchorless prion protein results in infectious amyloid disease without clinical scrapie. *Science* 308: 1435-1439.
[17] Bueler H, Fischer M, Lang Y, Bluethmann H, Lipp HP, et al. (1992) Normal development and behavior of mice lacking the neuronal cell-surface PrP protein. *Nature* 356: 577-582.
[18] Mallucci GR, Ratte S, Asante EA, Linehan J, Gowland I, et al. (2002) Post-natal knockout of prion protein alters hippocampal CA1 properties, but does not result in neurodegeneration. *Embo Journal* 21: 202-210.
[19] Bueler H, Aguzzi A, Sailer A, Greiner RA, Autenried P, et al. (1993) Mice devoid of PrP are resistant to scrapie. *Cell* 73: 1339-1347.
[20] Manson JC, Clarke AR, McBride PA, McConnell I, Hope J (1994) PrP gene dosage determines the timing but not the final intensity or distribution of lesions in scrapie pathology. *Neurodegeneration* 3: 331-340.
[21] Brandner S, Isenmann S, Raeber A, Fischer M, Sailer A, et al. (1996) Normal host prion protein necessary for scrapie-induced neurotoxicity. *Nature* 379: 339-343.
[22] Mallucci G, Dickinson A, Linehan J, Klohn PC, Brandner S, et al. (2003) Depleting neuronal PrP in prion infection prevents disease and reverses spongiosis. *Science* 302: 871-874.
[23] Mallucci GR, White MD, Farmer M, Dickinson A, Khatun H, et al. (2007) Targeting cellular prion protein reverses early coanitive deficits and neurophysiological dysfunction in prion-infected mice. *Neuron* 53: 325-335.
[24] Kimberlin RH, Walker CA (1978) Evidence that transmission of one source of scrapie agent to hamsters involves separation of agent strains from a mixture. *Journal of General Virology* 39: 487-496.

[25] Hill AF, Joiner S, Linehan J, Desbruslais M, Lantos PL, et al. (2000) Species-barrier-independent prion replication in apparently resistant species. *Proceedings of the National Academy of Sciences of the United States of America* 97: 10248-10253.
[26] Thackray AM, Klein MA, Aguzzi A, Bujdoso R (2002) Chronic subclinical prion disease induced by low-dose inoculum. *Journal of Virology* 76: 2510-2517.
[27] Thackray AM, Klein MA, Bujdoso R (2003) Subclinical prion disease induced by oral inoculation. *Journal of Virology* 77: 7991-7998.
[28] Race R, Raines A, Raymond GJ, Caughey B, Chesebro B (2001) Long-term subclinical carrier state precedes scrapie replication and adaptation in a resistant species: Analogies to bovine spongiform encephalopathy and variant Creutzfeldt-Jakob disease in humans. *Journal of Virology* 75: 10106-10112.
[29] Collins SJ, Lewis V, Brazier MW, Hill AF, Lawson VA, et al. (2005) Extended period of asymptomatic prion disease after low dose inoculation: Assessment of detection methods and implications for infection control. *Neurobiology of Disease* 20: 336-346.
[30] Weissmann C (1991) Spongiform encephalopathies - The prion's progress. *Nature* 349: 569-571.
[31] Cohen FE, Pan KM, Huang Z, Baldwin M, Fletterick RJ, et al. (1994) Structual clues to prion replication. *Science* 264: 530-531.
[32] Hill AF, Collinge J (2003) Subclinical prion infection. *Trends in Microbiology* 11: 578-584.
[33] Collinge J, Clarke AR (2007) A general model of prion strains and their pathogenicity. *Science* 318: 930-936.
[34] Baringer JR, Bowman KA, Prusiner SB (1983) Replication of the scrapie agent in hamster brain precedes neuronal vacuolation. *Journal of Neuropathology and Experimental Neurology* 42: 539-547.
[35] Sandberg MK, Al-Doujaily H, Sharps B, Clarke AR, Collinge J (2011) Prion propagation and toxicity in vivo occur in two distinct mechanistic phases. *Nature* 470: 540-542.
[36] Sandberg MK, Al-Doujaily H, Sharps B, De Oliveira MW, Schmidt C, et al. (2014) Prion neuropathology follows the accumulation of alternate prion protein isoforms after infective titre has peaked. *Nature Communications* 5.
[37] Fischer M, Rulicke T, Raeber A, Sailer A, Moser M, et al. (1996) Prion protein (PrP) with amino-proximal deletions restoring susceptibility of PrP knockout mice to scrapie. *Embo Journal* 15: 1255-1264.
[38] Li JL, Browning S, Mahal SP, Oelschlegel AM, Weissmann C (2010) Darwinian evolution of prions in cell culture. *Science* 327: 869-872.
[39] Pastrana MA, Sajnani G, Onisko B, Castilla J, Morales R, et al. (2006) Isolation and characterization of a proteinase K-sensitive PrPSc fraction. *Biochemistry* 45: 15710-15717.
[40] Coleman BM, Harrison CF, Guo B, Masters CL, Barnham KJ, et al. (2014) Pathogenic mutations within the hydrophobic domain of the prion protein lead to the formation of protease-sensitive prion species with increased lethality. *Journal of Virology* 88: 2690-2703.
[41] Hwang D, Lee IY, Yoo H, Gehlenborg N, Cho JH, et al. (2009) A systems approach to prion disease. *Molecular Systems Biology* 5.

[42] Zampieri M, Legname G, Segre D, Altafini C (2011) A system-level approach for deciphering the transcriptional response to prion infection. *Bioinformatics* 27: 3407-3414.

[43] Mays CE, Kim C, Haldiman T, van der Merwe J, Lau A, et al. (2014) Prion disease tempo determined by host-dependent substrate reduction. *Journal of Clinical Investigation* 124: 847-858.

[44] Bueler H, Raeber A, Sailer A, Fischer M, Aguzzi A, et al. (1994) High prion and PrPSc levels but delayed-onset of disease in scrapie-inoclulated mice heterozygous for a disrupted PrP gene. *Molecular Medicine* 1: 19-30.

[45] Schulz-Schaeffer WJ, Tschoke S, Kranefuss N, Drose W, Hause-Reitner D, et al. (2000) The paraffin-embedded tissue blot detects PrPSC early in the incubation time in prion diseases. *American Journal of Pathology* 156: 51-56.

[46] Moreno JA, Radford H, Peretti D, Steinert JR, Verity N, et al. (2012) Sustained translational repression by eIF2 alpha-P mediates prion neurodegeneration. *Nature* 485: 507-U119.

[47] Giannakopoulos P, Herrmann FR, Bussiere T, Bouras C, Kovari E, et al. (2003) Tangle and neuron numbers, but not amyloid load, predict cognitive status in Alzheimer's disease. *Neurology* 60: 1495-1500.

[48] Bennett DA, Schneider JA, Wilson RS, Bienias JL, Arnold SE (2004) Neurofibrillary tangles mediate the association of amyloid load with clinical Alzheimer disease and level of cognitive function. *Archives of Neurology* 61: 378-384.

[49] Carlson GA, Borchelt DR, Dake A, Turner S, Danielson V, et al. (1997) Genetic modification of the phenotypes produced by amyloid precursor protein overexpression in transgenic mice. *Human Molecular Genetics* 6: 1951-1959.

[50] McLean CA, Cherny RA, Fraser FW, Fuller SJ, Smith MJ, et al. (1999) Soluble pool of A beta amyloid as a determinant of severity of neurodegeneration in Alzheimer's disease. *Annals of Neurology* 46: 860-866.

[51] Mc Donald JM, Savva GM, Brayne C, Welzel AT, Forster G, et al. (2010) The presence of sodium dodecyl sulphate-stable A beta dimers is strongly associated with Alzheimer-type dementia. *Brain* 133: 1328-1341.

[52] Lesne S, Koh MT, Kotilinek L, Kayed R, Glabe CG, et al. (2006) A specific amyloid-beta protein assembly in the brain impairs memory. *Nature* 440: 352-357.

[53] Lacor PN, Buniel MC, Furlow PW, Clemente AS, Velasco PT, et al. (2007) A beta oligomer-induced aberrations in synapse composition, shape, and density provide a molecular basis for loss of connectivity in Alzheimer's disease. *Journal of Neuroscience* 27: 796-807.

[54] Shankar GM, Bloodgood BL, Townsend M, Walsh DM, Selkoe DJ, et al. (2007) Natural oligomers of the Alzheimer amyloid-beta protein induce reversible synapse loss by modulating an NMDA-type glutamate receptor-dependent signaling pathway. *Journal of Neuroscience* 27: 2866-2875.

[55] Walsh DM, Klyubin I, Fadeeva JV, Cullen WK, Anwyl R, et al. (2002) Naturally secreted oligomers of amyloid beta protein potently inhibit hippocampal long-term potentiation in vivo. *Nature* 416: 535-539.

[56] Shankar GM, Li SM, Mehta TH, Garcia-Munoz A, Shepardson NE, et al. (2008) Amyloid-beta protein dimers isolated directly from Alzheimer's brains impair synaptic plasticity and memory. *Nature Medicine* 14: 837-842.

[57] Nilsberth C, Westlind-Danielsson A, Eckman CB, Condron MM, Axelman K, et al. (2001) The 'Arctic' APP mutation (E693G) causes Alzheimer's disease by enhanced A beta protofibril formation. *Nature Neuroscience* 4: 887-893.
[58] Cerf E, Gustot A, Goormaghtigh E, Ruysschaert JM, Raussens V (2011) High ability of apolipoprotein E4 to stabilize amyloid-beta peptide oligomers, the pathological entities responsible for Alzheimer's disease. *Faseb Journal* 25: 1585-1595.
[59] Lauren J, Gimbel DA, Nygaard HB, Gilbert JW, Strittmatter SM (2009) Cellular prion protein mediates impairment of synaptic plasticity by amyloid-beta oligomers. *Nature* 457: 1128-U1184.
[60] Hu NW, Nicoll AJ, Zhang DN, Mably AJ, O'Malley T, et al. (2014) mGlu5 receptors and cellular prion protein mediate amyloid-beta-facilitated synaptic long-term depression in vivo. *Nature Communications* 5.
[61] Klyubin I, Nicoll AJ, Khalili-Shirazi A, Farmer M, Canning S, et al. (2014) Peripheral administration of a humanized anti-PrP antibody blocks Alzheimer's disease A Beta synaptotoxicity. *Journal of Neuroscience* 34: 6140-6145.
[62] Handoko M, Grant M, Kuskowski M, Zahs KR, Wallin A, et al. (2013) Correlation of specific Amyloid-beta oligomers with tau in cerebrospinal fluid From cognitively normal older adults. *Jama Neurology* 70: 594-599.
[63] Lesne SE, Sherman MA, Grant M, Kuskowski M, Schneider JA, et al. (2013) Brain amyloid-beta oligomers in ageing and Alzheimer's disease. *Brain* 136: 1383-1398.
[64] Hughes AJ, Daniel SE, Kilford L, Lees AJ (1992) Accuracy of clinical diagnosis of idiopathic Parkinson's disease: a clinicopathological study of 100 cases. *Journal of Neurology Neurosurgery and Psychiatry* 55: 181-184.
[65] Tompkins MM, Hill WD (1997) Contribution of somal Lewy bodies to neuronal death. *Brain Research* 775: 24-29.
[66] Parkkinen L, Kauppinen T, Pirttila T, Autere JM, Alafuzoff I (2005) alpha-Synuclein pathology does not predict extrapyramidal symptoms or dementia. *Annals of Neurology* 57: 82-91.
[67] Auluck PK, Chan HYE, Trojanowski JQ, Lee VMY, Bonini NM (2002) Chaperone suppression of alpha-synuclein toxicity in a Drosophila model for Parkinson's disease. *Science* 295: 865-868.
[68] Masliah E, Rockenstein E, Veinbergs I, Mallory M, Hashimoto M, et al. (2000) Dopaminergic loss and inclusion body formation in alpha-synuclein mice: Implications for neurodegenerative disorders. *Science* 287: 1265-1269.
[69] Kramer ML, Schulz-Schaeffer WJ (2007) Presynaptic alpha-synuclein aggregates, not Lewy bodies, cause neurodegeneration in dementia with Lewy bodies. *Journal of Neuroscience* 27: 1405-1410.
[70] Danzer KM, Haasen D, Karow AR, Moussaud S, Habeck M, et al. (2007) Different species of alpha-synuclein oligomers induce calcium influx and seeding. *Journal of Neuroscience* 27: 9220-9232.
[71] Kahle PJ, Neumann M, Ozmen L, Muller V, Jacobsen H, et al. (2000) Subcellular localization of wild-type and Parkinson's disease-associated mutant alpha-synuclein in human and transgenic mouse brain. *Journal of Neuroscience* 20: 6365-6373.
[72] Feany MB, Bender WW (2000) A Drosophila model of Parkinson's disease. *Nature* 404: 394-398.

[73] van der Putten H, Wiederhold KH, Probst A, Barbieri S, Mistl C, et al. (2000) Neuropathology in mice expressing human alpha-synuclein. *Journal of Neuroscience* 20: 6021-6029.

[74] Karpinar DP, Balija MBG, Kugler S, Opazo F, Rezaei-Ghaleh N, et al. (2009) Pre-fibrillar alpha-synuclein variants with impaired beta-structure increase neurotoxicity in Parkinson's disease models. *Embo Journal* 28: 3256-3268.

[75] Winner B, Jappelli R, Maji SK, Desplats PA, Boyer L, et al. (2011) In vivo demonstration that alpha-synuclein oligomers are toxic. Proceedings of the National Academy of Sciences of the United States of America 108: 4194-4199.

[76] Pountney DL, Lowe R, Quilty M, Vickers JC, Voelcker NH, et al. (2004) Annular alpha-synuclein species from purified multiple system atrophy inclusions. *Journal of Neurochemistry* 90: 502-512.

[77] Volles MJ, Lansbury PT (2003) Zeroing in on the pathogenic form of alpha-synuclein and its mechanism of neurotoxicity in Parkinson's disease. *Biochemistry* 42: 7871-7878.

[78] Gosavi N, Lee HJ, Lee JS, Patel S, Lee SJ (2002) Golgi fragmentation occurs in the cells with prefibrillar alpha-synuclein aggregates and precedes the formation of fibrillar inclusion. *Journal of Biological Chemistry* 277: 48984-48992.

[79] Luth ES, Stavrovskaya IG, Bartels T, Kristal BS, Selkoe DJ (2014) Soluble, Prefibrillar alpha-Synuclein Oligomers Promote Complex I-dependent, Ca2+-induced Mitochondrial Dysfunction. *Journal of Biological Chemistry* 289: 21490-21507.

[80] Schapira AHV, Cooper JM, Dexter D, Jenner P, Clark JB, et al. (1989) Mitochondrial complex I deficiency in Parkinson's Disease. *Lancet* 1: 1269-1269.

[81] Parker WD, Boyson SJ, Parks JK (1989) Abnormalities of the electron transport chain in idiopathic Parkinson's Disease. *Annals of Neurology* 26: 719-723.

[82] Janetzky B, Hauck S, Youdim MBH, Riederer P, Jellinger K, et al. (1994) Unaltered aconitase activity, but decreased complex I activity is substantia nigra pars compacta of patients with Parkinson's Disease. *Neuroscience Letters* 169: 126-128.

[83] Langston JW, Ballard PA (1983) Parkinson's Disease in a chemist working with 1-methyl-4-phenyl-1,2,5,6-tetrahydropyridine. *New England Journal of Medicine* 309: 310-310.

[84] Burns RS, Chiueh CC, Markey SP, Ebert MH, Jacobowitz DM, et al. (1983) A primate model of Parkinsonism: Selective destruction of dopaminergic neurons in the pars compacta of the substantia nigra by n-methyl-4-phenyl-1,2,3,6-tetrahydropyridine. *Proceedings of the National Academy of Sciences of the United States of America-Biological Sciences* 80: 4546-4550.

[85] Betarbet R, Sherer TB, MacKenzie G, Garcia-Osuna M, Panov AV, et al. (2000) Chronic systemic pesticide exposure reproduces features of Parkinson's disease. *Nature* Neuroscience 3: 1301-1306.

[86] Camilleri A, Vassallo N (2014) The centrality of mitochondria in the pathogenesis and treatment of Parkinson's disease. *Cns Neuroscience & Therapeutics* 20: 591-602.

[87] Kayed R, Head E, Thompson JL, McIntire TM, Milton SC, et al. (2003) Common structure of soluble amyloid oligomers implies common mechanism of pathogenesis. *Science* 300: 486-489.

[88] Chiti F, Dobson CM (2006) Protein misfolding, functional amyloid, and human disease. *Annual Review of Biochemistry*. pp. 333-366.

[89] Kazlauskaite J, Young A, Gardner CE, Macpherson JV, Venien-Bryan C, et al. (2005) An unusual soluble beta-turn-rich conformation of prion is involved in fibril formation and toxic to neuronal cells. *Biochemical and Biophysical Research Communications* 328: 292-305.

[90] Novitskaya V, Bocharova OV, Bronstein I, Baskakov IV (2006) Amyloid fibrils of mammalian prion protein are highly toxic to cultured cells and primary neurons. *Journal of Biological Chemistry* 281: 13828-13836.

[91] Simoneau S, Rezaei H, Sales N, Kaiser-Schulz G, Lefebvre-Roque M, et al. (2007) In vitro and in vivo neurotoxicity of prion protein oligomers. *Plos Pathogens* 3: 1175-1186.

[92] Jansen K, Schafer O, Birkmann E, Post K, Serban H, et al. (2001) Structural intermediates in the putative pathway from the cellular prion protein to the pathogenic form. *Biological Chemistry* 382: 683-691.

[93] Zhou MH, Ottenberg G, Sferrazza GF, Lasmezas CI (2012) Highly neurotoxic monomeric alpha-helical prion protein. *Proceedings of the National Academy of Sciences of the United States of America* 109: 3113-3118.

[94] Silveira JR, Raymond GJ, Hughson AG, Race RE, Sim VL, et al. (2005) The most infectious prion protein particles. *Nature* 437: 257-261.

[95] Kristiansen M, Deriziotis P, Dimcheff DE, Jackson GS, Ovaa H, et al. (2007) Disease-associated prion protein oligomers inhibit the 26S proteasome. *Molecular Cell* 26: 175-188.

[96] Deriziotis P, Andre R, Smith DM, Goold R, Kinghorn KJ, et al. (2011) Misfolded PrP impairs the UPS by interaction with the 20S proteasome and inhibition of substrate entry. *Embo Journal* 30: 3065-3077.

[97] O'Nuallain B, Freir DB, Nicoll AJ, Risse E, Ferguson N, et al. (2010) Amyloid beta-protein dimers rapidly form stable synaptotoxic protofibrils. *Journal of Neuroscience* 30: 14411-14419.

[98] Bitan G, Fradinger EA, Spring SM, Teplow DB (2005) Neurotoxic protein oligomers - what you see is not always what you get. *Amyloid-Journal of Protein Folding Disorders* 12: 88-95.

[99] Giehm L, Pinto Oliveira CL, Christiansen G, Pedersen JS, Otzen DE (2010) SDS-induced fibrillation of alpha-synuclein: An alternative fibrillation pathway. *Journal of Molecular Biology* 401: 115-133.

[100] Shmerling D, Hegyi I, Fischer M, Blattler T, Brandner S, et al. (1998) Expression of amino-terminally truncated PrP in the mouse leading to ataxia and specific cerebellar lesions. *Cell* 93: 203-214.

[101] Baumann F, Tolnay M, Brabeck C, Pahnke J, Kloz U, et al. (2007) Lethal recessive myelin toxicity of prion protein lacking its central domain. *Embo Journal* 26: 538-547.

[102] Schatzl HM, Dacosta M, Taylor L, Cohen FE, Prusiner SB (1995) Prion protein gene variation among primates. *Journal of Molecular Biology* 245: 362-374.

[103] Harrison CF, Lawson VA, Coleman BM, Kim YS, Masters CL, et al. (2010) Conservation of a glycine-rich region in the prion protein is required for uptake of prion infectivity. *Journal of Biological Chemistry* 285: 20213-20223.

[104] Peretz D, Williamson RA, Matsunaga Y, Serban H, Pinilla C, et al. (1997) A conformational transition at the N terminus of the prion protein features in formation of the scrapie isoform. *Journal of Molecular Biology* 273: 614-622.

[105] Moore RC, Mastrangelo P, Bouzamondo E, Heinrich C, Legname G, et al. (2001) Doppel-induced cerebellar degeneration in transgenic mice. *Proceedings of the National Academy of Sciences of the United States of America* 98: 15288-15293.
[106] Hoshino S, Inoue K, Yokoyama T, Kobayashi S, Asakura T, et al. (2003) Prions prevent brain damage after experimental brain injury: a preliminary report. In: Kuroiwa T, Baethmann A, Czernicki Z, Hoff JT, Ito U et al., editors. *Brain Edema* Xii. pp. 297-299.
[107] Weise J, Crome O, Sandau R, Schulz-Schaeffer W, Bahr M, et al. (2004) Upregulation of cellular prion protein (PrPc) after focal cerebral ischemia and influence of lesion severity. *Neuroscience Letters* 372: 146-150.
[108] Sakurai-Yamashita Y, Sakaguchi S, Yoshikawa D, Okimura N, Masuda Y, et al. (2005) Female-specific neuroprotection against transient brain ischemia observed in mice devoid of prion protein is abolished by ectopic expression of prion protein-like protein. *Neuroscience* 136: 281-287.
[109] McLennan NF, Brennan PM, McNeill A, Davies I, Fotheringham A, et al. (2004) Prion protein accumulation and neuroprotection in hypoxic brain damage. *American Journal of Pathology* 165: 227-235.
[110] Kuwahara C, Takeuchi AM, Nishimura T, Haraguchi K, Kubosaki A, et al. (1999) Prions prevent neuronal cell-line death. *Nature* 400: 225-226.
[111] Bounhar Y, Zhang Y, Goodyer CG, LeBlanc A (2001) Prion protein protects human neurons against Bax-mediated apoptosis. *Journal of Biological Chemistry* 276: 39145-39149.
[112] Mitteregger G, Vosko M, Krebs B, Xiang W, Kohlmannsperger V, et al. (2007) The role of the octarepeat region in neuroprotective function of the cellular prion protein. *Brain Pathology* 17: 174-183.
[113] Sakudo A, Lee DC, Nishimura T, Li SM, Tsuji S, et al. (2005) Octapeptide repeat region and N-terminal half of hydrophobic region of prion protein (PrP) mediate PrP-dependent activation of superoxide dismutase. *Biochemical and Biophysical Research Communications* 326: 600-606.
[114] Palmer MS, Mahal SP, Campbell TA, Hill AF, Sidle KC, et al. (1993) Deletions in the prion protein gene are not associated with CJD. *Human Molecular Genetics* 2: 541-544.
[115] Krasemann S, Zerr I, Weber T, Poser S, Kretzschmar H, et al. (1995) Prion disease associated with a novel nine octapeptide repeat insertion in the PRNP gene. *Molecular Brain Research* 34: 173-176.
[116] Mead S, Poulter M, Beck J, Webb TEF, Campbell TA, et al. (2006) Inherited prion disease with six octapeptide repeat insertional mutation - molecular analysis of phenotypic heterogeneity. *Brain* 129: 2297-2317.
[117] Pietrini V, Puoti G, Limido L, Rossi G, Di Fede G, et al. (2003) Creutzfeldt-Jakob disease with a novel extra-repeat insertional mutation in the PRNP gene. *Neurology* 61: 1288-1291.
[118] Campbell TA, Palmer MS, Will RG, Gibb WRG, Luthert PJ, et al. (1996) A prion disease with a novel 96-base pair insertional mutation in the prion protein gene. *Neurology* 46: 761-766.

[119] Flechsig E, Shmerling D, Hegyi I, Raeber AJ, Fischer M, et al. (2000) Prion protein devoid of the octapeptide repeat region restores susceptibility to scrapie in PrP knockout mice. *Neuron* 27: 399-408.

[120] Scalabrino G, Mutti E, Veber D, Menendez VR, Novembrino C, et al. (2011) The octapeptide repeat region and cobalamin-deficient polyneuropathy of the rat. *Muscle & Nerve* 44: 957-967.

[121] Yoshikawa D, Yamaguchi N, Ishibashi D, Yamanaka H, Okimura N, et al. (2008) Dominant-negative effects of the N-terminal half of prion protein on neurotoxicity of prion protein-like protein/doppel in mice. *Journal of Biological Chemistry* 283: 24202-24211.

[122] Solforosi L, Criado JR, McGavern DB, Wirz S, Sanchez-Alavez M, et al. (2004) Cross-linking cellular prion protein triggers neuronal apoptosis in vivo. *Science* 303: 1514-1516.

[123] Sonati T, Reimann RR, Falsig J, Baral PK, O'Connor T, et al. (2013) The toxicity of antiprion antibodies is mediated by the flexible tail of the prion protein. *Nature* 501: 102-+.

[124] Falsig J, Sonati T, Herrmann US, Saban D, Li B, et al. (2012) Prion pathogenesis is faithfully reproduced in cerebellar organotypic slice cultures. P*los Pathogens* 8.

[125] Herrmann US, Sonati T, Falsig J, Reimann RR, Dametto P, et al. (2015) Prion infections and anti-PrP antibodies trigger converging neurotoxic pathways. *PLoS Pathog* 11: e1004662.

[126] Swayampakula M, Baral PK, Aguzzi A, Kav NNV, James MNG (2013) The crystal structure of an octapeptide repeat of the Prion protein in complex with a Fab fragment of the POM2 antibody. *Protein Science* 22: 893-903.

[127] Ron D, Walter P (2007) Signal integration in the endoplasmic reticulum unfolded protein response. *Nature Reviews Molecular Cell Biology* 8: 519-529.

[128] Hegde RS, Mastrianni JA, Scott MR, DeFea KA, Tremblay P, et al. (1998) A transmembrane form of the prion protein in neurodegenerative disease. *Science* 279: 827-834.

[129] Hegde RS, Tremblay P, Groth D, DeArmond SJ, Prusiner SB, et al. (1999) Transmissible and genetic prion diseases share a common pathway of neurodegeneration. *Nature* 402: 822-826.

[130] Stewart RS, Drisaldi B, Harris DA (2001) A transmembrane form of the prion protein contains an uncleaved signal peptide and is retained in the endoplasmic reticululm. *Molecular Biology of the Cell* 12: 881-889.

[131] Stewart RS, Piccardo P, Ghetti B, Harris DA (2005) Neurodegenerative illness in transgenic mice expressing a transmembrane form of the prion protein. *Journal of Neuroscience* 25: 3469-3477.

[132] Drisaldi B, Stewart RS, Adles C, Stewart LR, Quaglio E, et al. (2003) Mutant PrP is delayed in its exit from the endoplasmic reticulum, but neither wild-type nor mutant PrP undergoes retrotranslocation prior to proteasomal degradation. *Journal of Biological Chemistry* 278: 21732-21743.

[133] Rane NS, Yonkovich JL, Hegde RS (2004) Protection from cytosolic prion protein toxicity by modulation of protein translocation. *Embo Journal* 23: 4550-4559.

[134] Ma JY, Lindquist S (2001) Wild-type PrP and a mutant associated with prion disease are subject to retrograde transport and proteasome degradation. P*roceedings of the National Academy of Sciences of the United States of America* 98: 14955-14960.

[135] Yedidia Y, Horonchik L, Tzaban S, Yanai A, Taraboulos A (2001) Proteasomes and ubiquitin are involved in the turnover of the wild-type prion protein. *Embo Journal* 20: 5383-5391.

[136] Ma JY, Lindquist S (2002) Conversion of PrP to a self-perpetuating PrPSc-like conformation in the cytosol. *Science* 298: 1785-1788.

[137] Ma JY, Wollmann R, Lindquist S (2002) Neurotoxicity and neurodegeneration when PrP accumulates in the cytosol. *Science* 298: 1781-1785.

[138] Grenier C, Bissonnette C, Volkov L, Roucou X (2006) Molecular morphology and toxicity of cytoplasmic prion protein aggregates in neuronal and non-neuronal cells. *Journal of Neurochemistry* 97: 1456-1466.

[139] Chakrabarti O, Hegde RS (2009) Functional depletion of mahogunin by cytosolically exposed prion protein contributes to neurodegeneration. *Cell* 137: 1136-1147.

[140] He L, Lu XY, Jolly AF, Eldridge AG, Watson SJ, et al. (2003) Spongiform degeneration in mahoganoid mutant mice. *Science* 299: 710-712.

[141] Silvius D, Pitstick R, Ahn M, Meishery D, Oehler A, et al. (2013) Levels of the mahogunin ring finger 1 E3 ubiquitin ligase do not influence prion disease. *Plos One* 8.

[142] Gunn TM, Carlson GA (2013) RML prions act through Mahogunin and Attractin-independent pathways. *Prion* 7: 267-271.

[143] Yost CS, Lopez CD, Prusiner SB, Myers RM, Lingappa VR (1990) Non-hydrophobic extracytoplasmic determinant of stop transfer in the prion protein. *Nature* 343: 669-672.

[144] Rane NS, Kang SW, Chakrabarti O, Feigenbaum L, Hegde RS (2008) Reduced translocation of nascent prion protein during ER stress contributes to neurodegeneration. *Developmental Cell* 15: 359-370.

[145] Roucou X, Guo Q, Zhang Y, Goodyer CG, LeBlanc AC (2003) Cytosolic prion protein is not toxic and protects against Bax-mediated cell death in human primary neurons. *Journal of Biological Chemistry* 278: 40877-40881.

[146] Thackray AM, Zhang C, Arndt T, Bujdoso R (2014) Cytosolic PrP can participate in prion-mediated toxicity. *Journal of Virology* 88: 8129-8138.

[147] Bertolotti A, Zhang YH, Hendershot LM, Harding HP, Ron D (2000) Dynamic interaction of BiP and ER stress transducers in the unfolded-protein response. *Nature Cell Biology* 2: 326-332.

[148] Shen JS, Snapp EL, Lippincott-Schwartz J, Prywes R (2005) Stable binding of ATF6 to BiP in the endoplasmic reticulum stress response. *Molecular and Cellular Biology* 25: 921-932.

[149] Hetz C, Russelakis-Carneiro M, Maundrell K, Castilla J, Soto C (2003) Caspase-12 and endoplasmic reticulum stress mediate neurotoxicity of pathological prion protein. *Embo Journal* 22: 5435-5445.

[150] Ferreiro E, Resende R, Costa R, Oliveira CR, Pereira CMF (2006) An endoplasmic-reticulum-specific apoptotic pathway is involved in prion and amyloid-beta peptides neurotoxicity. *Neurobiology of Disease* 23: 669-678.

[151] Moreno JA, Halliday M, Molloy C, Radford H, Verity N, et al. (2013) Oral treatment targeting the unfolded protein response prevents neurodegeneration and clinical disease in prion-infected mice. *Science Translational Medicine* 5.

[152] Halliday M, Radford H, Sekine Y, Moreno J, Verity N, et al. (2015) Partial restoration of protein synthesis rates by the small molecule ISRIB prevents neurodegeneration without pancreatic toxicity. *Cell Death & Disease* 6: e1672-e1672.

[153] Kober L, Zehe C, Bode J (2012) Development of a novel ER stress based selection system for the isolation of highly productive clones. *Biotechnology and Bioengineering* 109: 2599-2611.

[154] Steele AD, Hetz C, Yi CH, Jackson WS, Borkowski AW, et al. (2007) Prion Pathogenesis is Independent of Caspase-12. *Prion* 1: 243-247.

[155] Steele AD, King OD, Jackson WS, Hetz CA, Borkowski AW, et al. (2007) Diminishing apoptosis by deletion of bax or overexpression of Bcl-2 does not protect against infectious prion toxicity in vivo. *Journal of Neuroscience* 27: 13022-13027.

[156] Harding HP, Zhang YH, Zeng HQ, Novoa I, Lu PD, et al. (2003) An integrated stress response regulates amino acid metabolism and resistance to oxidative stress. *Molecular Cell* 11: 619-633.

[157] Hoozemans JJM, van Haastert ES, Eikelenboom P, de Vos RAI, Rozemuller JM, et al. (2007) Activation of the unfolded protein response in Parkinson's disease. *Biochemical and Biophysical Research Communications* 354: 707-711.

[158] Bellucci A, Navarria L, Zaltieri M, Falarti E, Bodei S, et al. (2011) Induction of the unfolded protein response by alpha-synuclein in experimental models of Parkinson's disease. *Journal of Neurochemistry* 116: 588-605.

[159] Xu B, Wu SW, Lu CW, Deng Y, Liu W, et al. (2013) Oxidative stress involvement in manganese-induced alpha-synuclein oligomerization in organotypic brain slice cultures. *Toxicology* 305: 71-78.

[160] Xu B, Wang F, Wu SW, Deng Y, Liu W, et al. (2014) Alpha-synuclein is involved in manganese-induced ER stress via PERK signal pathway in organotypic brain slice cultures. *Molecular Neurobiology* 49: 399-412.

[161] Smith WW, Jiang HB, Pei Z, Tanaka Y, Morita H, et al. (2005) Endoplasmic reticulum stress and mitochondrial cell death pathways mediate A53T mutant alpha-synuclein-induced toxicity. *Human Molecular Genetics* 14: 3801-3811.

[162] Colla E, Coune P, Liu Y, Pletnikova O, Troncoso JC, et al. (2012) Endoplasmic reticulum stress is important for the manifestations of alpha-synucleinopathy in vivo. *Journal of Neuroscience* 32: 3306-3320.

[163] Hoozemans JJM, van Haastert ES, Nijholt DAT, Rozemuller AJM, Eikelenboom P, et al. (2009) The unfolded protein response is activated in pretangle neurons in Alzheimer's disease hippocampus. *American Journal of Pathology* 174: 1241-1251.

[164] Hoozemans JJM, Veerhuis R, Van Haastert ES, Rozemuller JM, Baas F, et al. (2005) The unfolded protein response is activated in Alzheimer's disease. *Acta Neuropathologica* 110: 165-172.

[165] Segev Y, Michaelson DM, Rosenblum K (2013) ApoE epsilon 4 is associated with eIF2 alpha phosphorylation and impaired learning in young mice. *Neurobiology of Aging* 34: 863-872.

[166] Ma T, Trinh MA, Wexler AJ, Bourbon C, Gatti E, et al. (2013) Suppression of eIF2 alpha kinases alleviates Alzheimer's disease-related plasticity and memory deficits. *Nature Neuroscience* 16: 1299-U1185.

[167] O'Connor T, Sadleir KR, Maus E, Velliquette RA, Zhao J, et al. (2008) Phosphorylation of the translation initiation factor eIF2 alpha increases BACE1 levels and promotes amyloidogenesis. *Neuron* 60: 988-1009.

[168] Mihailovich M, Thermann R, Grohovaz F, Hentze MW, Zacchetti D (2007) Complex translational regulation of BACE1 involves upstream AUGs and stimulatory elements within the 5 ' untranslated region. *Nucleic Acids Research* 35: 2975-2985.

[169] Lammich S, Schobel S, Zimmer AK, Lichtenthaler SF, Haass C (2004) Expression of the Alzheimer protease BACE1 is suppressed via its 5 '-untranslated region. *Embo Reports* 5: 620-625.

[170] Devi L, Ohno M (2010) Phospho-eIF2 alpha level is important for determining abilities of BACE1 reduction to rescue cholinergic neurodegeneration and memory defects in 5XFAD mice. *Plos One* 5.

[171] Tonelli DD, Mihailovich M, Di Cesare A, Codazzi F, Grohovaz F, et al. (2004) Translational regulation of BACE-1 expression in neuronal and non-neuronal cells. *Nucleic Acids Research* 32: 1808-1817.

[172] Devi L, Ohno M (2014) PERK mediates eIF2 alpha phosphorylation responsible for BACE1 elevation, CREB dysfunction and neurodegeneration in a mouse model of Alzheimer's disease. *Neurobiology of Aging* 35: 2272-2281.

[173] Nijholt DAT, van Haastert ES, Rozemuller AJM, Scheper W, Hoozemans JJM (2012) The unfolded protein response is associated with early tau pathology in the hippocampus of tauopathies. *Journal of Pathology* 226: 693-702.

[174] Hoglinger GU, Melhem NM, Dickson DW, Sleiman PMA, Wang LS, et al. (2011) Identification of common variants influencing risk of the tauopathy progressive supranuclear palsy. *Nature Genetics* 43: 699-U125.

[175] Abisambra JF, Jinwal UK, Blair LJ, O'Leary JC, Li QY, et al. (2013) Tau accumulation activates the unfolded protein response by impairing endoplasmic reticulum-associated degradation. *Journal of Neuroscience* 33: 9498-9507.

[176] Kim AJ, Shi YY, Austin RC, Werstuck GH (2005) Valproate protects cells from ER stress-induced lipid accumulation and apoptosis by inhibiting glycogen synthase kinase-3. *Journal of Cell Science* 118: 89-99.

[177] Song L, De Sarno P, Jope RS (2002) Central role of glycogen synthase kinase-3 beta in endoplasmic reticulum stress-induced caspase-3 activation. *Journal of Biological Chemistry* 277: 44701-44708.

[178] Atkin JD, Farg MA, Turner BJ, Tomas D, Lysaght JA, et al. (2006) Induction of the unfolded protein response in familial amyotrophic lateral sclerosis and association of protein-disulfide isomerase with superoxide dismutase 1. *Journal of Biological Chemistry* 281: 30152-30165.

[179] Tobisawa S, Hozumi Y, Arawaka S, Koyama S, Wada M, et al. (2003) Mutant SOD1 linked to familial amyotrophic lateral sclerosis, but not wild-type SOD1, induces ER stress in COS7 cells and transgenic mice. *Biochemical and Biophysical Research Communications* 303: 496-503.

[180] Kim HJ, Raphael AR, LaDow ES, McGurk L, Weber RA, et al. (2014) Therapeutic modulation of eIF2 alpha phosphorylation rescues TDP-43 toxicity in amyotrophic lateral sclerosis disease models. *Nature Genetics* 46: 152-+.

[181] Matus S, Lopez E, Valenzuela V, Nassif M, Hetz C (2013) Functional contribution of the transcription factor ATF4 to the pathogenesis of Amyotrophic Lateral Sclerosis. *Plos One* 8.

[182] Wang LJ, Popko B, Roos RP (2011) The unfolded protein response in familial amyotrophic lateral sclerosis. *Human Molecular Genetics* 20: 1008-1015.

[183] Vaccaro A, Patten SA, Aggad D, Julien C, Maios C, et al. (2013) Pharmacological reduction of ER stress protects against TDP-43 neuronal toxicity in vivo. *Neurobiology of Disease* 55: 64-75.

[184] Quaglio E, Restelli E, Garofoli A, Dossena S, De Luigi A, et al. (2011) Expression of Mutant or Cytosolic PrP in Transgenic Mice and Cells Is Not Associated with Endoplasmic Reticulum Stress or Proteasome Dysfunction. *Plos One* 6.

[185] Korth C, May BCH, Cohen FE, Prusiner SB (2001) Acridine and phenothiazine derivatives as pharmacotherapeutics for prion disease. *Proceedings of the National Academy of Sciences of the United States of America* 98: 9836-9841.

[186] Kocisko DA, Baron GS, Rubenstein R, Chen JC, Kuizon S, et al. (2003) New inhibitors of scrapie-associated prion protein formation in a library of 2,000 drugs and natural products. *Journal of Virology* 77: 10288-10294.

[187] Doh-Ura K, Iwaki T, Caughey B (2000) Lysosomotropic agents and cysteine protease inhibitors inhibit scrapie-associated prion protein accumulation. *Journal of Virology* 74: 4894-4897.

[188] Collinge J, Gorham M, Hudson F, Kennedy A, Keogh G, et al. (2009) Safety and efficacy of quinacrine in human prion disease (PRION-1 study): a patient-preference trial. *Lancet Neurology* 8: 334-344.

[189] Geschwind MD, Kuo AL, Wong KS, Haman A, Devereux G, et al. (2013) Quinacrine treatment trial for sporadic Creutzfeldt-Jakob disease. *Neurology* 81: 2015-2023.

[190] Haik S, Brandel JP, Salomon D, Sazdovitch V, Delasnerie-Laupretre N, et al. (2004) Compassionate use of quinacrine in Creutzfeldt-Jakob disease fails to show significant effects. *Neurology* 63: 2413-2415.

[191] Martinez-Lage JF, Rabano A, Bermejo J, Perez MM, Guerrero MC, et al. (2005) Creutzfeldt-Jakob disease acquired via a dural graft: failure of therapy with quinacrine and chlorpromazine. *Surgical Neurology* 64: 542-545.

[192] Benito-Leon J (2004) Combined quinacrine and chlorpromazine therapy in fatal familial insomnia. *Clinical Neuropharmacology* 27: 201-203.

[193] Collins SJ, Lewis V, Brazier M, Hill AF, Fletcher A, et al. (2002) Quinacrine does not prolong survival in a murine Creutzfeldt-Jakob disease model. *Annals of Neurology* 52: 503-506.

[194] Doh-Ura K, Ishikawa K, Murakami-Kubo I, Sasaki K, Mohri S, et al. (2004) Treatment of transmissible spongiform encephalopathy by intraventricular drug infusion in animal models. *Journal of Virology* 78: 4999-5006.

[195] Ghaemmaghami S, Ahn M, Lessard P, Giles K, Legname G, et al. (2009) Continuous quinacrine treatment results in the formation of drug-resistant prions. *Plos Pathogens* 5.

[196] Bian JF, Kang HE, Telling GC (2014) Quinacrine promotes replication and conformational mutation of chronic wasting disease prions. *Proceedings of the National Academy of Sciences of the United States of America* 111: 6028-6033.

[197] Diringer H, Ehlers B (1991) Chemoprophylaxis of scrapie in mice. *Journal of General Virology* 72: 457-460.

[198] Ehlers B, Diringer H (1984) Dextran sulfate-500 delays and prevents mouse scrapie by impairment of agent replication in spleen. *Journal of General Virology* 65: 1325-1330.

[199] Ladogana A, Casaccia P, Ingrosso L, Cibati M, Salvatore M, et al. (1992) Sulphate polyanions prolong the incubation period of scrapie-infected hamsters. *Journal of General Virology* 73: 661-665.

[200] Farquhar C, Dickinson A, Bruce M (1999) Prophylactic potential of pentosan polysulphate in transmissible spongiform encephalopathies. *Lancet* 353: 117-117.

[201] Tsuboi Y, Doh-ura K, Yamada T (2009) Continuous intraventricular infusion of pentosan polysulfate: Clinical trial against prion diseases. *Neuropathology* 29: 632-636.

[202] Bone I, Belton L, Walker AS, Darbyshire J (2008) Intraventricular pentosan polysulphate in human prion disease: An observational study in the UK. *European Journal of Neurology* 15: 458-464.

[203] Newman PK, Todd NV, Scoones D, Mead S, Knight RSG, et al. (2014) Postmortem findings in a case of variant Creutzfeldt-Jakob disease treated with intraventricular pentosan polysulfate. *Journal of Neurology Neurosurgery and Psychiatry* 85: 919-922.

[204] Parry A, Baker I, Stacey R, Wimalaratna S (2007) Long term survival in a patient with variant Creutzfeldt-Jakob disease treated with intraventricular pentosan polysulphate. *Journal of Neurology Neurosurgery and Psychiatry* 78: 733-734.

[205] Terada T, Tsuboi Y, Obi T, Doh-ura K, Murayama S, et al. (2010) Less protease-resistant PrP in a patient with sporadic CJD treated with intraventricular pentosan polysulphate. *Acta Neurologica Scandinavica* 121: 127-130.

[206] Whittle IR, Knight RSG, Will RG (2006) Unsuccessful intraventricular pentosan polysulphate treatment of variant Creutzfeldt-Jakob disease. *Acta Neurochirurgica* 148: 677-679.

[207] Kawasaki Y, Kawagoe K, Chen C-j, Teruya K, Sakasegawa Y, et al. (2007) Orally administered amyloidophilic compound is effective in prolonging the incubation periods of animals cerebrally infected with prion diseases in a prion strain-dependent manner. *Journal of Virology* 81: 12889-12898.

[208] Hwu JR, Lin CC, Chuang SH, King KY, Sue TR, et al. (2004) Aminyl and iminyl radicals from arylhydrazones in the photo-induced DNA cleavage. *Bioorganic & Medicinal Chemistry* 12: 2509-2515.

[209] Lu D, Giles K, Li Z, Rao S, Dolghih E, et al. (2013) Biaryl Amides and Hydrazones as Therapeutics for Prion Disease in Transgenic Mice. *Journal of Pharmacology and Experimental Therapeutics* 347: 325-338.

[210] Berry DB, Lu D, Geva M, Watts JC, Bhardwaj S, et al. (2013) Drug resistance confounding prion therapeutics. *Proceedings of the National Academy of Sciences of the United States of America* 110: E4160-E4169.

[211] Aslund A, Sigurdson CJ, Klingstedt T, Grathwohl S, Bolmont T, et al. (2009) Novel Pentameric Thiophene Derivatives for in Vitro and in Vivo Optical Imaging of a

Plethora of Protein Aggregates in Cerebral Amyloidoses. *Acs Chemical Biology* 4: 673-684.

[212] Margalith I, Suter C, Ballmer B, Schwarz P, Tiberi C, et al. (2012) Polythiophenes inhibit prion propagation by stabilizing prion protein (PrP) aggregates. *Journal of Biological Chemistry* 287: 18872-18887.

[213] Kimberlin RH, Walker CA (1979) Antiviral compound effective against experimental scrapie. *Lancet* 2: 591-592.

[214] Tateishi J (1981) Antibiotics and antivirals do not modify experimentally-induced Creutzfeldt-Jakob disease in mice. *Journal of Neurology Neurosurgery and Psychiatry* 44: 723-724.

[215] Terzano MG, Montanari E, Calzetti S, Mancia D, Lechi A (1983) The effect of amantadine on arousal and EEG patterns in Creutzfeldt-Jakob Disease. *Archives of Neurology* 40: 555-559.

[216] Neri G, Figa-Talamanca L, Di Battista GC, Lo Russo F (1984) Amantadine in Creutzfeldt-Jakob disease. Review of the literature and case contribution. *Riv Neurobiol* 30: 47-56.

[217] Otto M, Cepek L, Ratzka P, Doehlinger S, Boekhoff I, et al. (2004) Efficacy of flupirtine on cognitive function in patients with CJD - A double-blind study. *Neurology* 62: 714-718.

[218] Barret A, Tagliavini F, Forloni G, Bate C, Salmona M, et al. (2003) Evaluation of quinacrine treatment for prion diseases. *Journal of Virology* 77: 8462-8469.

[219] De Luigi A, Colombo L, Diomede L, Capobianco R, Mangieri M, et al. (2008) The efficacy of tetracyclines in peripheral and intracerebral prion infection. *Plos One* 3.

[220] Tagliavini F (2008) Prion therapy: Tetracyclic compounds in animal models and patients with Creutzfeldt-Jakob disease. *Alzheimer's & Dementia* 4: T149-T150.

[221] Zerr I (2009) Therapeutic trials in human Transmissible Spongiform Encephalopathies: Recent advances and problems to address. *Infectious Disorders - Drug Targets* 9: 92-99.

[222] Haik S, Marcon G, Mallet A, Tettamanti M, Welaratne A, et al. (2014) Doxycycline in Creutzfeldt-Jakob disease: a phase 2, randomised, double-blind, placebo-controlled trial. *Lancet Neurology* 13: 150-158.

[223] Wagner J, Ryazanov S, Leonov A, Levin J, Shi S, et al. (2013) Anle138b: a novel oligomer modulator for disease-modifying therapy of neurodegenerative diseases such as prion and Parkinson's disease. *Acta Neuropathologica* 125: 795-813.

[224] Axten JM, Medina JR, Feng YH, Shu A, Romeril SP, et al. (2012) Discovery of 7-Methyl-5-(1-{3-(trifluoromethyl)phenylacetyl}-2,3-dihydro-1H-indol-5-yl)-7H-pyrrolo 2,3-d pyrimidin-4-amine (GSK2606414), a Potent and Selective First-in-Class Inhibitor of Protein Kinase R (PKR)-like Endoplasmic Reticulum Kinase (PERK). *Journal of Medicinal Chemistry* 55: 7193-7207.

[225] Kadowaki H, Nishitoh H (2013) Signaling pathways from the endoplasmic reticulum and their roles in disease. *Genes* (Basel) 4: 306-333.

[226] Harding HP, Zhang YH, Bertolotti A, Zeng HQ, Ron D (2000) Perk is essential for translational regulation and cell survival during the unfolded protein response. *Molecular Cell* 5: 897-904.

[227] Scheuner D, Song BB, McEwen E, Liu C, Laybutt R, et al. (2001) Translational control is required for the unfolded protein response and in vivo glucose homeostasis. *Molecular Cell* 7: 1165-1176.

[228] Harding HP, Zeng HQ, Zhang YH, Jungries R, Chung P, et al. (2001) Diabetes mellitus and exocrine pancreatic dysfunction in Perk-/- mice reveals a role for translational control in secretory cell survival. *Molecular Cell* 7: 1153-1163.

[229] Ozcan U, Yilmaz E, Ozcan L, Furuhashi M, Vaillancourt E, et al. (2006) Chemical chaperones reduce ER stress and restore glucose homeostasis in a mouse model of type 2 diabetes. *Science* 313: 1137-1140.

[230] Enari M, Flechsig E, Weissmann C (2001) Scrapie prion protein accumulation by scrapie-infected neuroblastoma cells abrogated by exposure to a prion protein antibody. *Proceedings of the National Academy of Sciences of the United States of America* 98: 9295-9299.

[231] Horiuchi M, Caughey B (1999) Specific binding of normal prion protein to the scrapie form via a localized domain initiates its conversion to the protease-resistant state. *Embo Journal* 18: 3193-3203.

[232] Feraudet C, Morel N, Simon S, Volland H, Frobert Y, et al. (2005) Screening of 145 anti-PrP monoclonal antibodies for their capacity to inhibit PrPSc replication in infected cells. *Journal of Biological Chemistry* 280: 11247-11258.

[233] Pankiewicz J, Prelli F, Sy MS, Kascsak RJ, Kascsak RB, et al. (2006) Clearance and prevention of prion infection in cell culture by anti-PrP antibodies. *European Journal of Neuroscience* 23: 2635-2647.

[234] Peretz D, Williamson RA, Kaneko K, Vergara J, Leclerc E, et al. (2001) Antibodies inhibit prion propagation and clear cell cultures of prion infectivity. *Nature* 412: 739-743.

[235] Perrier V, Solassol J, Crozet C, Frobert Y, Mourton-Gilles C, et al. (2004) Anti-PrP antibodies block PrPSc replication in prion-infected cell cultures by accelerating PrP degradation. *Journal of Neurochemistry* 89: 454-463.

[236] White AR, Enever P, Tayebi M, Mushens R, Linehan J, et al. (2003) Monoclonal antibodies inhibit prion replication and delay the development of prion disease. *Nature* 422: 80-83.

[237] Klohn PC, Farmer M, Linehan JM, O'Malley C, de Marco MF, et al. (2012) PrP antibodies do not trigger mouse hippocampal neuron apoptosis. *Science* 335: 52-52.

[238] Antonyuk SV, Trevitt CR, Strange RW, Jackson GS, Sangar D, et al. (2009) Crystal structure of human prion protein bound to a therapeutic antibody. *Proceedings of the National Academy of Sciences of the United States of America* 106: 2554-2558.

[239] Chung E, Ji Y, Sun Y, Kascsak RJ, Kascsak RB, et al. (2010) Anti-PrPC monoclonal antibody infusion as a novel treatment for cognitive deficits in an alzheimer's disease model mouse. *Bmc Neuroscience* 11.

[240] Bard F, Cannon C, Barbour R, Burke RL, Games D, et al. (2000) Peripherally administered antibodies against amyloid beta-peptide enter the central nervous system and reduce pathology in a mouse model of Alzheimer disease. *Nature Medicine* 6: 916-919.

[241] Banks WA, Terrell B, Farr SA, Robinson SA, Nonaka N, et al. (2002) Passage of amyloid beta protein antibody across the blood-brain barrier in a mouse model of Alzheimer's disease. *Peptides* 23: 2223-2226.

[242] Chung YL, Williams A, Beech JS, Williams SCR, Bell JD, et al. (1995) MRI assessment of the blood-brain-barrier in a hamster model of scrapie. *Neurodegeneration* 4: 203-207.
[243] Brandner S, Isenmann S, Kuhne G, Aguzzi A (1998) Identification of the end stage of scrapie using infected neural grafts. *Brain Pathology* 8: 19-27.
[244] Sadowski MJ, Pankiewicz J, Prelli F, Scholtzova H, Spinner DS, et al. (2009) Anti-PrP Mab 6D11 suppresses PrPSc replication in prion infected myeloid precursor line FDC-P1/22L and in the lymphoreticular system in vivo. *Neurobiology of Disease* 34: 267-278.
[245] Petsch B, Muller-Schiffmann A, Lehle A, Zirdum E, Prikulis I, et al. (2011) Biological effects and use of PrPSc- and PrP-specific antibodies generated by immunization with purified full-length native mouse prions. *Journal of Virology* 85: 4538-4546.
[246] Baral PK, Swayampakula M, Rout MK, Kav NNV, Spyracopoulos L, et al. (2014) Structural basis of prion inhibition by phenothiazine compounds. *Structure* 22: 291-303.
[247] White MD, Farmer M, Mirabile I, Brandner S, Collinge J, et al. (2008) Single treatment with RNAi against prion protein rescues early neuronal dysfunction and prolongs survival in mice with prion disease. *Proceedings of the National Academy of Sciences of the United States of America* 105: 10238-10243.
[248] Feng XR, Zhao P, He YX, Zuo ZY (2006) Allele-specific silencing of Alzheimer's disease genes - The amyloid precursor protein genes with Swedish or London mutations. *Gene* 371: 68-74.
[249] de Ynigo-Mojado L, Martin-Ruiz I, Sutherland JD (2011) Efficient allele-specific targeting of LRRK2 R1441 mutations mediated by RNAi. *Plos One* 6.
[250] Wang HY, Ghosh A, Baigude H, Yang CS, Qiu LH, et al. (2008) Therapeutic gene silencing delivered by a chemically modified small interfering RNA against mutant SOD1 slows amyotrophic lateral sclerosis progression. *Journal of Biological Chemistry* 283: 15845-15852.
[251] Carroll JB, Warby SC, Southwell AL, Doty CN, Greenlee S, et al. (2011) Potent and selective antisense oligonucleotides targeting single-nucleotide polymorphisms in the Huntington disease gene/allele-specific silencing of mutant huntingtin. *Molecular Therapy* 19: 2178-2185.
[252] Schwank G, Koo BK, Sasselli V, Dekkers JF, Heo I, et al. (2013) Functional repair of CFTR by CRISPR/Cas9 in intestinal stem cell organoids of Cystic Fibrosis patients. *Cell Stem Cell* 13: 653-658.
[253] Gauczynski S, Nikles D, El-Gogo S, Papy-Garcia D, Rey C, et al. (2006) The 37-kDa/67-kDa laminin receptor acts as a receptor for infectious prions and is inhibited by polysulfated glycanes. *Journal of Infectious Diseases* 194: 702-709.
[254] Gauczynski S, Peyrin JM, Haik S, Leucht C, Hundt C, et al. (2001) The 37-kDa/67-kDa laminin receptor acts as the cell-surface receptor for the cellular prion protein. *Embo Journal* 20: 5863-5875.
[255] Leucht C, Simoneau S, Rey C, Vana K, Rieger R, et al. (2003) The 37 kDa/67 kDa laminin receptor is required for PrPSc propagation in scrapie-infected neuronal cells. *Embo Reports* 4: 290-295.
[256] Pflanz H, Vana K, Mitteregger G, Pace C, Messow D, et al. (2009) Microinjection of lentiviral vectors expressing small interfering RNAs directed against laminin receptor

precursor mRNA prolongs the pre-clinical phase in scrapie-infected mice. *Journal of General Virology* 90: 269-274.

[257] Bellingham SA, Coleman LA, Masters CL, Camakaris J, Hill AF (2009) Regulation of prion gene expression by transcription factors SP1 and Metal Transcription Factor-1. *Journal of Biological Chemistry* 284: 1291-1301.

[258] Saba R, Goodman CD, Huzarewich R, Robertson C, Booth SA (2008) A miRNA signature of prion induced neurodegeneration. *Plos One* 3.

[259] Montag J, Hitt R, Opitz L, Schulz-Schaeffer WJ, Hunsmann G, et al. (2009) Upregulation of miRNA hsa-miR-342-3p in experimental and idiopathic prion disease. *Molecular Neurodegeneration* 4.

[260] Bellingham SA, Coleman BM, Hill AF (2012) Small RNA deep sequencing reveals a distinct miRNA signature released in exosomes from prion-infected neuronal cells. *Nucleic Acids Research* 40: 10937-10949.

[261] Boudreau RL, McBride JL, Martins I, Shen SH, Xing Y, et al. (2009) Nonallele-specific silencing of mutant and wild-type huntingtin demonstrates therapeutic efficacy in Huntington's disease mice. *Molecular Therapy* 17: 1053-1063.

[262] Kang SG, Roh YM, Lau A, Westaway D, McKenzie D, et al. (2011) Establishment and characterization of Prnp knockdown neuroblastoma cells using dual microRNA-mediated RNA interference. *Prion* 5: 93-102.

[263] Boese AS, Majer A, Saba R, Booth SA (2013) Small RNA drugs for prion disease: a new frontier. *Expert Opinion on Drug Discovery* 8: 1265-1284.

[264] Alvarez-Erviti L, Seow YQ, Yin HF, Betts C, Lakhal S, et al. (2011) Delivery of siRNA to the mouse brain by systemic injection of targeted exosomes. *Nature Biotechnology* 29: 341-U179.

[265] Zhuang XY, Xiang XY, Grizzle W, Sun DM, Zhang SQ, et al. (2011) Treatment of brain inflammatory diseases by delivering exosome encapsulated anti-inflammatory drugs from the nasal region to the brain. *Molecular Therapy* 19: 1769-1779.

[266] Paterson RW, Torres-Chae CC, Kuo AL, Ando T, Nguyen EA, et al. (2012) Differential diagnosis of Jakob-Creutzfeldt disease. *Archives of Neurology* 69: 1578-1582.

[267] Craig-Schapiro R, Fagan AM, Holtzman DM (2009) Biomarkers of Alzheimer's disease. *Neurobiology of Disease* 35: 128-140.

[268] Cheng L, Doecke JD, Sharples RA, Villemagne VL, Fowler CJ, et al. (2014) Prognostic serum miRNA biomarkers associated with Alzheimer's disease shows concordance with neuropsychological and neuroimaging assessment. *Molecular Psychiatry.*

In: The Prion Phenomena in Neurodegenerative Diseases ISBN: 978-1-63483-399-8
Editors: Giuseppe Legname and Gabriele Giachin

Chapter 4

GLYCOSAMINOGLYCANS IN PRION AND PRION-LIKE DISEASES

***Tuane C. R. G. Vieira*[1,*] *and Jerson L. Silva*[2,*]**
[1]Instituto Federal do Rio de Janeiro, Rio de Janeiro, Brazil
[2]Centro Nacional de Ressonância Magnética Nuclear Jiri Jonas, Instituto de Bioquímica Médica Leopoldo De Meis, Instituto Nacional de Ciência e Tecnologia de Biologia Estrutural e Bioimagem, Universidade Federal do Rio de Janeiro, Rio de Janeiro, Brazil

ABSTRACT

Glycosaminoglycans (GAGs) comprise an important group of polysaccharides that are found inside and outside animal cells and that act as tissue organizers, modulate growth factor activity, and regulate neurite outgrowth, among many other functions. Amyloid deposits were first found to contain polysaccharides in 1854 by Virchow, but the association of GAGs with amyloid deposits gained much attention after the 1980s, when GAGs were implicated in many conformational diseases (prion diseases, Alzheimer's disease, Parkinson's disease, and others). The role of GAGs in prion-like diseases and amyloidoses has been related to amyloid fiber nucleation and formation *via* a passive role as a component of amyloid deposits and an active role by promoting aggregation-prone protein conformations. In the case of prion pathology, GAGs are important cofactors and receptors in prion infections. These molecules may serve as cofactors by acting as adjuvants for prion conversion, whereas others demonstrated that these molecules serve as inhibitors of conversion. Alternatively, GAGs may serve as the primary cell surface receptor for the pathological isoform of the cellular prion protein (PrP^C), although some studies reported contrasting results. GAGs play paradoxical roles in prion and prion-like diseases. In this chapter, we discuss how these molecules regulate protein conformation to provide crucial guidance for the development of therapeutic drugs for many amyloid diseases. Recent studies have shown that the interaction of low-molecular-weight heparin (LMWHep) with the N- or C-terminal domain of PrP^C affects the extent and kinetics of PrP^C fibrillization. These findings explain the protective effect of heparin in different models of prion and prion-like neurodegenerative diseases and establish the foundation for developing therapeutic strategies based on GAGs.

[*] Corresponding Authors addresses. Emails: tuane.vieira@ifrj.edu.br and jerson@bioqmed.ufrj.br

INTRODUCTION

Transmissible spongiform encephalopathies (TSEs) have either a genetic, infectious or sporadic nature and have been found in several species such as humans (kuru and Creutzfeldt-Jakob disease), sheep (scrapie) and cattle (bovine spongiform encephalopathy, also known as "mad cow disease") [1]. Although rare, these diseases are unavoidably fatal. The primary TSE symptoms are paralysis, ataxia and dementia [1]. A '*prion*', which is a term created as a contraction of '*proteinaceous infectious particle*' lacks the codifying nucleic acid [1]. Although this particle alone accounts for the transmission of these diseases [2], cofactors have been suggested to catalyze, initiate or modulate the conversion of PrP^{C} to PrP^{Sc} [3, 4]: nucleic acids [5, 6, 7, 8, 9, 10, 11, 12, 13, 14, 15], lipids [14, 16, 17, 18, 19] or polysaccharides [9, 20, 21, 22, 23, 24].

Mature PrP^{C} comprises 208-209 amino acids and is attached to the outer leaflet of the plasma membrane through a glycosylphosphatidylinositol (GPI) anchor [25]. The first half of the PrP^{C} protein is an intrinsically disordered peptide containing four repeats of an eight-amino acid sequence (PHGGGWGQ) termed the octapeptide or octarepeat domain, which is related to copper binding [26] as well as to the binding of glycosaminoglycans and nucleic acids, especially RNA [12]. The C-terminal region of PrP^{C} is globular and contains three alpha-helices at positions 144-154, 173-194 and 200-228. A disulfide bond is formed between cysteine residues 179 and 214 [27]. The conversion of PrP^{C} to its misfolded isoform, PrP^{Sc}, is characterized by an increase in beta sheet content [1]. PrP^{Sc} has a high propensity to form protease-resistant aggregates, which tends to accumulate in the brains of TSE patients.

Here, we review the role of GAGs in TSEs and prion-like diseases. GAGs appear to play paradoxical roles by either attenuating or stimulating prion conversion. We review how GAGs affect protein misfolding and the potential of GAGs as therapeutic agents against these diseases and discuss the protective effects of low-molecular-weight heparin (LMWHep) against prion and prion-like neurodegenerative diseases.

PROTEOGLYCANS AND GLYCOSAMINOGLYCANS

Proteoglycans (PGs) are a group of glycoconjugates comprising a protein portion and an unbranched polysaccharide portion termed as glycosaminoglycan (GAG). GAGs comprise the largest group of sulfated polysaccharides found in animal tissues. These compounds possess a negative charge due to the presence of carboxylated and/or sulfated sugar residues. In these carboxylated polysaccharides, one sugar (a hexuronic acid) alternates *via* an O-glycosidic bond with an amino sugar (one hexosamine), forming repeating disaccharide units along the chain [28, 29].

PGs act as tissue organizers, influence the growth and maturation of cells from specialized tissues, perform functions such as biological filtration, modulate the growth factor activity, regulate collagen fibrillogenesis, affect tumor cell growth and invasion, regulate neurite growth, attract cations, and mediate blood coagulation and pressure variation absorption. GAG chains are primarily responsible for the functions of PGs [28, 29, 30].

GAGs are classified according to their structural organization (disaccharide units) and to the extent and nature of their modifications after polymerization (N-sulfation, O-sulfation and epimerization). According to the Jeanloz (1960) nomenclature [31], naturally occurring GAGs can be divided into the following groups: hyaluronic acid (HA), dermatan sulfate (DS)/chondroitin sulfate (CS), keratan sulfate (KS), and heparan sulfate (HS)/heparin (Hep).

HA shows greater simplicity in its structural composition. The disaccharide units of HA comprise a glucuronic acid (GlcA) connected to an N-acetylglucosamine (GlcNAc) linked β 1 $\rightarrow$ 4. HA is not sulfonated; therefore, the anionic property of HA is provided only by its carboxyl groups [32]. In contrast to other GAGs, HA is not covalently attached to the protein chain and is therefore simply classified as a GAG. HA forms high-molecular-weight polymers that are important extracellular matrix components [32] and plays important functional roles in signaling during embryonic morphogenesis, cell repair, and joint lubrication, among others [32].

CS and DS are considered as GAGs belonging to the same family, also referred to as galactosaminoglycans [33], due to their identical disaccharide units of N-acetylgalactosamine (GalNAc). CS contains a disaccharide unit comprising a GalNAc linked to GlcA as β 1 $\rightarrow$ 4 or β 1 $\rightarrow$ 3, and its GalNAc may be sulfonated at position 4 or 6, forming chondroitin 4 (chondroitin A) or 6 (chondroitin C) sulfate, respectively. DS contains alternating GalNAc residues with a variable number of GlcAs and iduronic acid (IdoA) residues; these residues are formed from the epimerization of GlcA during polymerization and the subsequent sulfation of GalNAc at position 4. DS is considered as a variant of chondroitin 4 sulfate and is also referred to as B chondroitin. Additionally, DS is often sulfated at position 2 of IdoA and is occasionally sulfated at position 6 of GalNAc [34]. CS and DS play roles in central nervous system development, tissue repair, infection, growth factor signaling, morphogenesis and cell division, among others [34].

KS has β 1 $\rightarrow$ 3-linked disaccharide units comprising GlcNAc and the neutral sugar galactose (Gal) in place of hexuronic acid. This polysaccharide is found in a wide variety of sizes and sulfation patterns and is present in the cornea, cartilage, dermis and zona pellucida [35].

HS and Hep GAGs have closely related structures. They form another group of GAGs in which the amino sugar is glucosamine with a hexosamine bond in the α 1 $\rightarrow$ 4 configuration. Glucosamine can be N- or 6-sulfated ($GlcNSO_3$), N-acetylated (GlcNAc), or N-free ($GlcNH_2$). The hexuronic acid may be GlcA or IdoA, O-sulfated at position 2 [36, 37]. Approximately 40-50% of the glucosamines in HS are N-sulfated [37]. Approximately 80% of the glucosamines in Hep are sulfated, and this polysaccharide primarily comprises trisulfated disaccharides [38].

Notably, Hep can be isolated from different animal tissues, including those of vertebrates and invertebrates [39]. In mammals, Hep is synthesized and stored in cytoplasmic granules of mast cells and is released as protein-free chains following mast cell activation and degranulation. HS is synthesized by a variety of cell types, is secreted as either a free GAG or a PG chain, and is found on the cell surface and basement membrane [40, 41].

Depending on its localization, HS interacts with several proteins. These interactions are physiologically important as they modulate the function of various proteins such as growth factors, extracellular matrix proteins, and lipolytic enzymes, among others, to regulate different biological activities such as cell signaling, cytoskeletal organization, migration, inflammation, metastasis and synapse formation [41]. In addition to its known anticoagulant activity, Hep displays activities such as of lipid metabolism regulation and antiproliferative activity [41].

GAGs and Amyloids

Protein aggregation has been suggested as a generic feature of the polypeptide chain [42]. This aggregation can occur *via* two processes, one of which involves the formation of species with well-ordered morphological and structural features such as amyloid fibers, and the other one involves the formation of disordered structures such as amorphous aggregates [43]. Aggregation can occur slowly *via* an orderly process in which partially unfolded proteins combine to form a stable core. This core then acts as a template by recruiting other intermediates that are then added to the growing aggregated protein filament (protofibril). The sequential addition of intermediates leads to the formation of a highly structured insoluble protein structure known as an amyloid fiber. The kinetics of amyloid fiber formation include a lag phase, which involves the formation of a stable nucleus, and an elongation phase [44, 45, 46].

Many diseases, including Parkinson's (PD) and Alzheimer's diseases (AD), TSEs, systemic AA amyloidosis (AA) and type II diabetes, are directly associated with extracellular or intracellular aggregate formation. In each disease, these aggregates are primarily formed by a major protein such as Aβ and Tau in AD, α-synuclein in PD, prion scrapie or resistant prion protein (PrP^{Sc} or PrP^{res}, respectively) in TSEs, serum amyloid A (SAA) in AA, and islet amyloid polypeptide (IAPP) in type II diabetes.

PrP^{Sc} is able to convert the cellular prion (PrP^{C}) form into the misfolded protein form and to seed PrP fibrillization. Acting as a template, PrP^{Sc} is able to transmit its pathological structural information. Over the last decade, many authors have shown that aggregated proteins associated with diseases other than TSEs show the same characteristics; therefore, these diseases have been termed prion-like diseases [47, 48].

Amyloid deposits were first found to contain polysaccharides in 1854 by Virchow [49]. GAGs and PGs have been implicated in many conformational diseases and have been detected in different types of amyloid deposits. Furthermore, the importance of these molecules is not restricted to the deposition space but also to time [50] and induction of conformational changes [20] in amyloidogenesis.

Among all GAGs, HS and DS are predominantly found in amyloid deposits [51]. In addition to several extracellular amyloid deposits, GAGs are associated with intracellular proteins, which form deposits such as Lewy bodies in patients with PD [52]. The role of GAGs in amyloidoses is related to the nucleation and formation of amyloid fibers. These molecules stabilize mature amyloid fibers from dissociation [53] and proteolytic degradation [54] and interact with various amyloid proteins to facilitate fiber formation [55]. HS/Hep were shown to promote the fibrillization of transthyretin [56] and the polymerization of amyloidogenic light chain (AL) [57], IAPP [58], Aβ peptide [59], Tau protein [60] and α-synuclein [52]. GAGs may play an active role in amyloid deposition by promoting protein conformations that are likely to fibrillize [52, 55].

GAGs in Prion Metabolism

GAGs, especially HS, have been the subject of many prion disease studies. Snow et al., first demonstrated the presence of heparan sulfate in prion-based amyloid plaques in diseases such as Creutzfeldt-Jakob disease (CJD), Gerstmann-Sträussler-Scheinker syndrome, and scrapie [61, 62]. Since then, studies have focused on the function of these carbohydrates in the pathogenesis of TSEs.

Much evidence shows the interaction of GAGs with PrP^C both in its soluble form and on the cell surface [20, 63, 64, 65, 66, 67, 68]. These findings emphasize two primary roles for these molecules in prion pathology: as receptors and as cofactors.

GAGs as Receptors

PrP^C is primarily localized to the cell surface *via* its attachment to a glycosylphosphatidylinositol (GPI) anchor [25] in lipid raft microdomains [69]; in this environment, PrP^C likely interacts with cell surface proteoglycans (HS proteoglycans (-HSPGs) such as syndecans and glypicans) and the extracellular matrix (Figure 1). The ability of PrP^C to interact with GAGs appears to be involved in not only prion pathogenesis but also the normal functions of PrP^C and HS [70, 71, 72]. The GPI-anchored GAG glypican-1 (Gpc-1) mediates PrP^C localization to lipid rafts [73]; thus, HSPG and PrP^C trafficking are closely related. PrP^C controls Gpc-1 internalization and self-processing, although Gpc-1 expression does not influence PrP^C endocytosis [72]. Additionally, PrP^C loaded with copper (Cu(II)) is able to sustain Gpc-1 autodegradation catalyzed by nitric oxide *in vitro* [71], and sulfated polysaccharides and Cu(II) ions stimulate PrP^C endocytosis [74, 75].

PrP^C conversion likely occurs at a location at which the two PrP isoforms can physically interact. At present, the specific intracellular compartment in which this event occurs remains controversial [76, 77, 78, 79]. In some studies, the entry of PrP^{Sc} into cells was shown to be an essential event for its conversion, because the inhibition of endocytosis prevented its formation [80, 81], whereas others showed that the plasma membrane is the initial site of prion conversion and is able to act alone to support this event [82, 83].

Although PrP^C must be present at the cell surface to enable infection [82, 84], other molecules have been indicated as receptors or co-receptors of PrP^{Sc} [85, 86, 87, 88, 89]. Many studies have suggested that HS may be the primary receptor of PrP^{Sc} on the cell surface [74, 85, 86, 90], whereas others [91] have not, representing a paradoxical effect of HS (Figure 1). HS is responsible for the binding and uptake of prion rods (PrP 27-30 purified from prion-infected hamster tissues) in neurons [85] and of PrP^{Sc} from hamster-infected brain homogenates in Chinese hamster ovary (CHO) cells [86]. The specific depletion of Gpc-1 reduced the formation of PrP^{Sc} by 55% in persistently infected N2a cells [73, 90]. Moreover, sheep strain propagation in mice was suggested to be internalized in epithelial Rov cells independent of HS binding, although HS was important for infection during the steps after uptake [91]. These controversial results may be due to differences in prion strains, PrP^{Sc} preparations and cell lineages analyzed and due to the presence of components other than PrP^{Sc} in brain homogenates. Thus, a single mechanism of PrP^{Sc} uptake (Figure 1) must not exist, depending on factors that remain unknown.

During the last decade, many authors have shown that other aggregated proteins such as amyloid-β, Tau protein, and α-synuclein are able to seed the aggregation of the corresponding soluble protein [92, 93, 94, 95]. This capacity was also shown for other proteins that are not related to neurodegenerative diseases, including p53, a protein related to cell cycle control, the aggregation of which appears to be associated with cancer development [96, 97, 98, 99,

100]. Aβ peptide forms extracellular aggregates, but proteins that form intracellular aggregates must enter the cell to propagate. HSPG mediates the uptake of Tau and α-synuclein aggregates but not of huntingtin fibrils in cell culture [93]. Intracellular Aβ accumulation induces neurotoxic and inflammatory activity, and its uptake is cooperatively mediated by HSPG and low-density lipoprotein receptor-related protein 1 (LRP1) [94].

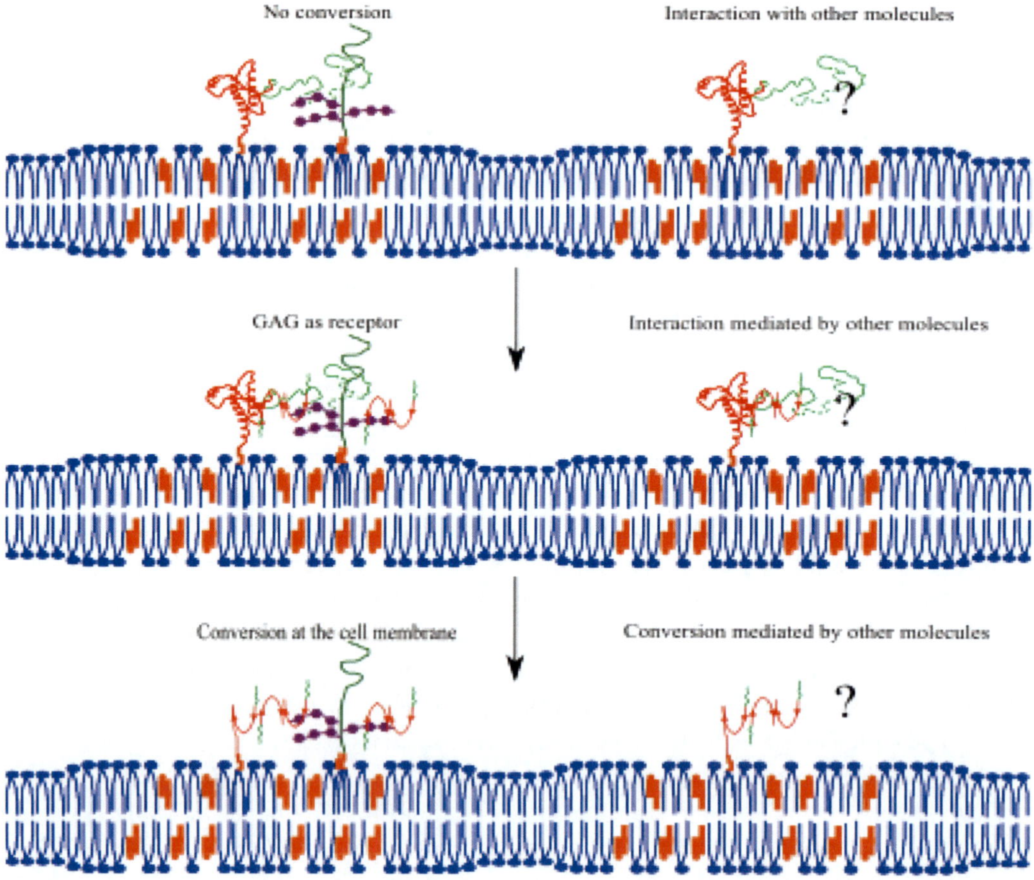

Figure 1. Cell surface PG may interact with PrP^C. This interaction is insufficient to trigger prion conversion, but PG may act as a receptor of PrP^{Sc}, thereby bringing isoforms together. Because PrP^{Sc} is able to convert PrP^C, this conversion may occur at the cell surface. However, PG is not the only molecule at the cell surface that interacts with PrP^C. Thus, other ligands may interact with PrP^{Sc} to mediate its conversion.

GAGs As Cofactors

The "protein-only" hypothesis is the most accepted theory for prion protein conversion [1]. Nevertheless, brain homogenates and polyanions (including HS) have been shown to generate more efficiently prion conversion than purified prion proteins [9, 101, 102, 103]. Thus, other molecules may promote important changes in protein structure that induce or facilitate prion conversion. The following classes of molecules have been shown to act as an adjuvant factor for prion conversion: nucleic acids [5, 6, 7, 8, 9, 10, 11, 12, 13, 14, 15], lipids [14, 16, 17, 18, 19] and polysaccharides [9, 20, 21, 22, 23, 24].

As GAGs are significant components of amyloid aggregates and share the PrP^{C} microenvironment, these molecules serve as excellent candidate receptors and cofactors. Using a cell-free conversion assay, Wong et al., [20] suggested that sulfated carbohydrates induce conformational changes in PrP^{sen} and stimulate conversion to the PrP^{res} isoform. Moreover, in another study, exogenous GAGs were able to reconstitute PrP^{Sc} formation in cells in association with a large reduction in cell membrane-associated GAGs [22]. HSPG also stimulated the amplification of PrP^{res} *in vitro* [9], and Hep enhanced the amplification of variant CJD seeds *via* protein misfolding cyclic amplification (PMCA) [24], increased prion protein fragment (PrP185-208) aggregation and induced toxic amyloid aggregate formation in neurons [104, 105]. In contrast, studies have shown that sulfated polysaccharides suppressed PrP^{res} accumulation in scrapie-infected cells [63, 106, 107, 108] and inhibited its endocytosis [109]. GAGs inhibited the polymerization of synthetic prion peptides into amyloid fibrils, thereby decreasing their neurotoxicity [110], and Hep significantly inhibited lipid-induced PrP (106-126) fibrillization [111]. Moreover, intraventricular pentosan polysulfate (iPPS) infusion was shown to modify the accumulation of PrP oligomers in the brains of patients with prion diseases [112] and to extend the life of mice infected with bovine spongiform encephalopathy [113]. Additionally, HS mimetics decreased PrP^{res} accumulation in infected mice and prolonged infected hamster survival [108]. This contradiction in the literature regarding the ability of sulfated polysaccharides to stimulate PrP^{C} conversion represents another paradoxical effect of these molecules.

One hypothesis explaining the protective effect of these sulfated polysaccharides postulates that the interaction of PrP (PrP^{C} and/or PrP^{Sc}) with endogenous GAGs is necessary for PrP^{Sc} propagation and that exogenous GAGs act as inhibitors to block the interaction of PrP with endogenous PGs (Figure 2B). Thus, distinct from endogenous GAGs, exogenous polysaccharides alone may not play an important role in facilitating PrP^{Sc} formation/propagation (Figure 2A).

The suggestion that GAGs may promote changes in PrP^{C} structure to induce prion conversion have primarily been derived from *in vitro* studies using spectroscopic techniques [20, 114], but protein aggregation renders the interpretation of these results difficult. We showed that the interaction of PrP^{C} with LMWHep leads to protein aggregation but that this effect is transitory and highly influenced by the salt concentration and pH [67]. LMWHep showed a dissociation constant for PrP^{C} of 31.5 nM at pH 5.5 and 120.3 nM at pH 7.4 [67]. After disaggregation, a complex was observed, and *via* nuclear magnetic resonance (NMR) we found that LMWHep alone was insufficient to induce prion conversion [67].

The interaction of PrP with Hep was shown to protect PrP from aggregation induced by other known cofactors (Figure 3A). The soluble complex LMWHep-PrP was shown to be resistant to RNA-induced aggregation [67]. Similarly, Hep inhibited lipid-induced PrP(106-126) fibrillization [111]. The binding of PrP to LMWHep modulates PrP fibrillization thermodynamics (decreasing the amount of fibrils) and kinetics (affecting fibril nucleation and growth) [68]. LMWHep inhibits PrP seeding by Syrian hamster ShaPrP(109-149) aggregates and modulates the seeding activity of mouse- and hamster-infected brain homogenates in real-time quaking-induced conversion (RT-QuIC) assays [68] (Figure 3A). LMWHep-PrP also failed to form amyloid fibrils under denaturing conditions [68].

Stabilization of the PrP monomer may modulate its tendency to aggregate [68], and this activity may explain the protective effects of GAGs.

This paradoxical effect was also observed for molecules other than PrP. Although HS and CS promoted Aβ peptide fibrillization [59], they protected neuronal cultures from the neurotoxic effects of Aβ [115, 116]. The same result was observed for the interaction of HS or Hep with IAPP [58, 117]. CS but not HS showed an inhibitory effect on AL fibrillization [57].

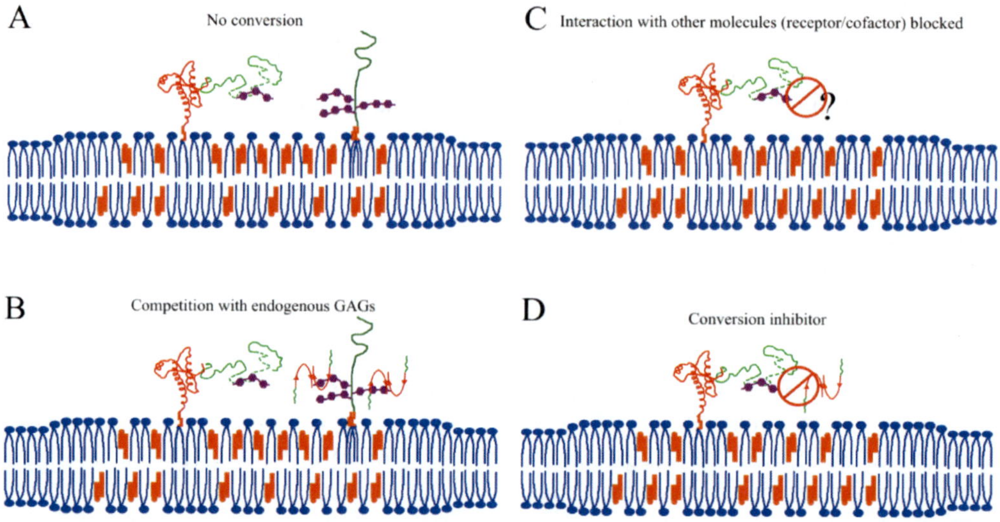

Figure 2. Exogenous GAGs exert protective effects in different models. These molecules have not been shown to facilitate PrP^{Sc} formation alone (A). Their protective effect may be explained by different mechanisms: these molecules may act as inhibitors to block the interaction of PrP^{C} with endogenous PG (B), may compete with other adjuvant cofactors (C), and/or may promote the stabilization of the PrP^{C} monomer.

GAGs at the cell surface in the form of PGs are immobilized on the cell membrane as PrP^{C}. Aggregation induced by these molecules in this environment may be a sporadic event that is rare due to spatial restriction and the influence of ions (Figure 1). Monsellier et al., [118] collected data from articles in PubMed showing the kinetic data of protein aggregation in the presence of GAGs under detailed experimental conditions. They developed a mathematical aggregation prediction tool, which determined that the sulfation state of the GAG, the solute molarity and the protein/GAG molar ratio are determinants of the effect of the GAG on amyloid formation. They found a correlation between the sulfation degree and accelerated amyloid formation, with no effect caused by the molecular weight of the GAG. At salt concentrations identical to those in the extracellular space, GAGs weakly affected aggregation. The protein/GAG molar ratio showed a bell-shaped dependency, as a low or a high molar ratio (as found at the basement membrane and cell surface) exerted a small effect. Therefore, GAGs may not directly convert and/or aggregate PrP or other amyloidogenic proteins in the cellular context (Figure 1). However, these polysaccharides are able to interact with not only well-folded proteins but also misfolded proteins, oligomers and fibrils, and these interactions may be important for the establishment of related diseases (Figure 1). The protective effects of exogenous GAGs may arise from their competition for binding with endogenous PGs that may facilitate protein aggregation (Figure 2B). Exogenous GAGs may also compete with other cofactors (Figure 2C); for example, Hep might block the interaction of PrP with membrane lipids, thereby decreasing its amyloid toxicity [111]. The increase in protein stability observed for the LMWHep-PrP interaction [68] may also explain the protective effect of this molecule (Figure 2D). Evaluating whether interaction with PrP^{Sc} stabilizes the scrapie isoform remains necessary.

HEP/HS BINDING SITES

GAGs are negatively charged molecules due to the presence of sulfate and carboxylic groups. For this reason, its interactions with proteins are primarily ionic, with basic amino groups. This interaction, although appearing random, shows specificity for certain sequences. Cardin and Weintraub in 1989 [119] were the first to demonstrate the presence of certain patterns in Hep-binding domains in four investigated proteins. They characterized two consensus sequences, XBBXBX and XBBBXXBX, where B is a basic residue and X is any amino acid. Sobel et al., [120] proposed a third consensus sequence, XBBBXXBBBXXBBX. These motifs are not always found in characterized Hep-binding regions; therefore, a distinct spatial pattern might also be important in determining the ability of a protein to interact with Hep [121, 122, 123]. Torrent et al., when analyzing the protein structures bound to Hep in the Protein Data Bank, recently reported a novel motif referred to as a cation-polar-cation (CPC) clip-like structure, which contained two cationic residues and a polar residue displaying conserved distances between the α carbons and the side chains [123].

Lysine and arginine are basic amino acids that show the highest affinity for Hep, although the affinity of arginine is 2.5-fold higher than that of lysine [124]. Alternatively, histidine residues are important for the interaction of Hep with some proteins, which was strongly dependent on pH and cation binding [125, 126, 127].

Prion proteins contain a conserved region in their N-terminal domain termed an octapeptide region with the consensus sequence PHGGGWGQ [26]. This region binds to Cu(II), and repetitions of this region are associated with prion diseases [128, 129]. Although this region does not contain a Hep consensus sequence, some studies have indicated this motif as the Hep-binding region of prion proteins. This interaction may be mediated by divalent ions in histidine side chains [21, 130, 131]. Synthetic peptides comprising amino acids 53-93 interact with HS/Hep, as measured by biosensor analyses [65] and NMR [131]. Experiments using peptides cannot always be extrapolated to the entire protein. Using the full-length protein in fast kinetic experiments, we found that the number of binding sites in PrP^C for LMWHep was two at pH 5.5 and one at pH 7.4 [67]. Using a PrP mutant in which amino acids 51-90 were deleted, we observed no interaction at pH 7.4 but did find an interaction at pH 5.5 at a stoichiometry of 1:1 (PrPΔ51-90:LMWHep), suggesting that the octarepeat is the binding site for LMWHep at pH 7.4 and that a second region is responsible for LMWHep binding at pH 5.5 [67]. The interaction with the octarepeat at the N-terminus was shown to be important for the LMWHep-mediated modulation of PrP conversion and fibrillization induced by infected seeds [68].

In addition to the octapeptide region, Warner et al., [65] identified two additional synthetic peptides comprising amino acids 23-52 and 110-128 that independently interact with Hep/HS. The first region contains a Cardin-Weintraub sequence with four basic residues,

KKRPK. Pan et al., [66], using the synthetic peptide 23-35, identified this region as the only site that was able to interact with GAGs. Subsequently, they found that deleting the first 12 amino acids in the prion protein was sufficient to abolish its interaction with GAGs. Another Cardin-Weintraub sequence is present in the N-terminus of PrP comprising amino acids 112-121, which are included in the third sequence identified by Warner et al., [65]. The 185-208 amino acid fragment of the prion protein was also able to interact with Hep/HS, and this interaction led to amyloid aggregate formation [104, 105].

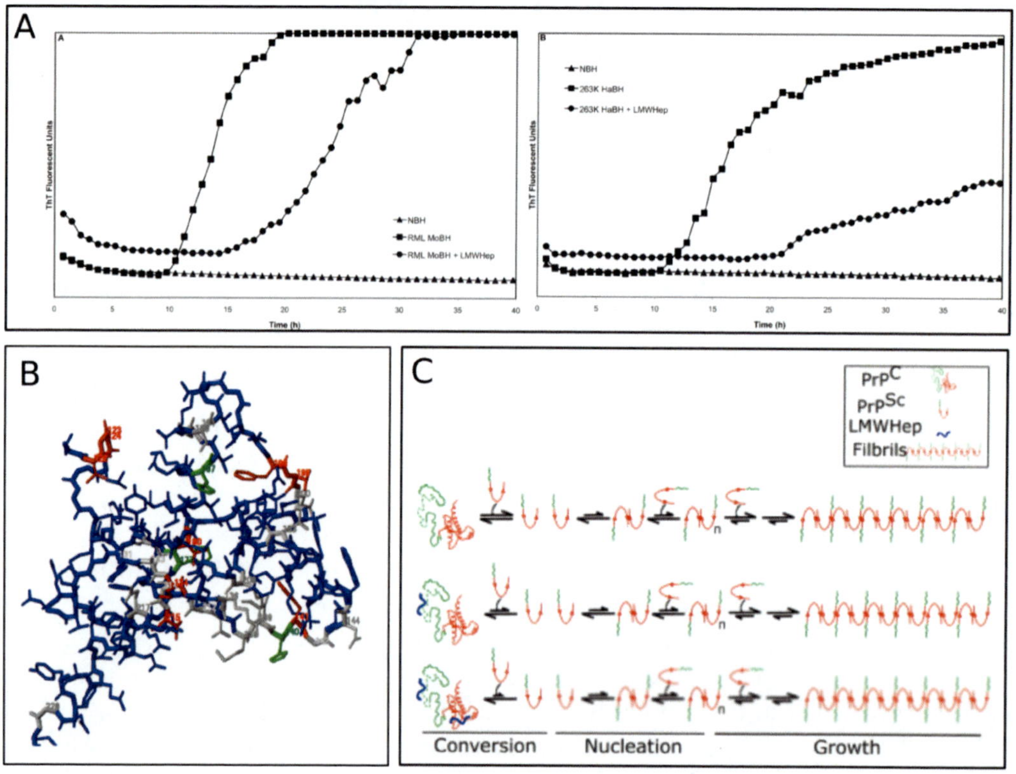

Figure 3. LMWHep was shown to protect PrP from aggregation induced PrP^{Sc} seeds from mouse- and hamster-infected brain homogenates in real-time quaking-induced conversion (RT-QuIC) assays. Modified from [68] (A). LMWHep was shown to bind PrP C-terminal near histidine 187 in the tertiary structure of PrP, between helix 2 (H2) and helix 3 (H3) at acid pH. Modified from [67] (B). The binding of LMWHep to PrP at acidic pH, likely at the octarepeat and H2H3 regions, impaired PrP conversion and fibrillization. Modified from [68] (C).

The conformational properties of PrP are modulated by pH [132, 133]. The presence of a binding site for LMWHep only at acidic pH [67] might be justified by changes causing increased exposure of the N-terminus and/or motifs that are typically hidden from the solvent. Another possible reason for this pH dependence is the protonation state of histidine residues. Histidine is the only amino acid with a side chain that can function as either an acid or a base at physiological pH; thus, these side chains may be responsible for this interaction. The pK(a) of His155 and His187 is approximately 5.5 [133, 134]. We showed that PrP treatment with DEPC (known to modify histidine side chains) blocks its interaction with LMWHep at pH 5.5 [67]. In NMR experiments, we also observed chemical shift differences from the PrP C-terminus at pH 5.5, which occurred near histidine 187 in the tertiary structure of PrP, suggesting a second binding site near helix 2 (H2) and helix 3 (H3) at this pH (Figure 3B). The binding of LMWHep to PrP at acidic pH, likely at the octarepeat and H2H3 regions, impaired PrP conversion and fibrillization [68].

GAGS AS THERAPEUTIC DRUGS FOR MANY AMYLOID DISEASES

A number of therapeutic strategies have been used to identify effective treatments against amyloidosis. In this setting, the therapeutic agent should be effective and eliminate protein accumulation, targeted to the sites affected within a specific time window, and tolerated by the body. Because the aggregates accumulate and the resulting damage occurs prior to the clinical signs of the disease, developing an effective therapy is a major challenge. Compounds that affect the amyloid nucleation and growth steps are termed true inhibitors [135]. Preventing the formation of oligomeric species is a very interesting effect because several studies have demonstrated the toxic effect of soluble species, pre-fibrillar dimers and trimers, or other oligomers produced during the nucleation step of amyloid fiber formation [136]. Affecting the kinetics of these steps might be important for halting the progression of these diseases.

Sulfated sugars, which were originally used as antivirals, were the first drugs used against TSEs that were demonstrated to prolong the incubation period of the disease and to prevent symptoms when prophylactically administered in mice [137, 138, 139, 140]. As noted above, these molecules show protective effects *in vitro* and *in vivo* [63, 106, 107, 108, 109, 110, 111, 112, 113]. PPS has been the main glycan used as treatment for prion diseases in clinical trials. iPPS treatment of patients with vCJD showed no definite clinical benefit in a 39-year-old female [141], but was suggested to prolong survival of a 22-year-old male [142]. 11 Japanese patients receiving long-term iPPS including familial CJD, iatrogenic CJD and sporadic CJD also showed no clinical improvements and extended survival [143]. The explanation for the longer survival observed in different patients [142, 143, 144, 145] still has to be uncovered. A case report of sporadic CJD suggested that prolonged survival might be associated with a decrease on the level of protease-resistant PrP [145]. However, brain examination of vCJD treated patients showed no neuropathological changes [146].

In the setting of neurodegenerative diseases, although intraventricular infusion was shown to be safe, complication from the surgical procedure may arise [144]. Hence, the therapeutic agent must be able to cross the blood-brain barrier (BBB); therefore the size and charge of the drug are issues. Many sulfated polysaccharides cannot cross the BBB [147]. For this reason, LMW drugs have been developed to overcome this challenge [148]. LMWHep was shown to cross the BBB, inhibit Aβ precursor protein secretion [149] and play a protective role against AD and AA in animal models [150, 151]. LMWHep limited SAA [151], Aβ [151] and PrP [68] fibril formation *in vitro.* We showed that LMWHep acts as a true inhibitor to modulate PrP fibrillization kinetics and thermodynamics; these results are very interesting regarding disease progression. As PGs act as receptors in many of these diseases, the putative inhibitory activity of these exogenous polysaccharides displays therapeutic potential.

Hep has been used for a century, primarily as an anticoagulant drug. Hep is obtained from animal tissues, and LMWHep is essentially prepared *via* the controlled depolymerization of unfractionated Hep. After the Hep crisis in 2008, due to its contamination with an oversulfated CS that exerted severe side effects, new approaches for obtaining synthetic Hep became urgent [152]. Recently, a chemoenzymatic process was successfully developed to synthesize Hep using *Escherichia coli* [153]; this method represents a good strategy for the near future.

REFERENCES

[1] Prusiner SB (1998) Prions. *Proc Natl Acad Sci U S A* 95: 13363-13383.

[2] Kim JI, Cali I, Surewicz K, Kong Q, Raymond GJ, et al. (2010) Mammalian prions generated from bacterially expressed prion protein in the absence of any mammalian cofactors. *J Biol Chem* 285: 14083-14087.

[3] Caughey B, Baron GS (2006) Prions and their partners in crime. *Nature* 443: 803-810.

[4] Silva JL, Vieira TC, Gomes MP, Rangel LP, Scapin SM, et al. (2011) Experimental approaches to the interaction of the prion protein with nucleic acids and glycosaminoglycans: Modulators of the pathogenic conversion. *Methods* 53: 306-317.

[5] Cordeiro Y, Machado F, Juliano L, Juliano MA, Brentani RR, et al. (2001) DNA converts cellular prion protein into the beta-sheet conformation and inhibits prion peptide aggregation. *J Biol Chem* 276: 49400-49409.

[6] Nandi PK, Leclerc E, Nicole JC, Takahashi M (2002) DNA-induced partial unfolding of prion protein leads to its polymerisation to amyloid. *J Mol Biol* 322: 153-161.

[7] Adler V, Zeiler B, Kryukov V, Kascsak R, Rubenstein R, et al. (2003) Small, highly structured RNAs participate in the conversion of human recombinant PrP(Sen) to PrP(Res) in vitro. *J Mol Biol* 332: 47-57.

[8] Deleault NR, Lucassen RW, Supattapone S (2003) RNA molecules stimulate prion protein conversion. *Nature* 425: 717-720.

[9] Deleault NR, Geoghegan JC, Nishina K, Kascsak R, Williamson RA, et al. (2005) Protease-resistant prion protein amplification reconstituted with partially purified substrates and synthetic polyanions. *J Biol Chem* 280: 26873-26879.

[10] Lima LM, Cordeiro Y, Tinoco LW, Marques AF, Oliveira CL, et al. (2006) Structural insights into the interaction between prion protein and nucleic acid. *Biochemistry* 45: 9180-9187.

[11] Gomes MP, Millen TA, Ferreira PS, e Silva NL, Vieira TC, et al. (2008) Prion protein complexed to N2a cellular RNAs through its N-terminal domain forms aggregates and is toxic to murine neuroblastoma cells. *J Biol Chem* 283: 19616-19625.

[12] Silva JL, Lima LM, Foguel D, Cordeiro Y (2008) Intriguing nucleic-acid-binding features of mammalian prion protein. *Trends Biochem* Sci 33: 132-140.

[13] Macedo B, Millen TA, Braga CA, Gomes MP, Ferreira PS, et al. (2012) Nonspecific prion protein-nucleic acid interactions lead to different aggregates and cytotoxic species. *Biochemistry* 51: 5402-5413.

[14] Timmes AG, Moore RA, Fischer ER, Priola SA (2013) Recombinant prion protein refolded with lipid and RNA has the biochemical hallmarks of a prion but lacks in vivo infectivity. *PLoS One* 8: e71081.

[15] Olsthoorn RC (2014) G-quadruplexes within prion mRNA: the missing link in prion disease? *Nucleic Acids Res* 42: 9327-9333.

[16] Deleault NR, Harris BT, Rees JR, Supattapone S (2007) Formation of native prions from minimal components in vitro. *Proc Natl Acad Sci U S A* 104: 9741-9746.

[17] Gilch S, Bach C, Lutzny G, Vorberg I, Schatzl HM (2009) Inhibition of cholesterol recycling impairs cellular PrP(Sc) propagation. *Cell Mol Life Sci* 66: 3979-3991.

[18] Tsiroulnikov K, Shchutskaya Y, Muronetz V, Chobert JM, Haertle T (2009) Phospholipids influence the aggregation of recombinant ovine prions. From rapid extensive aggregation to amyloidogenic conversion. *Biochim Biophys Acta* 1794: 506-511.

[19] Deleault NR, Piro JR, Walsh DJ, Wang F, Ma J, et al. (2012) Isolation of phosphatidylethanolamine as a solitary cofactor for prion formation in the absence of nucleic acids. *Proc Natl Acad Sci U S A* 109: 8546-8551.

[20] Wong C, Xiong LW, Horiuchi M, Raymond L, Wehrly K, et al. (2001) Sulfated glycans and elevated temperature stimulate PrP(Sc)-dependent cell-free formation of protease-resistant prion protein. *EMBO J* 20: 377-386.

[21] Gonzalez-Iglesias R, Pajares MA, Ocal C, Espinosa JC, Oesch B, et al. (2002) Prion protein interaction with glycosaminoglycan occurs with the formation of oligomeric complexes stabilized by Cu(II) bridges. *J Mol Biol* 319: 527-540.

[22] Ben-Zaken O, Tzaban S, Tal Y, Horonchik L, Esko JD, et al. (2003) Cellular heparan sulfate participates in the metabolism of prions. *J Biol Chem* 278: 40041-40049.

[23] Murayama Y, Yoshioka M, Masujin K, Okada H, Iwamaru Y, et al. (2010) Sulfated dextrans enhance in vitro amplification of bovine spongiform encephalopathy PrP(Sc) and enable ultrasensitive detection of bovine PrP(Sc). *PLoS One* 5.

[24] Yokoyama T, Takeuchi A, Yamamoto M, Kitamoto T, Ironside JW, et al. (2011) Heparin enhances the cell-protein misfolding cyclic amplification efficiency of variant Creutzfeldt-Jakob disease. *Neurosci Lett* 498: 119-123.

[25] Puig B, Altmeppen H, Glatzel M (2014) The GPI-anchoring of PrP: implications in sorting and pathogenesis. *Prion* 8: 11-18.

[26] Wopfner F, Weidenhofer G, Schneider R, von Brunn A, Gilch S, et al. (1999) Analysis of 27 mammalian and 9 avian PrPs reveals high conservation of flexible regions of the prion protein. *J Mol Biol* 289: 1163-1178.

[27] Zahn R, von Schroetter C, Wuthrich K (1997) Human prion proteins expressed in Escherichia coli and purified by high-affinity column refolding. *FEBS Lett* 417: 400-404.

[28] Iozzo RV (1998) Matrix proteoglycans: from molecular design to cellular function. *Annu Rev Biochem* 67: 609-652.

[29] Sasisekharan R, Raman R, Prabhakar V (2006) Glycomics approach to structure-function relationships of glycosaminoglycans. *Annu Rev Biomed Eng* 8: 181-231.

[30] Belting M (2003) Heparan sulfate proteoglycan as a plasma membrane carrier. *Trends Biochem Sci* 28: 145-151.

[31] Jeanloz RW (1960) The nomenclature of mucopolysaccharides. *Arthritis Rheum* 3: 233-237.

[32] Itano N (2008) Simple primary structure, complex turnover regulation and multiple roles of hyaluronan. *J Biochem* 144: 131-137.

[33] Sugahara K, Kitagawa H (2000) Recent advances in the study of the biosynthesis and functions of sulfated glycosaminoglycans. *Curr Opin Struct Biol* 10: 518-527.

[34] Sugahara K, Mikami T, Uyama T, Mizuguchi S, Nomura K, et al. (2003) Recent advances in the structural biology of chondroitin sulfate and dermatan sulfate. *Curr Opin Struct Biol* 13: 612-620.

[35] Funderburgh JL (2000) Keratan sulfate: structure, biosynthesis, and function. *Glycobiology* 10: 951-958.

[36] Silva ME, Dietrich CP (1975) Structure of heparin. Characterization of the products formed from heparin by the action of a heparinase and a heparitinase from Flavobacterium heparinum. *J Biol Chem* 250: 6841-6846.

[37] Gallagher JT (2001) Heparan sulfate: growth control with a restricted sequence menu. *J Clin Invest* 108: 357-361.

[38] Mulloy B, Forster MJ (2000) Conformation and dynamics of heparin and heparan sulfate. *Glycobiology* 10: 1147-1156.

[39] Nader HB, Chavante SF, dos-Santos EA, Oliveira TW, de-Paiva JF, et al. (1999) Heparan sulfates and heparins: similar compounds performing the same functions in vertebrates and invertebrates? *Braz J Med Biol Res* 32: 529-538.

[40] Capila I, Linhardt RJ (2002) Heparin-protein interactions. *Angew Chem Int Ed Engl* 41: 391-412.

[41] Bishop JR, Schuksz M, Esko JD (2007) Heparan sulphate proteoglycans fine-tune mammalian physiology. *Nature* 446: 1030-1037.

[42] Dobson CM (1999) Protein misfolding, evolution and disease. *Trends Biochem Sci* 24: 329-332.

[43] Dobson CM (2003) Protein folding and misfolding. *Nature* 426: 884-890.

[44] Lomakin A, Chung DS, Benedek GB, Kirschner DA, Teplow DB (1996) On the nucleation and growth of amyloid beta-protein fibrils: detection of nuclei and quantitation of rate constants. *Proc Natl Acad Sci U S A* 93: 1125-1129.

[45] Harper JD, Lansbury PT, Jr. (1997) Models of amyloid seeding in Alzheimer's disease and scrapie: mechanistic truths and physiological consequences of the time-dependent solubility of amyloid proteins. *Annu Rev Biochem* 66: 385-407.

[46] Kelly JW (2000) Mechanisms of amyloidogenesis. *Nat Struct Biol* 7: 824-826.

[47] Rangel LP, Costa DC, Vieira TC, Silva JL (2014) The aggregation of mutant p53 produces prion-like properties in cancer. *Prion* 8: 75-84.

[48] Fraser PE (2014) Prions and prion-like proteins. *J Biol Chem* 289: 19839-19840.

[49] Virchow R (1855) Zur Cellulose-Frage. *Archiv für pathologische Anatomie und Physiologie und für klinische Medicin* 8: 140-144.

[50] McBride PA, Wilson MI, Eikelenboom P, Tunstall A, Bruce ME (1998) Heparan sulfate proteoglycan is associated with amyloid plaques and neuroanatomically targeted PrP pathology throughout the incubation period of scrapie-infected mice. *Exp Neurol* 149: 447-454.

[51] Hirschfield GM, Hawkins PN (2003) Amyloidosis: new strategies for treatment. *Int J Biochem Cell Biol* 35: 1608-1613.

[52] Cohlberg JA, Li J, Uversky VN, Fink AL (2002) Heparin and other glycosaminoglycans stimulate the formation of amyloid fibrils from alpha-synuclein in vitro. *Biochemistry* 41: 1502-1511.

[53] Yamaguchi I, Suda H, Tsuzuike N, Seto K, Seki M, et al. (2003) Glycosaminoglycan and proteoglycan inhibit the depolymerization of beta2-microglobulin amyloid fibrils in vitro. *Kidney Int* 64: 1080-1088.

[54] Gupta-Bansal R, Frederickson RC, Brunden KR (1995) Proteoglycan-mediated inhibition of A beta proteolysis. A potential cause of senile plaque accumulation. *J Biol Chem* 270: 18666-18671.

[55] Ancsin JB (2003) Amyloidogenesis: historical and modern observations point to heparan sulfate proteoglycans as a major culprit. *Amyloid* 10: 67-79.

[56] Noborn F, O'Callaghan P, Hermansson E, Zhang X, Ancsin JB, et al. (2011) Heparan sulfate/heparin promotes transthyretin fibrillization through selective binding to a basic motif in the protein. *Proc Natl Acad Sci U S A* 108: 5584-5589.

[57] Blancas-Mejia LM, Hammernik J, Marin-Argany M, Ramirez-Alvarado M (2015) Differential effects on light chain amyloid formation depend on mutations and type of glycosaminoglycans. *J Biol Chem* 290: 4953-4965.

[58] Meng F, Abedini A, Song B, Raleigh DP (2007) Amyloid formation by pro-islet amyloid polypeptide processing intermediates: examination of the role of protein heparan sulfate interactions and implications for islet amyloid formation in type 2 diabetes. *Biochemistry* 46: 12091-12099.

[59] Castillo GM, Lukito W, Wight TN, Snow AD (1999) The sulfate moieties of glycosaminoglycans are critical for the enhancement of beta-amyloid protein fibril formation. *J Neurochem* 72: 1681-1687.

[60] Goedert M, Jakes R, Spillantini MG, Hasegawa M, Smith MJ, et al. (1996) Assembly of microtubule-associated protein tau into Alzheimer-like filaments induced by sulphated glycosaminoglycans. *Nature* 383: 550-553.

[61] Snow AD, Kisilevsky R, Willmer J, Prusiner SB, DeArmond SJ (1989) Sulfated glycosaminoglycans in amyloid plaques of prion diseases. *Acta Neuropathol* 77: 337-342.

[62] Snow AD, Wight TN, Nochlin D, Koike Y, Kimata K, et al. (1990) Immunolocalization of heparan sulfate proteoglycans to the prion protein amyloid plaques of Gerstmann-Straussler syndrome, Creutzfeldt-Jakob disease and scrapie. *Lab Invest* 63: 601-611.

[63] Gabizon R, Meiner Z, Halimi M, Ben-Sasson SA (1993) Heparin-like molecules bind differentially to prion-proteins and change their intracellular metabolic fate. *J Cell Physiol* 157: 319-325.

[64] Caughey B, Brown K, Raymond GJ, Katzenstein GE, Thresher W (1994) Binding of the protease-sensitive form of PrP (prion protein) to sulfated glycosaminoglycan and congo red [corrected]. *J Virol* 68: 2135-2141.

[65] Warner RG, Hundt C, Weiss S, Turnbull JE (2002) Identification of the heparan sulfate binding sites in the cellular prion protein. *J Biol Chem* 277: 18421-18430.

[66] Pan T, Wong BS, Liu T, Li R, Petersen RB, et al. (2002) Cell-surface prion protein interacts with glycosaminoglycans. *Biochem J* 368: 81-90.

[67] Vieira TC, Reynaldo DP, Gomes MP, Almeida MS, Cordeiro Y, et al. (2011) Heparin binding by murine recombinant prion protein leads to transient aggregation and formation of RNA-resistant species. *J Am Chem Soc* 133: 334-344.

[68] Vieira TC, Cordeiro Y, Caughey B, Silva JL (2014) Heparin binding confers prion stability and impairs its aggregation. *FASEB J* 28: 2667-2676.

[69] Taylor DR, Hooper NM (2006) The prion protein and lipid rafts. *Mol Membr Biol* 23: 89-99.

[70] Praus M, Kettelgerdes G, Baier M, Holzhutter HG, Jungblut PR, et al. (2003) Stimulation of plasminogen activation by recombinant cellular prion protein is conserved in the NH2-terminal fragment PrP23-110. *Thromb Haemost* 89: 812-819.

[71] Mani K, Cheng F, Havsmark B, Jonsson M, Belting M, et al. (2003) Prion, amyloid beta-derived Cu(II) ions, or free Zn(II) ions support S-nitroso-dependent autocleavage of glypican-1 heparan sulfate. *J Biol Chem* 278: 38956-38965.

[72] Cheng F, Lindqvist J, Haigh CL, Brown DR, Mani K (2006) Copper-dependent co-internalization of the prion protein and glypican-1. *J Neurochem* 98: 1445-1457.

[73] Taylor DR, Whitehouse IJ, Hooper NM (2009) Glypican-1 mediates both prion protein lipid raft association and disease isoform formation. PLoS Pathog 5: e1000666.

[74] Shyng SL, Lehmann S, Moulder KL, Harris DA (1995) Sulfated glycans stimulate endocytosis of the cellular isoform of the prion protein, PrPC, in cultured cells. *J Biol Chem* 270: 30221-30229.

[75] Pauly PC, Harris DA (1998) Copper stimulates endocytosis of the prion protein. *J Biol Chem* 273: 33107-33110.

[76] Caughey B, Raymond GJ, Ernst D, Race RE (1991) N-terminal truncation of the scrapie-associated form of PrP by lysosomal protease(s): implications regarding the site of conversion of PrP to the protease-resistant state. *J Virol* 65: 6597-6603.

[77] Barmada SJ, Harris DA (2005) Visualization of prion infection in transgenic mice expressing green fluorescent protein-tagged prion protein. *J Neurosci* 25: 5824-5832.

[78] Godsave SF, Wille H, Kujala P, Latawiec D, DeArmond SJ, et al. (2008) Cryo-immunogold electron microscopy for prions: toward identification of a conversion site. *J Neurosci* 28: 12489-12499.

[79] Marijanovic Z, Caputo A, Campana V, Zurzolo C (2009) Identification of an intracellular site of prion conversion. *PLoS Pathog* 5: e1000426.

[80] Borchelt DR, Taraboulos A, Prusiner SB (1992) Evidence for synthesis of scrapie prion proteins in the endocytic pathway. *J Biol Chem* 267: 16188-16199.

[81] Campana V, Sarnataro D, Zurzolo C (2005) The highways and byways of prion protein trafficking. *Trends Cell Biol* 15: 102-111.

[82] Goold R, Rabbanian S, Sutton L, Andre R, Arora P, et al. (2011) Rapid cell-surface prion protein conversion revealed using a novel cell system. *Nat Commun* 2: 281.

[83] Rouvinski A, Karniely S, Kounin M, Moussa S, Goldberg MD, et al. (2014) Live imaging of prions reveals nascent PrPSc in cell-surface, raft-associated amyloid strings and webs. *J Cell Biol* 204: 423-441.

[84] McNally KL, Ward AE, Priola SA (2009) Cells expressing anchorless prion protein are resistant to scrapie infection. *J Virol* 83: 4469-4475.

[85] Horonchik L, Tzaban S, Ben-Zaken O, Yedidia Y, Rouvinski A, et al. (2005) Heparan sulfate is a cellular receptor for purified infectious prions. *J Biol Chem* 280: 17062-17067.

[86] Hijazi N, Kariv-Inbal Z, Gasset M, Gabizon R (2005) PrPSc incorporation to cells requires endogenous glycosaminoglycan expression. *J Biol Chem* 280: 17057-17061.

[87] Jen A, Parkyn CJ, Mootoosamy RC, Ford MJ, Warley A, et al. (2010) Neuronal low-density lipoprotein receptor-related protein 1 binds and endocytoses prion fibrils via receptor cluster 4. *J Cell Sci* 123: 246-255.

[88] Taylor DR, Hooper NM (2007) The low-density lipoprotein receptor-related protein 1 (LRP1) mediates the endocytosis of the cellular prion protein. *Biochem J* 402: 17-23.

[89] Gauczynski S, Peyrin JM, Haik S, Leucht C, Hundt C, et al. (2001) The 37-kDa/67-kDa laminin receptor acts as the cell-surface receptor for the cellular prion protein. *EMBO J* 20: 5863-5875.

[90] Hooper NM (2011) Glypican-1 facilitates prion conversion in lipid rafts. *J Neurochem* 116: 721-725.

[91] Paquet S, Daude N, Courageot MP, Chapuis J, Laude H, et al. (2007) PrPc does not mediate internalization of PrPSc but is required at an early stage for de novo prion infection of Rov cells. *J Virol* 81: 10786-10791.

[92] Clavaguera F, Bolmont T, Crowther RA, Abramowski D, Frank S, et al. (2009) Transmission and spreading of tauopathy in transgenic mouse brain. *Nat Cell Biol* 11: 909-913.

[93] Holmes BB, DeVos SL, Kfoury N, Li M, Jacks R, et al. (2013) Heparan sulfate proteoglycans mediate internalization and propagation of specific proteopathic seeds. *Proc Natl Acad Sci U S A* 110: E3138-3147.

[94] Kanekiyo T, Zhang J, Liu Q, Liu CC, Zhang L, et al. (2011) Heparan sulphate proteoglycan and the low-density lipoprotein receptor-related protein 1 constitute major pathways for neuronal amyloid-beta uptake. *J Neurosci* 31: 1644-1651.

[95] Rosen RF, Fritz JJ, Dooyema J, Cintron AF, Hamaguchi T, et al. (2012) Exogenous seeding of cerebral beta-amyloid deposition in betaAPP-transgenic rats. *J Neurochem* 120: 660-666.

[96] Forget KJ, Tremblay G, Roucou X (2013) p53 Aggregates penetrate cells and induce the co-aggregation of intracellular p53. *PLoS One* 8: e69242.

[97] Ano Bom AP, Rangel LP, Costa DC, de Oliveira GA, Sanches D, et al. (2012) Mutant p53 aggregates into prion-like amyloid oligomers and fibrils: implications for cancer. *J Biol Chem* 287: 28152-28162.

[98] Xu J, Reumers J, Couceiro JR, De Smet F, Gallardo R, et al. (2011) Gain of function of mutant p53 by coaggregation with multiple tumor suppressors. *Nat Chem Biol* 7: 285-295.

[99] Silva JL, Rangel LP, Costa DC, Cordeiro Y, De Moura Gallo CV (2013) Expanding the prion concept to cancer biology: dominant-negative effect of aggregates of mutant p53 tumour suppressor. *Biosci Rep* 33.

[100] Silva JL, De Moura Gallo CV, Costa DC, Rangel LP (2014) Prion-like aggregation of mutant p53 in cancer. *Trends Biochem Sci* 39: 260-267.

[101] Lucassen R, Nishina K, Supattapone S (2003) In vitro amplification of protease-resistant prion protein requires free sulfhydryl groups. *Biochemistry* 42: 4127-4135.

[102] Saborio GP, Permanne B, Soto C (2001) Sensitive detection of pathological prion protein by cyclic amplification of protein misfolding. *Nature* 411: 810-813.

[103] Supattapone S (2014) Synthesis of high titer infectious prions with cofactor molecules. *J Biol Chem* 289: 19850-19854.

[104] Klajnert B, Cortijo-Arellano M, Bryszewska M, Cladera J (2006) Influence of heparin and dendrimers on the aggregation of two amyloid peptides related to Alzheimer's and prion diseases. *Biochem Biophys Res Commun* 339: 577-582.

[105] Cortijo-Arellano M, Ponce J, Durany N, Cladera J (2008) Amyloidogenic properties of the prion protein fragment PrP(185-208): comparison with Alzheimer's peptide Abeta(1-28), influence of heparin and cell toxicity. *Biochem Biophys Res Commun* 368: 238-242.

[106] Caughey B, Raymond GJ (1993) Sulfated polyanion inhibition of scrapie-associated PrP accumulation in cultured cells. *J Virol* 67: 643-650.

[107] Caughey B, Race RE (1994) Scrapie-associated PrP accumulation and its inhibition: revisiting the amyloid-glycosaminoglycan connection. *Ann N Y Acad Sci* 724: 290-295.

[108] Adjou KT, Simoneau S, Sales N, Lamoury F, Dormont D, et al. (2003) A novel generation of heparan sulfate mimetics for the treatment of prion diseases. *J Gen Virol* 84: 2595-2603.

[109] Schonberger O, Horonchik L, Gabizon R, Papy-Garcia D, Barritault D, et al. (2003) Novel heparan mimetics potently inhibit the scrapie prion protein and its endocytosis. *Biochem Biophys Res Commun* 312: 473-479.

[110] Perez M, Wandosell F, Colaco C, Avila J (1998) Sulphated glycosaminoglycans prevent the neurotoxicity of a human prion protein fragment. *Biochem J* 335 (Pt 2): 369-374.

[111] Bazar E, Sheynis T, Dorosz J, Jelinek R (2011) Heparin inhibits membrane interactions and lipid-induced fibrillation of a prion amyloidogenic determinant. *Chembiochem* 12: 761-767.

[112] Honda H, Sasaki K, Minaki H, Masui K, Suzuki SO, et al. (2012) Protease-resistant PrP and PrP oligomers in the brain in human prion diseases after intraventricular pentosan polysulfate infusion. *Neuropathology* 32: 124-132.

[113] Larramendy-Gozalo C, Barret A, Daudigeos E, Mathieu E, Antonangeli L, et al. (2007) Comparison of CR36, a new heparan mimetic, and pentosan polysulfate in the treatment of prion diseases. *J Gen Virol* 88: 1062-1067.

[114] Andrievskaia O, Potetinova Z, Balachandran A, Nielsen K (2007) Binding of bovine prion protein to heparin: a fluorescence polarization study. *Arch Biochem Biophys* 460: 10-16.

[115] Woods AG, Cribbs DH, Whittemore ER, Cotman CW (1995) Heparan sulfate and chondroitin sulfate glycosaminoglycan attenuate beta-amyloid(25-35) induced neurodegeneration in cultured hippocampal neurons. *Brain Res* 697: 53-62.

[116] Pollack SJ, Sadler, II, Hawtin SR, Tailor VJ, Shearman MS (1995) Sulfated glycosaminoglycans and dyes attenuate the neurotoxic effects of beta-amyloid in rat PC12 cells. *Neurosci Lett* 184: 113-116.

[117] De Carufel CA, Nguyen PT, Sahnouni S, Bourgault S (2013) New insights into the roles of sulfated glycosaminoglycans in islet amyloid polypeptide amyloidogenesis and cytotoxicity. *Biopolymers* 100: 645-655.

[118] Monsellier E, Ramazzotti M, Taddei N, Chiti F (2010) A computational approach for identifying the chemical factors involved in the glycosaminoglycans-mediated acceleration of amyloid fibril formation. *PLoS One* 5: e11363.

[119] Cardin AD, Weintraub HJ (1989) Molecular modeling of protein-glycosaminoglycan interactions. *Arteriosclerosis* 9: 21-32.

[120] Sobel M, Soler DF, Kermode JC, Harris RB (1992) Localization and characterization of a heparin binding domain peptide of human von Willebrand factor. *J Biol Chem* 267: 8857-8862.

[121] Margalit H, Fischer N, Ben-Sasson SA (1993) Comparative analysis of structurally defined heparin binding sequences reveals a distinct spatial distribution of basic residues. *J Biol Chem* 268: 19228-19231.

[122] Fromm JR, Hileman RE, Weiler JM, Linhardt RJ (1997) Interaction of fibroblast growth factor-1 and related peptides with heparan sulfate and its oligosaccharides. *Arch Biochem Biophys* 346: 252-262.

[123] Torrent M, Nogues MV, Andreu D, Boix E (2012) The "CPC clip motif": a conserved structural signature for heparin-binding proteins. *PLoS One* 7: e42692.

[124] Fromm JR, Hileman RE, Caldwell EE, Weiler JM, Linhardt RJ (1995) Differences in the interaction of heparin with arginine and lysine and the importance of these basic amino acids in the binding of heparin to acidic fibroblast growth factor. *Arch Biochem Biophys* 323: 279-287.

[125] Pixley RA, Lin Y, Isordia-Salas I, Colman RW (2003) Fine mapping of the sequences in domain 5 of high molecular weight kininogen (HK) interacting with heparin and zinc. *J Thromb Haemost* 1: 1791-1798.

[126] Hallgren J, Backstrom S, Estrada S, Thuveson M, Pejler G (2004) Histidines are critical for heparin-dependent activation of mast cell tryptase. *J Immunol* 173: 1868-1875.

[127] Sebollela A, Cagliari TC, Limaverde GS, Chapeaurouge A, Sorgine MH, et al. (2005) Heparin-binding sites in granulocyte-macrophage colony-stimulating factor. Localization and regulation by histidine ionization. *J Biol Chem* 280: 31949-31956.

[128] Goldfarb LG, Brown P, McCombie WR, Goldgaber D, Swergold GD, et al. (1991) Transmissible familial Creutzfeldt-Jakob disease associated with five, seven, and eight extra octapeptide coding repeats in the PRNP gene. *Proc Natl Acad Sci U S A* 88: 10926-10930.

[129] Yu S, Yin S, Li C, Wong P, Chang B, et al. (2007) Aggregation of prion protein with insertion mutations is proportional to the number of inserts. *Biochem J* 403: 343-351.

[130] Brimacombe DB, Bennett AD, Wusteman FS, Gill AC, Dann JC, et al. (1999) Characterization and polyanion-binding properties of purified recombinant prion protein. *Biochem J* 342 Pt 3: 605-613.

[131] Taubner LM, Bienkiewicz EA, Copie V, Caughey B (2010) Structure of the flexible amino-terminal domain of prion protein bound to a sulfated glycan. *J Mol Biol* 395: 475-490.

[132] Calzolai L, Zahn R (2003) Influence of pH on NMR structure and stability of the human prion protein globular domain. *J Biol Chem* 278: 35592-35596.

[133] Swietnicki W, Petersen R, Gambetti P, Surewicz WK (1997) pH-dependent stability and conformation of the recombinant human prion protein PrP(90-231). *J Biol Chem* 272: 27517-27520.

[134] Langella E, Improta R, Crescenzi O, Barone V (2006) Assessing the acid-base and conformational properties of histidine residues in human prion protein (125-228) by means of pK(a) calculations and molecular dynamics simulations. *Proteins* 64: 167-177.

[135] Martins PM (2013) True and apparent inhibition of amyloid fibril formation. Prion 7: 136-139.

[136] Chiti F, Dobson CM (2006) Protein misfolding, functional amyloid, and human disease. *Annu Rev Biochem* 75: 333-366.

[137] Kimberlin RH, Walker CA (1986) Suppression of scrapie infection in mice by heteropolyanion 23, dextran sulfate, and some other polyanions. *Antimicrob Agents Chemother* 30: 409-413.

[138] Farquhar CF, Dickinson AG (1986) Prolongation of scrapie incubation period by an injection of dextran sulphate 500 within the month before or after infection. *J Gen Virol* 67 (Pt 3): 463-473.

[139] Diringer H, Ehlers B (1991) Chemoprophylaxis of scrapie in mice. *J Gen Virol* 72 (Pt 2): 457-460.

[140] Ladogana A, Casaccia P, Ingrosso L, Cibati M, Salvatore M, et al. (1992) Sulphate polyanions prolong the incubation period of scrapie-infected hamsters. *J Gen Virol* 73 (Pt 3): 661-665.

[141] Whittle IR, Knight RS, Will RG (2006) Unsuccessful intraventricular pentosan polysulphate treatment of variant Creutzfeldt-Jakob disease. *Acta Neurochir* (Wien) 148: 677-679; discussion 679.

[142] Parry A, Baker I, Stacey R, Wimalaratna S (2007) Long term survival in a patient with variant Creutzfeldt-Jakob disease treated with intraventricular pentosan polysulphate. *J Neurol Neurosurg Psychiatry* 78: 733-734.

[143] Tsuboi Y, Doh-Ura K, Yamada T (2009) Continuous intraventricular infusion of pentosan polysulfate: clinical trial against prion diseases. *Neuropathology* 29: 632-636.

[144] Bone I, Belton L, Walker AS, Darbyshire J (2008) Intraventricular pentosan polysulphate in human prion diseases: an observational study in the UK. *Eur J Neurol* 15: 458-464.

[145] Terada T, Tsuboi Y, Obi T, Doh-ura K, Murayama S, et al. (2010) Less protease-resistant PrP in a patient with sporadic CJD treated with intraventricular pentosan polysulphate. *Acta Neurol Scand* 121: 127-130.

[146] Newman PK, Todd NV, Scoones D, Mead S, Knight RS, et al. (2014) Postmortem findings in a case of variant Creutzfeldt-Jakob disease treated with intraventricular pentosan polysulfate. *J Neurol Neurosurg Psychiatry* 85: 921-924.

[147] Caughey B, Caughey WS, Kocisko DA, Lee KS, Silveira JR, et al. (2006) Prions and transmissible spongiform encephalopathy (TSE) chemotherapeutics: A common mechanism for anti-TSE compounds? *Acc Chem Res* 39: 646-653.

[148] Ma Q, Dudas B, Hejna M, Cornelli U, Lee JM, et al. (2002) The blood-brain barrier accessibility of a heparin-derived oligosaccharides C3. *Thromb Res* 105: 447-453.

[149] Leveugle B, Ding W, Laurence F, Dehouck MP, Scanameo A, et al. (1998) Heparin oligosaccharides that pass the blood-brain barrier inhibit beta-amyloid precursor protein secretion and heparin binding to beta-amyloid peptide. *J Neurochem* 70: 736-744.

[150] Dudas B, Rose M, Cornelli U, Pavlovich A, Hanin I (2008) Neuroprotective properties of glycosaminoglycans: potential treatment for neurodegenerative disorders. *Neurodegener Dis* 5: 200-205.

[151] Zhu H, Yu J, Kindy MS (2001) Inhibition of amyloidosis using low-molecular-weight heparins. *Mol Med* 7: 517-522.

[152] Liu H, Zhang Z, Linhardt RJ (2009) Lessons learned from the contamination of heparin. *Nat Prod Rep* 26: 313-321.

[153] Xu Y, Masuko S, Takieddin M, Xu H, Liu R, et al. (2011) Chemoenzymatic synthesis of homogeneous ultralow molecular weight heparins. *Science* 334: 498-501.

In: The Prion Phenomena in Neurodegenerative Diseases ISBN: 978-1-63483-399-8
Editors: Giuseppe Legname and Gabriele Giachin

Chapter 5

COMPLEXITY OF AGGREGATION PATHWAY OF α -SYNUCLEIN

Leonid Breydo[1,2] and Vladimir N. Uversky[1,2,3,4,*]
[1]Department of Molecular Medicine and [2]Byrd Alzheimer's Research Institute, Morsani College of Medicine, University of South Florida, Tampa, Florida, US
[3]Institute for Biological Instrumentation, Russian Academy of Sciences, Pushchino, Moscow Region, Russia
[4]Department of Biological Science, Faculty of Science, King Abdulaziz University, Jeddah, Jeddah, Saudi Arabi
[5]Laboratory of Structural Dynamics, Stability and Folding of Proteins, Institute of Cytology, Russian Academy of Sciences, St. Petersburg, Russia

ABSTRACT

The molecular basis of Parkinson's disease appears to be tightly coupled to the aggregation of α-synuclein. Due to intermolecular interactions the same protein can form aggregates with a variety of different structures and morphologies. This is especially true for an intrinsically disordered protein like α-synuclein. These aggregates can differ in morphology, structure, stability, cytotoxicity, and ability to propagate their conformation in prion-like manner. This chapter examines the aggregation pathways of α-synuclein, and the influence of the crowded cellular environment on this process.

STRUCTURAL PROPERTIES OF α-SYNUCLEIN

α-synuclein is an abundant 140-amino acid neuron-specific protein localized in the presynaptic nerve terminals and nucleus [1, 2]. Several possible functions for α-synuclein have been suggested, including synaptic vesicle release and trafficking, fatty acid binding and physiological regulation of certain enzymes, transporters, and neurotransmitter vesicles, as

* Corresponding Author address. Email: vuversky@health.usf.edu

well as roles in neuronal survival [3]. The involvement of α-synuclein in the control of the neuronal apoptotic response and in the protection of neurons from various apoptotic stimuli was demonstrated [4]. Knockout of all synucleins (there are three members of the synuclein family in the vertebrata, α-, β-, and γ-synucleins) in mice lead to age-dependent neuronal disfunction indicating that synucleins are important contributors to long-term operation of the nervous system [5]. α-synuclein was shown to physically interact with at least 30 proteins underlying its important role in cell signaling [3, 6]. Subsequent proteomic analysis identified 324 α-synuclein-interacting proteins in the dopaminergic cells of the MES (mouse embryonic stem) cell line [7]. Almost half of these interactors (141 proteins) experienced a significant change in their relative abundance (increase or decrease) after the MES cell were treated with rotenone [7], a pesticide that produces parkinsonism in animals and induces LB-like inclusions in the remaining dopaminergic neurons [8]. Figure 1 represents the results of the evaluation of human α-synuclein interactivity by STRING (Search Tool for the Retrieval of Interacting Genes), which is the online database resource, that provides both experimental and predicted interaction information [9]. STRING produces the network of predicted associations for a particular group of proteins. The network nodes are proteins, whereas the edges represent the predicted or known functional associations. An edge may be drawn with up to 7 differently colored lines that represent the existence of the seven types of evidence used in predicting the associations. A red line indicates the presence of fusion evidence; a green line - neighborhood evidence; a blue line – co-occurrence evidence; a purple line - experimental evidence; a yellow line – text mining evidence; a light blue line - database evidence; a black line – co-expression evidence [9].

α-synuclein is an intrinsically disordered protein (IDP). Figure 2A represents the results of disorder prediction on human α-synuclein sequence using several disorder predictors: PONDR® VL3 [10, 11], VSL2 [12], RONN [13] and IUPred [14]. It can be seen that α-synuclein is predicted to be almost completely disordered by all these predictors (as disorder probability scores ≥0.5 correspond to a prediction of disorder), emphasizing that its sequence is typical of the intrinsically disordered proteins [15]. Figure 2B represents the results disorder evaluation in human α-synuclein together with important disorder-related functional information retrieved from D^2P^2 database (http://d2p2.pro/) [16]. D^2P^2 is a database of predicted disorder that represents a community resource for pre-computed disorder predictions on a large library of proteins from completely sequenced genomes [16]. D^2P^2 database uses outputs of PONDR® VLXT [10], IUPred [14], PONDR® VSL2B [12, 17], PrDOS [18], ESpritz [19], and PV2 [16]. This database is further enhanced by information on the curated sites of various posttranslational modifications and on the location of predicted disorder-based potential binding sites. Results of the application of this tool to human α-synuclein shown in Figure 2B provide further support for the abundance and functional importance of intrinsic disorder in this protein. In fact, Figure 2B shows that human α-synuclein contains long disordered regions, which are enriched in potential disorder-based binding motifs and numerous sites of posttranslational modifications, PTMs. The fact that the human α-synuclein is densely populated with various PTMs, including multiple phosphorylation sites is in agreement with the well-known notion that phosphorylation [20] and many other enzymatically catalyzed PTMs are preferentially located within the IDPRs [21].

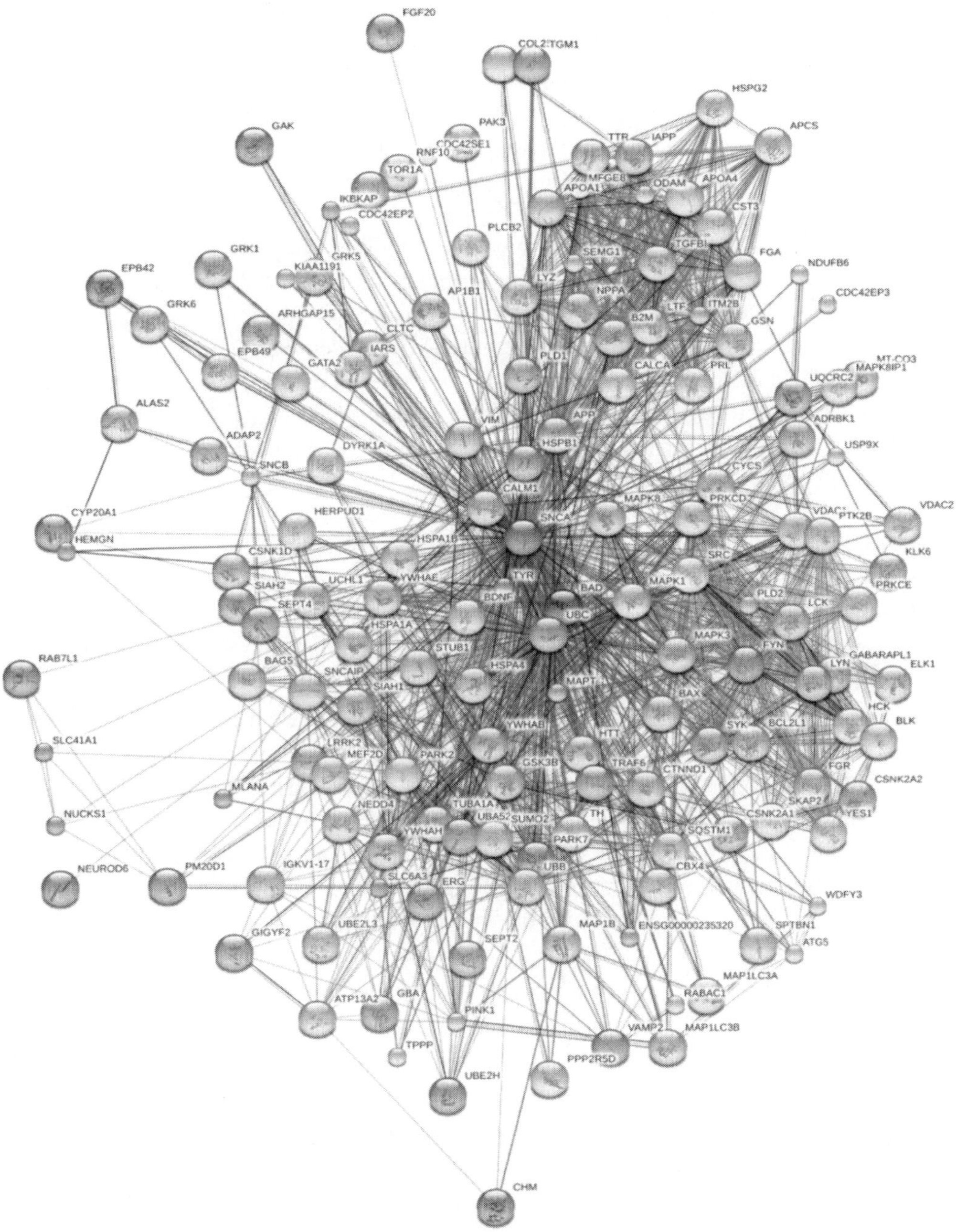

Figure 1. Analysis of the interactivity of the human α-synuclein (UniProt ID: P37840) by STRING [9]. STRING produces the network of predicted associations for a particular group of proteins. The network nodes are proteins, whereas the edges represent the predicted or known functional associations. An edge may be drawn with up to 7 differently colored lines that represent the existence of the seven types of evidence used in predicting the associations. A red line indicates the presence of fusion evidence; a green line - neighborhood evidence; a blue line – co-occurrence evidence; a purple line - experimental evidence; a yellow line – text mining evidence; a light blue line - database evidence; a black line – co-expression evidence [9].

The aforementioned high binding promiscuity and high levels of connectivity predicted for this intrinsically disordered protein indicates that human α-synuclein should be considered as disordered hub. In fact, in protein-protein interaction networks (PPI), there are several multitasking proteins. These multitasking proteins are promiscuous binders, have multiple links, and are known as hubs. With respect to the temporal structure of the PPI networks, some hub proteins have multiple simultaneous interactions ("party hubs"), while others have multiple sequential interactions ("date hubs") [22]. From a functional perspective, "date hubs" may connect biological modules to each other [23], whereas "party hubs" may form scaffolds that enable the assembly of functional modules [22]. Involvement of intrinsic disorder is one of the reasonable mechanisms for the description of the promiscuity of hub proteins [24, 25, 26, 27, 28, 29], where intrinsic disorder and related disorder-to-order transitions could enable one protein to interact with multiple partners (one-to-many signaling) or to enable multiple partners to bind to one protein (many-to-one signaling) [30]. In line with these considerations, intrinsically disordered nature of α-synuclein provides a plausible explanation for its potential roles as a hub protein.

α-synuclein attracted significant interest in 1997 after a mutation in its gene was found to be associated with the familial cases of early-onset Parkinson's disease [31], and its aggregates were found to be the major components of Lewy bodies, the hallmarks of PD [3, 32, 33, 34, 35]. These *in vivo* results have been supported by numerous studies that established that α-synuclein easily aggregates into amyloid fibrils and oligomers under a variety of conditions [36, 37, 38].

At the level of amino acid sequence, the structure of α-synuclein can be divided into three regions: residues 1–60, which contain four 11-amino acid imperfect repeats (coding for amphipathic α-helices) with a conserved motif (KTKEGV); residues 61–95, which contain the hydrophobic and highly amyloidogenic NAC region and three additional KTKEGV repeats; and the highly enriched in acidic residues and prolines C-terminal region, residues 96–140. The first two regions comprise a membrane-binding domain, whereas the C-terminal tail is thought to contain protein-protein and protein-small molecule interaction sites.

α-synuclein is more compact compared to what would be expected for a fully unfolded peptide chain [39, 40, 41, 42, 43, 44]. The compactness of α-synuclein has been confirmed by NMR studies, which demonstrated the presence of transient long-range contacts within the protein [43, 45, 46]. Like many IDPs, α-synuclein possesses remarkable conformational plasticity [47], being capable of adopt a variety of conformations, including the substantially unfolded "basic" state, an amyloidogenic partially folded conformation, and different α-helical or β-structural conformations folded to a different degree [47, 48, 49]. NMR studies suggest that residues 40-100 of both human [50] and mouse [51] α-synucleins exhibit propensity towards β-structure. X-ray crystallography data on the peptides derived from the N-terminal region of α-synuclein indicates that residues 1-13 and 20-34 of this protein possess higher propensity to form α-helices [52].

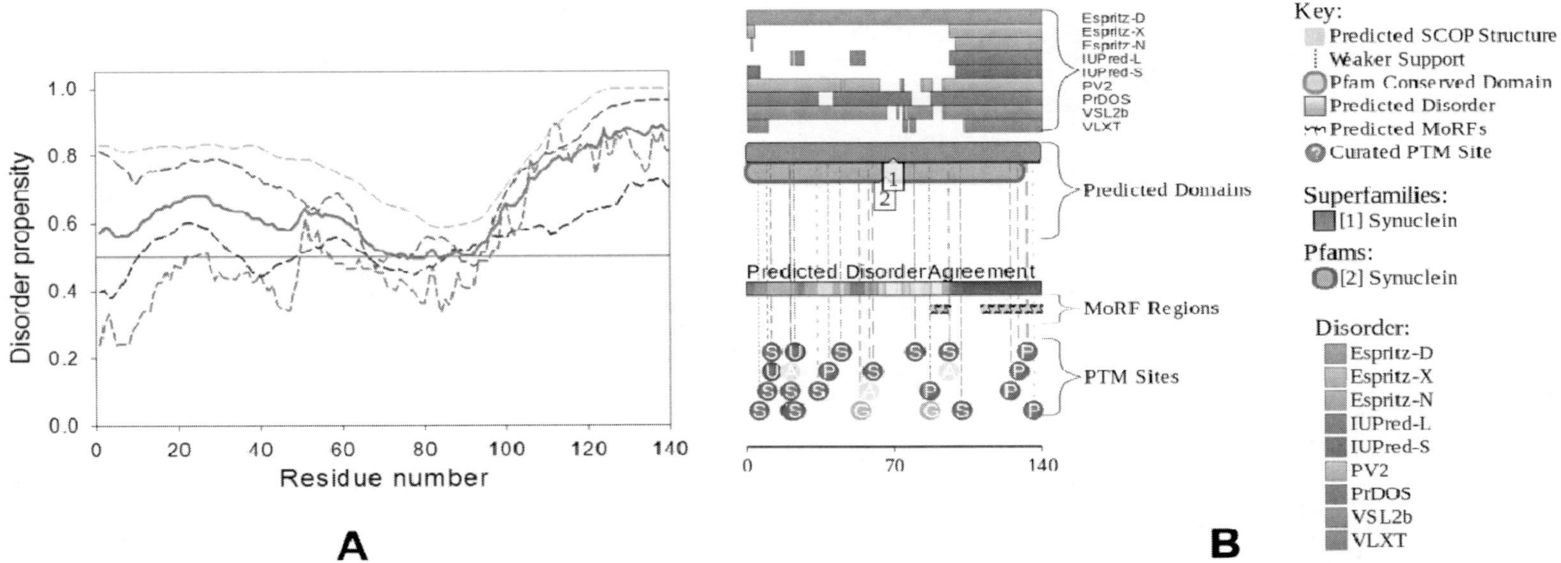

Figure 2. Evaluating disorder propensity of the human α-synuclein (UniProt ID: P37840). A. The per-residue disorder propensity plot represents the results of the intrinsic disorder prediction using IUPred (pink dashed line); RONN (blue dashed line); PONDR VSL2 (red dashed line) and PONDR VL3 (cyan dashed line). The results averaged over these for predictions are shown as a yellow solid line. B. Evaluation of the functional intrinsic disorder propensity of the human α-synuclein by D^2P^2 database (http://d2p2.pro/) [16]. In this plot, top nine colored bars represent location of disordered regions predicted by different disorder predictors (Espritz-D, Espritz-N, Espritz-X, IUPred-L, IUPred-S, PV2, PrDOS, PONDR® VSL2b, and PONDR® VLXT, see keys for the corresponding color codes). Light red bar and dark red bar shows the location of the functional domain "synuclein" found by the Superfamily and the Pfam platform, respectively. The Superfamily platform provides structural, functional and evolutionary information for proteins from all completely sequenced genomes, and large sequence collections such as UniProt [53]. Pfam is a database of protein families that includes their annotations and multiple sequence alignments generated using hidden Markov models [54, 55, 56]. Blue-and-white bar in the middle of the plot shows the predicted disorder agreement between these nine predictors, with green parts corresponding to disordered regions by consensus. Yellow bar shows the location of the predicted disorder-based binding site (MoRF region), whereas differently colored circles at the bottom of the plot show location of various PTMs. Here red, green, orange, yellow, and violet circles correspond to sites of phosphorylation, SUMOylation, glycosylation, acetylation, and ubiquitylation sites, respectively.

MECHANISM OF AGGREGATION OF INTRINSICALLY DISORDERED PROTEINS

Aggregation of IDPs tends to start from partially folded, pre-molten globule-like conformations that enable intramolecular interactions [57]. In some cases it has been shown that conversion of the monomeric protein into the amyloidogenic conformation is the slow step in the aggregation process and thus no stable oligomeric aggregation intermediates are formed [58, 59]. However, in other cases aggregation pathway for IDPs starts from formation of oligomers that may initially remain mostly unfolded [60, 61, 62]. Within these oligomers the protein molecules may form the metastable β-sheet conformations, and over time these oligomers become β-sheet rich [60, 61, 62, 63, 64]. At some point in this process, the structures capable of serving as nuclei for further propagation into oligomers or conversion to fibrils may be generated. Relative prevalence of *de novo* formation of aggregates from the monomers *vs.* conversion of monomers to the aggregates via seeding varies depending on the structure of the aggregates and reaction conditions. While fibrils have been consistently found to be capable of self-propagation by seeding, for oligomeric aggregates it may not always be the case as some oligomer populations could be incapable of seeding or have very low seeding efficiencies. Oligomer seeding has been shown for tau [65, 66], TDP-43 [67], lysozyme [68], prion protein [69], α-synuclein [70, 71] and is clearly a common phenomenon. Cross-seeding between oligomers of different proteins has been detected as well [66, 67, 72]. Multiple oligomer populations prepared from the Aβ40 peptide in different conditions faithfully propagated their respective conformations resulting in appearance of at least three distinct oligomer 'strains' [73, 74] while another population of oligomers didn't show effective self-propagation [75].

Amyloid fibrils are repetitive, β-sheet rich structures. However, subtle differences in arrangement of β-sheets both on local and global level can result in distinct self-propagating fibril populations ('strains') [76]. Fibrils can propagate by fragmentation followed by incorporation of monomers, and, in some cases, by secondary nucleation where fibrils present a catalytic surface for formation of new aggregates [77, 78]. Since more thermodynamically stable fibrils fragment less efficiently, efficiency of fibril propagation has been found to be inversely proportional to their thermodynamic stability [63, 79, 80]. Propagation of fibrils usually results in formation of 'daughter' fibrils with the same tertiary structure as the 'mother' fibrils. However, conformational changes in the fibrils sometimes occur during propagation [81, 82, 83, 84]. This may happen either by a rare spontaneous structural change in the fibril or due to lack of fidelity during the replication process [76, 81, 85, 86]. These changes are then amplified by the process akin to natural selection. Complexity of protein aggregation pathways allows proteins to access a great variety of conformations in the aggregated state.

α-SYNUCLEIN AGGREGATES *IN VITRO* AND *IN VIVO*

A partially folded conformation required for aggregation is induced in α-synuclein at various conditions, such as low pH [39], high temperature [39], low concentrations of organic solvents [49] or trimethylamine oxide (TMAO) [87] and other conditions. Destabilization of this conformation can prevent α-synuclein aggregation [88]. Partial folding of α-synuclein leads to appearance of sizable clusters of hydrophobic side chains on the protein surface. These patches facilitate intermolecular hydrophobic interactions and promote aggregation. Dimer formation has been proposed as a first step in the aggregation process of α-synuclein [89]. Aggregation can then proceed to a variety of structurally diverse oligomers and fibrils (Figure 3).

Fibrils

Proteolytic digestion [90] and EPR experiments [91] indicated that the region comprising residues 30-100 of α-synuclein represents the amyloid core. Structure of α-synuclein fibrils was determined by the X-ray crystallography of microcrystals of fibrils formed by fragments of α-synuclein [92, 93] and from solid state NMR of the fibrils [94, 95, 96, 97]. These studies revealed that α-synuclein fibrils are composed of several protofilaments containing a cross-β structure in which β-strands are arranged in parallel and the β-sheets are in-register with highly ordered amino acid side chain patterns exposed on the surface of the β-sheets (Figure 4). Amyloid core was found to comprise the residues 38-97 [94, 96].

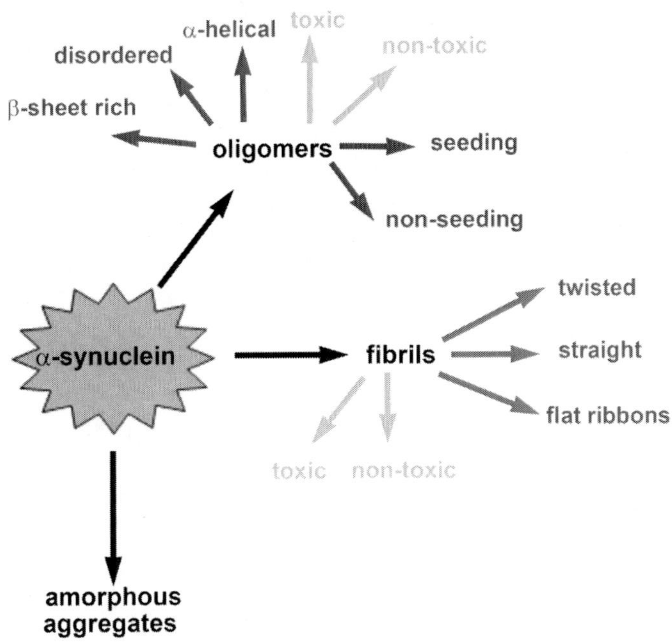

Figure 3. Classification of α-synuclein aggregates.

Subtle changes in buffer conditions such as the pH, temperature, ion concentration, and external variables such as agitation or toxins can drastically influence the folding and aggregation processes of α-synuclein. For example, cryo-electron microscopy and solid state NMR revealed that the morphology of both recombinant α-synuclein (30-110) fibrils and filaments extracted from PD patient brains can be classified as either 1) straight or 2) twisted ribbons [94, 97]. At the molecular level, both types of fibrils share a common parallel, in-register β-sheet core that consists of a five-layered β-sandwich [97, 98]. However, these two types of fibrils differ significantly in the arrangements of protofilaments. Solid state and quenched H/D exchange NMR further proposes that the straight fibrils have protofilaments (β4 and β5) aligned unidirectionally with each other to form a fibril, whereas in the twisted fibril type, two protofilaments twist around each other, giving rise to a sub-protofilament that can twist again with another sub-protofilament to form a fibril.

Other cases of structural polymorphism within α-synuclein fibrils have been described as well. In one case two fibril strains differed in morphology (fibrils *vs.* ribbons) and the size and location of the amyloid core [99]. These structural differences translated into significant differences in cytotoxicity. Addition of amyloid fibrils prepared from recombinant α-synuclein induced the PD-like pathology in wild-type mice indicating the ability of α-synuclein fibrils to propagate *in vivo* [100]. Cross-seeding between fibrils of α-synuclein and other amyloidogenic proteins and peptides (amyloid β, tau) has been observed both *in vitro* and *in vivo* [101, 102, 103, 104, 105].

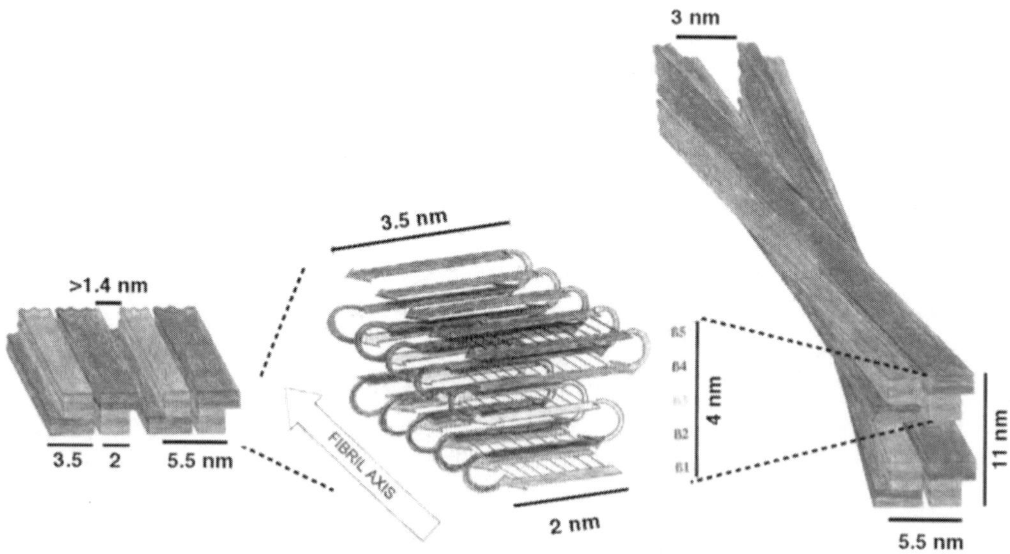

Figure 4. Proposed structure of α-synuclein fibrils (from [97]). Copyright (2008) National Academy of Sciences, U.S.A.

Oligomers

Early on it has been shown that α-synuclein oligomers can be generated by seeding with Aβ 25-35 [106] or oxidation with Cu^{2+} [107, 108]. Further studies have shown that a variety of chemical modifications (tyrosine nitration [109], methionine oxidation [110, 111], etc.) and small molecules (nicotine [112], rifampicin [113], baicalein [114], dopamine and its metabolites [115, 116, 117, 118] and others [119]) inhibited fibrillation of α-synuclein and thus resulted in formation of stable oligomer populations. Small molecules stopped aggregation of α-synuclein at the oligomeric stage either via chemical modification (usually at lysine residues [120, 121]) or via non-covalent binding to oligomers [118, 122]. In addition, oligomers can be generated by incubation of α-synuclein *in vitro* and have been isolated from *in vivo* sources [123].

Structural characterization of amyloid oligomers is complicated by their instability and conformational diversity and heterogeneity. Despite that, significant efforts to determine the structure of α-synuclein oligomers have been made and three broad classes of α-synuclein oligomers have been detected (Figure 3):

1. β-Sheet rich oligomers. These oligomers are usually prepared by incubation of α-synuclein in a variety of conditions in the absence of additives or chemical modifications.
2. Primarily disordered oligomers. Formation of these oligomers is induced by either small molecules (EGCG, dopamine derivatives, etc.) [124, 125, 126] or chemical modification of α-synuclein (e.g., methionine oxidation) [110, 127]. Oligomers of this type may also be present at the early stages of aggregation of α-synuclein [128, 129].
3. α-Helical oligomers. These oligomers are usually formed in the presence of lipid membranes or micelles.

Structural features of the β-sheet rich oligomers (degree of disorder, surface exposure of hydrophobic residues, extent of the β-structure, mechanical properties) were shown to be intermediate between monomers and fibrils [130, 131, 132, 133]. H/D exchange [134, 135] and fluorescence [136] measurements have shown that amyloid core (residues 40-90) in oligomers is consistently protected from the solvent and in some oligomer preparation this protection extents on all N-terminal half of the protein (residues 1-90). Investigation of a specific population of oligomers of this type has shown that they contain ~30 monomers, are ellipsoidal in shape (5x5x9 nm) and contain significant amount of β-structure [137, 138, 139, 140, 141]. Stable oligomers containing 13-15 monomers were also detected [142] along with smaller, metastable aggregates [143]. Arrangement of β-sheets in some of these oligomers was shown to be antiparallel [136, 144] but it's not clear if this is applicable to all oligomers from this structural class. Oligomers of this type tend to be cytotoxic [137, 145, 146] although the degree of their cytotoxicity varies [147]. Their toxicity is believed to derive from their ability to disrupt cellular membranes.

Polyphenols such as EGCG [124, 125, 126] and thioflavins [148] in addition to dopamine and the products of its oxidation [149, 150] were shown to induce formation of highly disordered α-synuclein oligomers. Similar oligomers were formed after oxidation of methionine residues in α-synuclein [110, 151]. In fact, it appears likely that dopamine induces formation of disordered α-synuclein oligomers primarily by triggering methionine oxidation [150, 152, 153]. In addition, quinone metabolites of dopamine can react with the lysine residues of α-synuclein [116, 154] further influencing the oligomer structure. While oligomers formed in the presence of EGCG were non-toxic [124, 125, 126], dopamine-induced oligomers appear to be cytotoxic [154, 155].

α-Helical oligomers of α-synuclein were observed upon incubation of this protein with lipid membranes [156] and isolated from *in vivo* sources [123, 157]. α-Helical trimers and tetramers of α-synuclein are believed to be present *in vivo* at low levels [123]. Formation of these oligomers exclusively in the presence of lipid membranes is likely due to induction of α-helical structure in α-synuclein by lipid membranes and fluorinated alcohols [49, 158, 159].

Self and cross-seeding has been observed for several populations of by α-synuclein oligomers. For example, three distinct types of oligomers were shown to seed their propagation in cultured human neuroblastoma (SH-SY5Y) cells [160] as well as in primary neuronal cell lines [70]. Primarily disordered α-synuclein oligomers produced in the presence of dopamine were able to propagate by seeding and seed formation of Aβ oligomers [161]. Aβ oligomers were also shown to seed aggregation of α-synuclein both *in vitro* and *in vivo* [72, 162, 163]. Newly formed α-synuclein oligomers were similar in structure to the Aβ oligomer seeds as indicated by their reactivity with conformational antibodies.

Role of Macromolecular Crowding in α-Synuclein Aggregation

Cellular environment is crowded with macromolecules, such as proteins, nucleic acids, and carbohydrates, which occupy up to 30% of the available volume. Macromolecular crowding increases the effective protein concentration, decreases the protein diffusion rate, promotes partial folding of IDPs and facilitates protein-protein interaction including protein aggregation [164, 165]. Macromolecular crowding has been believed to be one of the most important factors determining the structure and function of proteins in the cells. Thus, we have recently examined the effect of two model crowding agents (dextran and hydroxypropyl cellulose) on the secondary structure and aggregation of α-synuclein [166].

We found that at neutral pH the secondary structure of α-synuclein was not significantly affected by the presence of crowding agents [166, 167, 168]. Effect of crowding agents on α-synuclein secondary structure at pH 3.5 was more pronounced. In the presence of dextran we observed partial protein folding while in the presence of hydroxypropyl cellulose (HPC) the protein was further unfolded. Dextran significantly accelerated aggregation of α-synuclein at both pH values [166, 167, 168] while HPC inhibited aggregation [166]. α-Synuclein fibrils formed in the presence of either polysaccharide were also significantly less stable [166]. These results (Figure 5) indicate that secondary structure, aggregation kinetics and aggregate structures of α-synuclein are altered by macromolecular crowding, and the changes are strongly dependent on the nature of the crowding agent.

Conclusion

α-Synuclein forms a variety of aggregates. Specific aggregate populations (aka strains) often have distinct physical and biological properties, and many of them can be propagated by seeding. In this chapter we have attempted to describe the complexity of aggregation pathway of α-synuclein and proposed a classification of its aggregates depending on their structure.

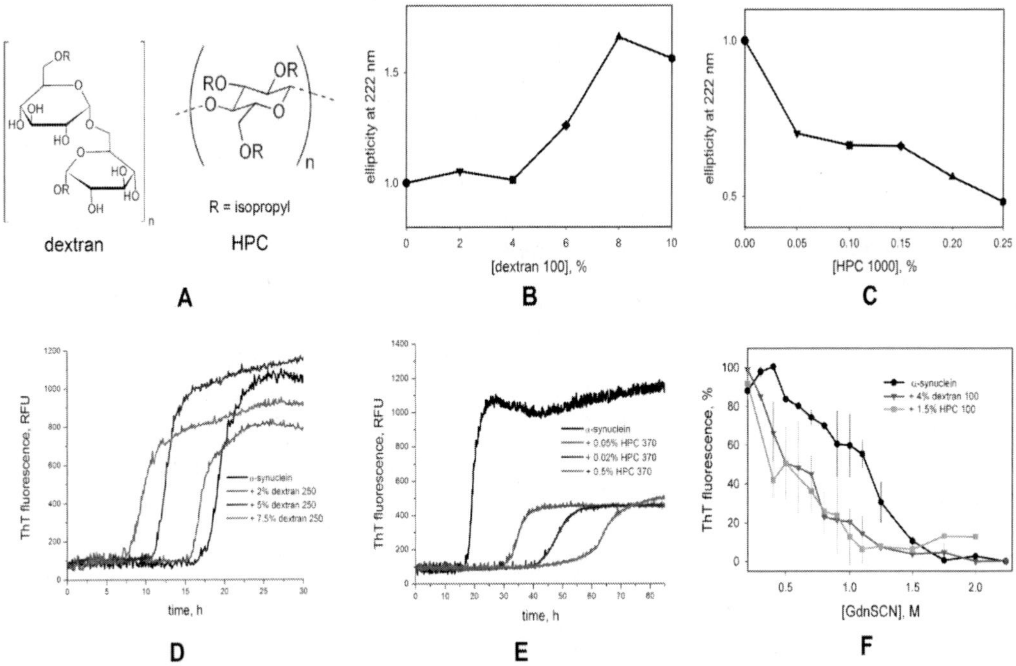

Figure 5. Effects of macromolecular crowding on α-synuclein structure and aggregation. (A) structures of polysaccharides; (B)-(C) – effects of polymers on the secondary structure of α-synuclein at pH 3.5; (D) – (E) - fibril formation from α-synuclein in the presence of dextran and HPC; (F) - denaturation of α-synuclein fibrils in the presence of guanidinium thiocyanate. Adapted from [166]

REFERENCES

[1] Maroteaux L, Campanelli JT, Scheller RH (1988) Synuclein: a neuron-specific protein localized to the nucleus and presynaptic nerve terminal. *J Neurosci* 8: 2804-2815.

[2] Iwai A, Masliah E, Yoshimoto M, Ge N, Flanagan L, et al. (1995) The precursor protein of non-A beta component of Alzheimer's disease amyloid is a presynaptic protein of the central nervous system. *Neuron* 14: 467-475.

[3] Dev KK, Hofele K, Barbieri S, Buchman VL, van der Putten H (2003) Part II: alpha-synuclein and its molecular pathophysiological role in neurodegenerative disease. *Neuropharmacology* 45: 14-44.

[4] da Costa CA, Ancolio K, Checler F (2000) Wild-type but not Parkinson's disease-related ala-53 --> Thr mutant alpha -synuclein protects neuronal cells from apoptotic stimuli. *J Biol Chem* 275: 24065-24069.

[5] Greten-Harrison B, Polydoro M, Morimoto-Tomita M, Diao L, Williams AM, et al. (2010) alphabetagamma-Synuclein triple knockout mice reveal age-dependent neuronal dysfunction. *Proc Natl Acad Sci U S A* 107: 19573-19578.

[6] Payton JE, Perrin RJ, Clayton DF, George JM (2001) Protein-protein interactions of alpha-synuclein in brain homogenates and transfected cells. *Brain Res Mol Brain Res* 95: 138-145.

[7] Jin J, Li GJ, Davis J, Zhu D, Wang Y, et al. (2006) Identification of novel proteins interacting with both a-synuclein and DJ-1. Mol Cell Proteomics.

[8] Betarbet R, Sherer TB, MacKenzie G, Garcia-Osuna M, Panov AV, et al. (2000) Chronic systemic pesticide exposure reproduces features of Parkinson's disease. *Nat Neurosci* 3: 1301-1306.

[9] Szklarczyk D, Franceschini A, Kuhn M, Simonovic M, Roth A, et al. (2011) The STRING database in 2011: functional interaction networks of proteins, globally integrated and scored. *Nucleic Acids Res* 39: D561-568.

[10] Romero P, Obradovic Z, Li X, Garner EC, Brown CJ, et al. (2001) Sequence complexity of disordered protein. *Proteins* 42: 38-48.

[11] Li X, Romero P, Rani M, Dunker AK, Obradovic Z (1999) Predicting Protein Disorder for N-, C-, and Internal Regions. *Genome Inform Ser Workshop Genome Inform* 10: 30-40.

[12] Obradovic Z, Peng K, Vucetic S, Radivojac P, Dunker AK (2005) Exploiting heterogeneous sequence properties improves prediction of protein disorder. *Proteins* 61 Suppl 7: 176-182.

[13] Yang ZR, Thomson R, McNeil P, Esnouf RM (2005) RONN: the bio-basis function neural network technique applied to the detection of natively disordered regions in proteins. *Bioinformatics* 21: 3369-3376.

[14] Dosztanyi Z, Csizmok V, Tompa P, Simon I (2005) IUPred: web server for the prediction of intrinsically unstructured regions of proteins based on estimated energy content. *Bioinformatics* 21: 3433-3434.

[15] Uversky VN (2008) Alpha-synuclein misfolding and neurodegenerative diseases. *Curr Protein Pept Sci* 9: 507-540.

[16] Oates ME, Romero P, Ishida T, Ghalwash M, Mizianty MJ, et al. (2013) D(2)P(2): database of disordered protein predictions. *Nucleic Acids Res* 41: D508-516.

[17] Peng K, Radivojac P, Vucetic S, Dunker AK, Obradovic Z (2006) Length-dependent prediction of protein intrinsic disorder. *Bmc Bioinformatics* 7.

[18] Ishida T, Kinoshita K (2007) PrDOS: prediction of disordered protein regions from amino acid sequence. *Nucleic Acids Res* 35: W460-464.

[19] Walsh I, Martin AJ, Di Domenico T, Tosatto SC (2012) ESpritz: accurate and fast prediction of protein disorder. *Bioinformatics* 28: 503-509.

[20] Iakoucheva LM, Radivojac P, Brown CJ, O'Connor TR, Sikes JG, et al. (2004) The importance of intrinsic disorder for protein phosphorylation. *Nucleic Acids Res* 32: 1037-1049.

[21] Pejaver V, Hsu WL, Xin F, Dunker AK, Uversky VN, et al. (2014) The structural and functional signatures of proteins that undergo multiple events of post-translational modification. *Protein Sci* 23: 1077-1093.

[22] Han JD, Bertin N, Hao T, Goldberg DS, Berriz GF, et al. (2004) Evidence for dynamically organized modularity in the yeast protein-protein interaction network. *Nature* 430: 88-93.

[23] Hartwell LH, Hopfield JJ, Leibler S, Murray AW (1999) From molecular to modular cell biology. *Nature* 402: C47-52.

[24] Uversky VN, Oldfield CJ, Dunker AK (2005) Showing your ID: intrinsic disorder as an ID for recognition, regulation and cell signaling. *J Mol Recognit* 18: 343-384.

[25] Patil A, Nakamura H (2006) Disordered domains and high surface charge confer hubs with the ability to interact with multiple proteins in interaction networks. *FEBS Lett* 580: 2041-2045.

[26] Haynes C, Oldfield CJ, Ji F, Klitgord N, Cusick ME, et al. (2006) Intrinsic disorder is a common feature of hub proteins from four eukaryotic interactomes. *PLoS Comput Biol* 2: e100.

[27] Ekman D, Light S, Bjorklund AK, Elofsson A (2006) What properties characterize the hub proteins of the protein-protein interaction network of Saccharomyces cerevisiae? *Genome Biol* 7: R45.

[28] Dosztanyi Z, Chen J, Dunker AK, Simon I, Tompa P (2006) Disorder and sequence repeats in hub proteins and their implications for network evolution. *J Proteome Res* 5: 2985-2995.

[29] Singh GP, Ganapathi M, Sandhu KS, Dash D (2006) Intrinsic unstructuredness and abundance of PEST motifs in eukaryotic proteomes. *Proteins* 62: 309-315.

[30] Dunker AK, Garner E, Guilliot S, Romero P, Albrecht K, et al. (1998) Protein disorder and the evolution of molecular recognition: theory, predictions and observations. *Pac Symp Biocomput:* 473-484.

[31] Polymeropoulos MH, Lavedan C, Leroy E, Ide SE, Dehejia A, et al. (1997) Mutation in the alpha-synuclein gene identified in families with Parkinson's disease. *Science* 276: 2045-2047.

[32] Spillantini MG, Schmidt ML, Lee VM, Trojanowski JQ, Jakes R, et al. (1997) Alpha-synuclein in Lewy bodies. *Nature* 388: 839-840.

[33] Goedert M (2001) Alpha-synuclein and neurodegenerative diseases. *Nat Rev Neurosci* 2: 492-501.

[34] Fink AL (2006) The aggregation and fibrillation of alpha-synuclein. *Acc Chem Res* 39: 628-634.

[35] Baba M, Nakajo S, Tu PH, Tomita T, Nakaya K, et al. (1998) Aggregation of alpha-synuclein in Lewy bodies of sporadic Parkinson's disease and dementia with Lewy bodies. *Am J Pathol* 152: 879-884.

[36] Breydo L, Wu JW, Uversky VN (2012) Alpha-synuclein misfolding and Parkinson's disease. *Biochim Biophys Acta* 1822: 261-285.

[37] Conway KA, Harper JD, Lansbury PT (1998) Accelerated in vitro fibril formation by a mutant alpha-synuclein linked to early-onset Parkinson disease. *Nat Med* 4: 1318-1320.

[38] El-Agnaf OM, Jakes R, Curran MD, Middleton D, Ingenito R, et al. (1998) Aggregates from mutant and wild-type alpha-synuclein proteins and NAC peptide induce apoptotic cell death in human neuroblastoma cells by formation of beta-sheet and amyloid-like filaments. *FEBS Lett* 440: 71-75.

[39] Uversky VN, Li J, Fink AL (2001) Evidence for a partially folded intermediate in alpha-synuclein fibril formation. *J Biol Chem* 276: 10737-10744.

[40] Cho MK, Kim HY, Bernado P, Fernandez CO, Blackledge M, et al. (2007) Amino acid bulkiness defines the local conformations and dynamics of natively unfolded alpha-synuclein and tau. *J Am Chem Soc* 129: 3032-3033.

[41] Allison JR, Varnai P, Dobson CM, Vendruscolo M (2009) Determination of the free energy landscape of alpha-synuclein using spin label nuclear magnetic resonance measurements. *J Am Chem Soc* 131: 18314-18326.

[42] Salmon L, Nodet G, Ozenne V, Yin G, Jensen MR, et al. (2010) NMR characterization of long-range order in intrinsically disordered proteins. *J Am Chem Soc* 132: 8407-8418.

[43] Bertoncini CW, Jung YS, Fernandez CO, Hoyer W, Griesinger C, et al. (2005) Release of long-range tertiary interactions potentiates aggregation of natively unstructured alpha-synuclein. *Proc Natl Acad Sci U S A* 102: 1430-1435.

[44] Rao JN, Jao CC, Hegde BG, Langen R, Ulmer TS (2010) A combinatorial NMR and EPR approach for evaluating the structural ensemble of partially folded proteins. *J Am Chem Soc* 132: 8657-8668.

[45] Dedmon MM, Lindorff-Larsen K, Christodoulou J, Vendruscolo M, Dobson CM (2005) Mapping long-range interactions in alpha-synuclein using spin-label NMR and ensemble molecular dynamics simulations. *J Am Chem Soc* 127: 476-477.

[46] Sung YH, Eliezer D (2007) Residual structure, backbone dynamics, and interactions within the synuclein family. *J Mol Biol* 372: 689-707.

[47] Uversky VN (2003) A protein-chameleon: conformational plasticity of alpha-synuclein, a disordered protein involved in neurodegenerative disorders. *J Biomol Struct Dyn* 21: 211-234.

[48] Uversky VN, Fink AL (2002) Biophysical properties of human alpha-synuclein and its role in Parkinson's disease. In: Pandalai SG, editor. Recent Research Developments in Proteins. Kerala, India: Transworld *Research Network.* pp. 153-186.

[49] Munishkina LA, Phelan C, Uversky VN, Fink AL (2003) Conformational behavior and aggregation of alpha-synuclein in organic solvents: modeling the effects of membranes. *Biochemistry* 42: 2720-2730.

[50] Kim HY, Heise H, Fernandez CO, Baldus M, Zweckstetter M (2007) Correlation of amyloid fibril beta-structure with the unfolded state of alpha-synuclein. *Chembiochem* 8: 1671-1674.

[51] Wu KP, Kim S, Fela DA, Baum J (2008) Characterization of conformational and dynamic properties of natively unfolded human and mouse alpha-synuclein ensembles by NMR: implication for aggregation. *J Mol Biol* 378: 1104-1115.

[52] Zhao M, Cascio D, Sawaya MR, Eisenberg D (2011) Structures of segments of α-synuclein fused to maltose-binding protein suggest intermediate states during amyloid formation. Protein Science: n/a-n/a.

[53] Wilson D, Pethica R, Zhou Y, Talbot C, Vogel C, et al. (2009) SUPERFAMILY--sophisticated comparative genomics, data mining, visualization and phylogeny. *Nucleic Acids Res* 37: D380-386.

[54] Bateman A, Coin L, Durbin R, Finn RD, Hollich V, et al. (2004) The Pfam protein families database. *Nucleic Acids Res* 32: D138-141.

[55] Finn RD, Mistry J, Schuster-Bockler B, Griffiths-Jones S, Hollich V, et al. (2006) Pfam: clans, web tools and services. *Nucleic Acids Res* 34: D247-251.

[56] Finn RD, Tate J, Mistry J, Coggill PC, Sammut SJ, et al. (2008) The Pfam protein families database. *Nucleic Acids Res* 36: D281-288.

[57] Uversky VN (2008) Amyloidogenesis of natively unfolded proteins. *Curr Alzheimer Res* 5: 260-287.

[58] Chen S, Ferrone FA, Wetzel R (2002) Huntington's disease age-of-onset linked to polyglutamine aggregation nucleation. *Proc Natl Acad Sci* U S A 99: 11884-11889.

[59] Ferrone FA (2015) Assembly of Abeta proceeds via monomeric nuclei. *J Mol Biol* 427: 287-290.
[60] Vitalis A, Caflisch A (2010) Micelle-like architecture of the monomer ensemble of Alzheimer's amyloid-beta peptide in aqueous solution and its implications for Abeta aggregation. *J Mol Biol* 403: 148-165.
[61] Vitalis A, Lyle N, Pappu RV (2009) Thermodynamics of beta-sheet formation in polyglutamine. *Biophys J* 97: 303-311.
[62] Ramachandran G, Milan-Garces EA, Udgaonkar JB, Puranik M (2014) Resonance Raman spectroscopic measurements delineate the structural changes that occur during tau fibril formation. *Biochemistry* 53: 6550-6565.
[63] Krishnan R, Lindquist SL (2005) Structural insights into a yeast prion illuminate nucleation and strain diversity. *Nature* 435: 765-772.
[64] Lee CC, Walters RH, Murphy RM (2007) Reconsidering the mechanism of polyglutamine peptide aggregation. *Biochemistry* 46: 12810-12820.
[65] Wu JW, Herman M, Liu L, Simoes S, Acker CM, et al. (2013) Small misfolded Tau species are internalized via bulk endocytosis and anterogradely and retrogradely transported in neurons. *J Biol Chem* 288: 1856-1870.
[66] Lasagna-Reeves CA, Castillo-Carranza DL, Sengupta U, Guerrero-Munoz MJ, Kiritoshi T, et al. (2012) Alzheimer brain-derived tau oligomers propagate pathology from endogenous tau. *Sci Rep* 2: 700.
[67] Fang YS, Tsai KJ, Chang YJ, Kao P, Woods R, et al. (2014) Full-length TDP-43 forms toxic amyloid oligomers that are present in frontotemporal lobar dementia-TDP patients. *Nat Commun* 5: 4824.
[68] Mulaj M, Foley J, Muschol M (2014) Amyloid oligomers and protofibrils, but not filaments, self-replicate from native lysozyme. *J Am Chem Soc* 136: 8947-8956.
[69] Hesketh S, Thompsett AR, Brown DR (2012) Prion protein polymerisation triggered by manganese-generated prion protein seeds. *J Neurochem* 120: 177-189.
[70] Danzer KM, Krebs SK, Wolff M, Birk G, Hengerer B (2009) Seeding induced by alpha-synuclein oligomers provides evidence for spreading of alpha-synuclein pathology. *J Neurochem* 111: 192-203.
[71] Danzer KM, Haasen D, Karow AR, Moussaud S, Habeck M, et al. (2007) Different species of alpha-synuclein oligomers induce calcium influx and seeding. *J Neurosci* 27: 9220-9232.
[72] Guerrero-Munoz MJ, Castillo-Carranza DL, Krishnamurthy S, Paulucci-Holthauzen AA, Sengupta U, et al. (2014) Amyloid-beta oligomers as a template for secondary amyloidosis in Alzheimer's disease. *Neurobiol Dis* 71: 14-23.
[73] Kayed R, Canto I, Breydo L, Rasool S, Lukacsovich T, et al. (2010) Conformation dependent monoclonal antibodies distinguish different replicating strains or conformers of prefibrillar Abeta oligomers. *Mol Neurodegener* 5: 57.
[74] Wu JW, Breydo L, Isas JM, Lee J, Kuznetsov YG, et al. (2010) Fibrillar Oligomers Nucleate the Oligomerization of Monomeric Amyloid {beta} but Do Not Seed Fibril Formation. *J Biol Chem* 285: 6071-6079.
[75] Lasagna-Reeves CA, Glabe CG, Kayed R (2011) Amyloid-beta annular protofibrils evade fibrillar fate in Alzheimer disease brain. *J Biol Chem* 286: 22122-22130.
[76] Breydo L (2013) Strain phenomenon in protein aggregation: interplay between sequence and conformation. *Intrinsically Disordered Proteins* 1: 39.

[77] Cohen SI, Linse S, Luheshi LM, Hellstrand E, White DA, et al. (2013) Proliferation of amyloid-beta42 aggregates occurs through a secondary nucleation mechanism. *Proc Natl Acad Sci U S A* 110: 9758-9763.

[78] Arosio P, Knowles TP, Linse S (2015) On the lag phase in amyloid fibril formation. *Phys Chem Chem Phys.*

[79] Colby DW, Giles K, Legname G, Wille H, Baskakov IV, et al. (2009) Design and construction of diverse mammalian prion strains. *Proc Natl Acad Sci U S A* 106: 20417-20422.

[80] Gonzalez-Montalban N, Makarava N, Savtchenko R, Baskakov IV (2011) Relationship between conformational stability and amplification efficiency of prions. *Biochemistry* 50: 7933-7940.

[81] Ghaemmaghami S, Colby DW, Nguyen HO, Hayashi S, Oehler A, et al. (2013) Convergent replication of mouse synthetic prion strains. *Am J Pathol* 182: 866-874.

[82] Weissmann C, Li J, Mahal SP, Browning S (2011) Prions on the move. *EMBO Rep* 12: 1109-1117.

[83] Giles K, Glidden DV, Patel S, Korth C, Groth D, et al. (2010) Human prion strain selection in transgenic mice. *Ann Neurol* 68: 151-161.

[84] Kochneva-Pervukhova NV, Chechenova MB, Valouev IA, Kushnirov VV, Smirnov VN, et al. (2001) [Psi(+)] prion generation in yeast: characterization of the 'strain' difference. *Yeast* 18: 489-497.

[85] Makarava N, Kovacs GG, Savtchenko R, Alexeeva I, Budka H, et al. (2011) Genesis of mammalian prions: from non-infectious amyloid fibrils to a transmissible prion disease. *PLoS Pathog* 7: e1002419.

[86] Makarava N, Baskakov IV (2012) Genesis of tramsmissible protein states via deformed templating. *Prion* 6: 252-255.

[87] Uversky VN, Li J, Fink AL (2001) Trimethylamine-N-oxide-induced folding of alpha-synuclein. *FEBS Lett* 509: 31-35.

[88] Acharya S, Safaie BM, Wongkongkathep P, Ivanova MI, Attar A, et al. (2014) Molecular basis for preventing alpha-synuclein aggregation by a molecular tweezer. *J Biol Chem* 289: 10727-10737.

[89] Krishnan S, Chi EY, Wood SJ, Kendrick BS, Li C, et al. (2003) Oxidative dimer formation is the critical rate-limiting step for Parkinson's disease alpha-synuclein fibrillogenesis. *Biochemistry* 42: 829-837.

[90] Miake H, Mizusawa H, Iwatsubo T, Hasegawa M (2002) Biochemical characterization of the core structure of alpha-synuclein filaments. *J Biol Chem* 277: 19213-19219.

[91] Der-Sarkissian A, Jao CC, Chen J, Langen R (2003) Structural organization of alpha-synuclein fibrils studied by site-directed spin labeling. *J Biol Chem* 278: 37530-37535.

[92] Sawaya MR, Sambashivan S, Nelson R, Ivanova MI, Sievers SA, et al. (2007) Atomic structures of amyloid cross-beta spines reveal varied steric zippers. *Nature* 447: 453-457.

[93] Nelson R, Sawaya MR, Balbirnie M, Madsen AO, Riekel C, et al. (2005) Structure of the cross-beta spine of amyloid-like fibrils. *Nature* 435: 773-778.

[94] Heise H, Hoyer W, Becker S, Andronesi OC, Riedel D, et al. (2005) Molecular-level secondary structure, polymorphism, and dynamics of full-length alpha-synuclein fibrils studied by solid-state NMR. *Proc Natl Acad Sci U S A* 102: 15871-15876.

[95] Lv G, Kumar A, Giller K, Orcellet ML, Riedel D, et al. (2012) Structural comparison of mouse and human alpha-synuclein amyloid fibrils by solid-state NMR. *J Mol Biol* 420: 99-111.

[96] Comellas G, Lemkau LR, Nieuwkoop AJ, Kloepper KD, Ladror DT, et al. (2011) Structured regions of alpha-synuclein fibrils include the early-onset Parkinson's disease mutation sites. *J Mol Biol* 411: 881-895.

[97] Vilar M, Chou HT, Luhrs T, Maji SK, Riek-Loher D, et al. (2008) The fold of alpha-synuclein fibrils. *Proc Natl Acad Sci U S A* 105: 8637-8642.

[98] Orcellet ML, Fernandez CO (2011) Structures Behind the Amyloid Aggregation of alpha-Synuclein: An NMR Based Approach. *Curr Protein Pept Sci* 12: 188-204.

[99] Bousset L, Pieri L, Ruiz-Arlandis G, Gath J, Jensen PH, et al. (2013) Structural and functional characterization of two alpha-synuclein strains. *Nat Commun* 4: 2575.

[100] Masuda-Suzukake M, Nonaka T, Hosokawa M, Oikawa T, Arai T, et al. (2013) Prion-like spreading of pathological alpha-synuclein in brain. *Brain* 136: 1128-1138.

[101] Guo JL, Covell DJ, Daniels JP, Iba M, Stieber A, et al. (2013) Distinct alpha-synuclein strains differentially promote tau inclusions in neurons. *Cell* 154: 103-117.

[102] Waxman EA, Giasson BI (2011) Induction of intracellular tau aggregation is promoted by alpha-synuclein seeds and provides novel insights into the hyperphosphorylation of tau. *J Neurosci* 31: 7604-7618.

[103] Sarell CJ, Stockley PG, Radford SE (2013) Assessing the causes and consequences of co-polymerization in amyloid formation. *Prion* 7.

[104] Ono K, Takahashi R, Ikeda T, Yamada M (2012) Cross-seeding effects of amyloid beta-protein and alpha-synuclein. *J Neurochem* 122: 883-890.

[105] Giasson BI, Forman MS, Higuchi M, Golbe LI, Graves CL, et al. (2003) Initiation and synergistic fibrillization of tau and alpha-synuclein. *Science* 300: 636-640.

[106] Paik SR, Lee JH, Kim DH, Chang CS, Kim YS (1998) Self-oligomerization of NACP, the precursor protein of the non-amyloid beta/A4 protein (A beta) component of Alzheimer's disease amyloid, observed in the presence of a C-terminal A beta fragment (residues 25-35). *Febs Letters* 421: 73-76.

[107] Paik SR, Shin HJ, Lee JH, Chang CS, Kim J (1999) Copper(II)-induced self-oligomerization of alpha-synuclein. *Biochem J* 340 (Pt 3): 821-828.

[108] Paik SR, Shin HJ, Lee JH (2000) Metal-catalyzed oxidation of alpha-synuclein in the presence of Copper(II) and hydrogen peroxide. *Arch Biochem Biophys* 378: 269-277.

[109] Yamin G, Uversky VN, Fink AL (2003) Nitration inhibits fibrillation of human alpha-synuclein in vitro by formation of soluble oligomers. FEBS Lett 542: 147-152.

[110] Uversky VN, Yamin G, Souillac PO, Goers J, Glaser CB, et al. (2002) Methionine oxidation inhibits fibrillation of human alpha-synuclein in vitro. *FEBS Lett* 517: 239-244.

[111] Carmo-Goncalves P, Pinheiro AS, Romao L, Cortines J, Follmer C (2014) UV-induced selective oxidation of Met5 to Met-sulfoxide leads to the formation of neurotoxic fibril-incompetent alpha-synuclein oligomers. *Amyloid* 21: 163-174.

[112] Hong DP, Fink AL, Uversky VN (2009) Smoking and Parkinson's disease: Does nicotine affect alpha-synuclein fibrillation? *Biochim Biophys Acta* 1794: 282-290.

[113] Li J, Zhu M, Rajamani S, Uversky VN, Fink AL (2004) Rifampicin inhibits alpha-synuclein fibrillation and disaggregates fibrils. *Chem Biol* 11: 1513-1521.

[114] Zhu M, Rajamani S, Kaylor J, Han S, Zhou F, et al. (2004) The flavonoid baicalein inhibits fibrillation of alpha-synuclein and disaggregates existing fibrils. *J Biol Chem* 279: 26846-26857.

[115] Li J, Zhu M, Manning-Bog AB, Di Monte DA, Fink AL (2004) Dopamine and L-dopa disaggregate amyloid fibrils: implications for Parkinson's and Alzheimer's disease. *Faseb J* 18: 962-964.

[116] Conway KA, Rochet JC, Bieganski RM, Lansbury PT, Jr. (2001) Kinetic stabilization of the alpha-synuclein protofibril by a dopamine-alpha-synuclein adduct. *Science* 294: 1346-1349.

[117] Cappai R, Leck SL, Tew DJ, Williamson NA, Smith DP, et al. (2005) Dopamine promotes alpha-synuclein aggregation into SDS-resistant soluble oligomers via a distinct folding pathway. *Faseb J* 19: 1377-1379.

[118] Norris EH, Giasson BI, Hodara R, Xu S, Trojanowski JQ, et al. (2005) Reversible inhibition of alpha-synuclein fibrillization by dopaminochrome-mediated conformational alterations. *J Biol Chem* 280: 21212-21219.

[119] Masuda M, Suzuki N, Taniguchi S, Oikawa T, Nonaka T, et al. (2006) Small molecule inhibitors of alpha-synuclein filament assembly. *Biochemistry* 45: 6085-6094.

[120] Li HT, Lin DH, Luo XY, Zhang F, Ji LN, et al. (2005) Inhibition of alpha-synuclein fibrillization by dopamine analogs via reaction with the amino groups of alpha-synuclein. Implication for dopaminergic neurodegeneration. *FEBS J* 272: 3661-3672.

[121] De Franceschi G, Frare E, Pivato M, Relini A, Penco A, et al. (2011) Structural and morphological characterization of aggregated species of {alpha}-synuclein induced by docosahexaenoic acid. *J Biol Chem*.

[122] Rao JN, Dua V, Ulmer TS (2008) Characterization of alpha-synuclein interactions with selected aggregation-inhibiting small molecules. *Biochemistry* 47: 4651-4656.

[123] Luth ES, Bartels T, Dettmer U, Kim NC, Selkoe DJ (2015) Purification of alpha-synuclein from human brain reveals an instability of endogenous multimers as the protein approaches purity. *Biochemistry* 54: 279-292.

[124] Ehrnhoefer DE, Bieschke J, Boeddrich A, Herbst M, Masino L, et al. (2008) EGCG redirects amyloidogenic polypeptides into unstructured, off-pathway oligomers. *Nat Struct Mol Biol* 15: 558-566.

[125] Bieschke J, Russ J, Friedrich RP, Ehrnhoefer DE, Wobst H, et al. (2010) EGCG remodels mature alpha-synuclein and amyloid-beta fibrils and reduces cellular toxicity. *Proc Natl Acad Sci U S A* 107: 7710-7715.

[126] Lorenzen N, Nielsen SB, Yoshimura Y, Vad BS, Andersen CB, et al. (2014) How epigallocatechin gallate can inhibit alpha-synuclein oligomer toxicity in vitro. *J Biol Chem* 289: 21299-21310.

[127] Glaser CB, Yamin G, Uversky VN, Fink AL (2005) Methionine oxidation, alpha-synuclein and Parkinson's disease. *Biochim Biophys Acta* 1703: 157-169.

[128] Apetri MM, Maiti NC, Zagorski MG, Carey PR, Anderson VE (2006) Secondary structure of alpha-synuclein oligomers: characterization by raman and atomic force microscopy. *J Mol Biol* 355: 63-71.

[129] Nath S, Meuvis J, Hendrix J, Carl SA, Engelborghs Y (2010) Early aggregation steps in alpha-synuclein as measured by FCS and FRET: evidence for a contagious conformational change. *Biophys J* 98: 1302-1311.

[130] Kim HY, Cho MK, Kumar A, Maier E, Siebenhaar C, et al. (2009) Structural properties of pore-forming oligomers of alpha-synuclein. *J Am Chem Soc* 131: 17482-17489.

[131] van Rooijen BD, van Leijenhorst-Groener KA, Claessens MM, Subramaniam V (2009) Tryptophan fluorescence reveals structural features of alpha-synuclein oligomers. *J Mol Biol* 394: 826-833.

[132] Kaylor J, Bodner N, Edridge S, Yamin G, Hong DP, et al. (2005) Characterization of oligomeric intermediates in alpha-synuclein fibrillation: FRET studies of Y125W/Y133F/Y136F alpha-synuclein. *J Mol Biol* 353: 357-372.

[133] Ruggeri FS, Adamcik J, Jeong JS, Lashuel HA, Mezzenga R, et al. (2015) Influence of the beta-Sheet Content on the Mechanical Properties of Aggregates during Amyloid Fibrillization. *Angew Chem Int Ed Engl* 54: 2462-2466.

[134] Paslawski W, Mysling S, Thomsen K, Jorgensen TJ, Otzen DE (2014) Co-existence of two different alpha-synuclein oligomers with different core structures determined by hydrogen/deuterium exchange mass spectrometry. *Angew Chem Int Ed Engl* 53: 7560-7563.

[135] Mysling S, Betzer C, Jensen PH, Jorgensen TJ (2013) Characterizing the dynamics of alpha-synuclein oligomers using hydrogen/deuterium exchange monitored by mass spectrometry. *Biochemistry* 52: 9097-9103.

[136] Gallea JI, Celej MS (2014) Structural insights into amyloid oligomers of the Parkinson disease-related protein alpha-synuclein. *J Biol Chem* 289: 26733-26742.

[137] Giehm L, Svergun DI, Otzen DE, Vestergaard B (2011) Low-resolution structure of a vesicle disrupting α-synuclein oligomer that accumulates during fibrillation. *Proc Natl Acad Sci U S A* 108: 3246-3251.

[138] Lorenzen N, Otzen DE (2014) Oligomers of alpha-synuclein: picking the culprit in the line-up. *Essays Biochem* 56: 137-148.

[139] Paslawski W, Andreasen M, Nielsen SB, Lorenzen N, Thomsen K, et al. (2014) High stability and cooperative unfolding of alpha-synuclein oligomers. *Biochemistry* 53: 6252-6263.

[140] Zijlstra N, Blum C, Segers-Nolten IM, Claessens MM, Subramaniam V (2012) Molecular composition of sub-stoichiometrically labeled alpha-synuclein oligomers determined by single-molecule photobleaching. *Angew Chem Int Ed Engl* 51: 8821-8824.

[141] Stockl MT, Zijlstra N, Subramaniam V (2013) alpha-Synuclein oligomers: an amyloid pore? Insights into mechanisms of alpha-synuclein oligomer-lipid interactions. *Mol Neurobiol* 47: 613-621.

[142] Zijlstra N, Claessens MM, Blum C, Subramaniam V (2014) Elucidating the aggregation number of dopamine-induced alpha-synuclein oligomeric assemblies. *Biophys J* 106: 440-446.

[143] Neupane K, Solanki A, Sosova I, Belov M, Woodside MT (2014) Diverse metastable structures formed by small oligomers of alpha-synuclein probed by force spectroscopy. *PLoS One* 9: e86495.

[144] Celej MS, Sarroukh R, Goormaghtigh E, Fidelio GD, Ruysschaert JM, et al. (2012) Toxic prefibrillar alpha-synuclein amyloid oligomers adopt a distinctive antiparallel beta-sheet structure. *Biochem J* 443: 719-726.

[145] Winner B, Jappelli R, Maji SK, Desplats PA, Boyer L, et al. (2011) In vivo demonstration that alpha-synuclein oligomers are toxic. *Proc Natl Acad Sci U S A* 108: 4194-4199.

[146] Hong DP, Han S, Fink AL, Uversky VN (2011) Characterization of the Non-Fibrillar alpha-Synuclein Oligomers. *Protein Pept Lett* 18: 230-240.

[147] Hong DP, Fink AL, Uversky VN (2008) Structural characteristics of alpha-synuclein oligomers stabilized by the flavonoid baicalein. *J Mol Biol* 383: 214-223.

[148] Grelle G, Otto A, Lorenz M, Frank RF, Wanker EE, et al. (2011) Black tea theaflavins inhibit formation of toxic amyloid-beta and alpha-synuclein fibrils. *Biochemistry* 50: 10624-10636.

[149] Lee HJ, Baek SM, Ho DH, Suk JE, Cho ED, et al. (2011) Dopamine promotes formation and secretion of non-fibrillar alpha-synuclein oligomers. *Exp Mol Med* 43: 216-222.

[150] Rekas A, Knott RB, Sokolova A, Barnham KJ, Perez KA, et al. (2010) The structure of dopamine induced alpha-synuclein oligomers. *Eur Biophys J* 39: 1407-1419.

[151] Zhou W, Long C, Reaney SH, Di Monte DA, Fink AL, et al. (2010) Methionine oxidation stabilizes non-toxic oligomers of alpha-synuclein through strengthening the auto-inhibitory intra-molecular long-range interactions. *Biochim Biophys Acta* 1802: 322-330.

[152] Zhou W, Gallagher A, Hong DP, Long C, Fink AL, et al. (2009) At low concentrations, 3,4-dihydroxyphenylacetic acid (DOPAC) binds non-covalently to alpha-synuclein and prevents its fibrillation. *J Mol Biol* 388: 597-610.

[153] Leong SL, Pham CL, Galatis D, Fodero-Tavoletti MT, Perez K, et al. (2009) Formation of dopamine-mediated alpha-synuclein-soluble oligomers requires methionine oxidation. *Free Radic Biol Med* 46: 1328-1337.

[154] Galvin JE (2006) Interaction of alpha-synuclein and dopamine metabolites in the pathogenesis of Parkinson's disease: a case for the selective vulnerability of the substantia nigra. *Acta Neuropathol* 112: 115-126.

[155] Jain MK, Bhat R (2014) Modulation of human alpha-synuclein aggregation by a combined effect of calcium and dopamine. *Neurobiol Dis* 63: 115-128.

[156] Varkey J, Mizuno N, Hegde BG, Cheng N, Steven AC, et al. (2013) alpha-Synuclein oligomers with broken helical conformation form lipoprotein nanoparticles. *J Biol Chem* 288: 17620-17630.

[157] Bartels T, Choi JG, Selkoe DJ (2011) alpha-Synuclein occurs physiologically as a helically folded tetramer that resists aggregation. *Nature* 477: 107-110.

[158] Weinreb PH, Zhen W, Poon AW, Conway KA, Lansbury PT, Jr. (1996) NACP, a protein implicated in Alzheimer's disease and learning, is natively unfolded. *Biochemistry* 35: 13709-13715.

[159] Maiti NC, Apetri MM, Zagorski MG, Carey PR, Anderson VE (2004) Raman spectroscopic characterization of secondary structure in natively unfolded proteins: alpha-synuclein. *J Am Chem Soc* 126: 2399-2408.

[160] Danzer KM, Haasen D, Karow AR, Moussaud S, Habeck M, et al. (2007) Different species of alpha-synuclein oligomers induce calcium influx and seeding. *J Neurosci* 27: 9220-9232.

[161] Planchard MS, Exley SE, Morgan SE, Rangachari V (2014) Dopamine-induced alpha-synuclein oligomers show self- and cross-propagation properties. *Protein Sci* 23: 1369-1379.

[162] Martin ZS, Neugebauer V, Dineley KT, Kayed R, Zhang W, et al. (2012) alpha-Synuclein oligomers oppose long-term potentiation and impair memory through a calcineurin-dependent mechanism: relevance to human synucleopathic diseases. *J Neurochem* 120: 440-452.

[163] Sengupta U, Guerrero-Munoz MJ, Castillo-Carranza DL, Lasagna-Reeves CA, Gerson JE, et al. (2015) Pathological Interface between Oligomeric Alpha-Synuclein and Tau in Synucleinopathies. *Biol Psychiatry.*

[164] Zhou HX, Rivas G, Minton AP (2008) Macromolecular crowding and confinement: biochemical, biophysical, and potential physiological consequences. *Annu Rev Biophys* 37: 375-397.

[165] Ellis RJ, Minton AP (2006) Protein aggregation in crowded environments. *Biol Chem* 387: 485-497.

[166] Breydo L, Reddy KD, Piai A, Felli IC, Pierattelli R, et al. (2014) The crowd you're in with: effects of different types of crowding agents on protein aggregation. *Biochim Biophys Acta* 1844: 346-357.

[167] Munishkina LA, Ahmad A, Fink AL, Uversky VN (2008) Guiding protein aggregation with macromolecular crowding. *Biochemistry* 47: 8993-9006.

[168] Munishkina LA, Cooper EM, Uversky VN, Fink AL (2004) The effect of macromolecular crowding on protein aggregation and amyloid fibril formation. *J Mol Recognit* 17: 456-464.

In: The Prion Phenomena in Neurodegenerative Diseases ISBN: 978-1-63483-399-8
Editors: Giuseppe Legname and Gabriele Giachin

Chapter 6

STRUCTURAL CHARACTERIZATION OF α-SYNUCLEIN AMYLOIDS

***Wolfgang Hoyer*[1], *Hamed Shaykhalishahi*[1], *Santhosh Ayalur-Karunakaran*[2] and *Henrike Heise*[1,2*]**

[1]Heinrich Heine University Düsseldorf, Institute of Physical Biology, Düsseldorf, Germany

[2]Forschungszentrum Jülich, Institute of Complex Systems (ICS), ICS-6: Structural Biochemistry, Jülich, Germany

ABSTRACT

The etiology of Parkinson's disease is closely linked to the appearance of Lewy Bodies in the substantia nigra and other regions of the nervous system. The major constituent of these Lewy bodies is the 140 amino acids containing protein α-synuclein in an aggregated form. While α-synuclein is natively unfolded, it has a strong propensity to attach to lipid bilayers or to form amyloid fibrils. In this chapter, we give an overview over different techniques used for structural studies on α-synuclein in free, lipid-bound and fibrillated form, such as NMR, EPR and FRET in solution and in the solid state. The conformational ensemble of the intrinsically unstructured protein in solution strongly depends on the environment, and even the natively unfolded monomeric state is under debate. Likewise, interaction with lipid bilayers results in an equilibrium between different binding modes. Fibrillation kinetics, morphological appearance of fibrils as well as details of the molecular conformation strongly depends on salt concentration, protein concentration as well as minor details in the aggregation pathway. As a consequence, structural investigations have revealed not only one isomorphic fibril conformation, but to date at least five different isomorphs have been reported in the literature. While the core region seems to vary between the different isomorphs, all conformations are consistent with a parallel in register arrangement of the β-sheets. Furthermore, the hydrophobic central part comprising residues 38-95 appears to be part of the core regions in all of the polymorphic forms, while the C-terminus appears unstructured and highly flexible.

* Corresponding Author address. Email: henrike.heise@uni-duesseldorf.de.

Introduction

The misfolding and aggregation of the presynaptic protein α-synuclein is a key event in the etiology of Parkinson's disease. This protein constitutes the major component of intraneuronal protein inclusions called Lewy bodies, a central hallmark of several neurodegenerative disorders [1]. Several genetic mutations leading to familial early-onset Parkinson are associated with the *SNCA* gene encoding for α-synuclein. Locus duplication [2] or triplication [3] lead to elevated expression levels and thus to an enhanced aggregation propensity. In addition, to date six single point mutations causative of early-onset Parkinson's disease have been identified: A53T [4], A30P [5], E46K [6], and, more recently, G51D [7, 8], H50Q [9, 10], and A53E [11]. The physiological role of α-synuclein may comprise the regulation of neurotransmitter release and modulation of synaptic plasticity [12]. As a cytosolic protein α-synuclein is localized close to synaptic nerve terminals. Upon interaction with membranes, the N-terminal repeat unit can form an amphipathic helix which attaches to membrane surfaces [13]. However, its exact mechanism of action is still elusive [14].

α-synuclein is characterized by its large flexibility and ability to adapt its structure to its surrounding, a property which has earned it the denomination "protein chameleon" [15]. The protein was first described as natively unfolded [16], however, with a distinct propensity to form α-helices in the N-terminus upon interaction with lipid vesicles or SDS micelles [13]. Upon aggregation and amyloid formation, in contrast, the protein adopts a β-sheet rich structure, with molecular details depending critically on the fibrillation conditions [17]. In addition, the nature of the native conformation has recently been under debate, when an α-helical tetramer was postulated as the native fold [18, 19] instead of the widely accepted natively unfolded monomeric conformation [20, 21]. Evidently, structural investigations of α-synuclein can typically cover only particular aspects of a multi-faceted manifold of possible structures or conformations. In this chapter, we will give an overview over different approaches to get a better understanding of α-synuclein, and we will first start with a brief outline of different methods and their underlying principles.

Methods

Due to its large versatility of states, the attempt of earning insight into the diverse structural intermediates and structures of α-synuclein has been made using a large arsenal of biophysical techniques for structural characterization. Besides microscopic and light scattering techniques which give insight into the shape of the molecule or molecular assembly, magnetic resonance and fluorescence spectroscopy are valuable tools for obtaining information about distances and dynamics at the molecular level; each technique with its intrinsic spectral time scale.

Free monomers in aqueous solution have a molecular tumbling rate which is sufficiently high for characterization by solution NMR-spectroscopy, which in absence of a defined tertiary structure may still give insight into dynamics and residual secondary structure under various conditions. By site-selective spin labeling with stable radicals, paramagnetic relaxation enhancement can be utilized to determine transient tertiary contacts in a dynamic ensemble [22, 23]. Further, interaction with large molecular assemblies as liposomes or oligomerization processes may be monitored by solution NMR *via* the broadening, damping or disappearance of NMR resonances from amino acid residues which lose their mobility upon such an interaction [13, 24, 25]. If a flexible protein conformation is in equilibrium with a less dynamic ordered state on the ms to s time scale, structural parameters of the "dark state" may be obtained via transfer NOEs, which are observed in the spectrum of the flexible fraction, but give structural information about the invisible state [26]. Regions which are protected by stable secondary structural elements (mostly β-sheets) in oligomeric or fibrillary assemblies may be detected indirectly by either solution state NMR or by mass spectrometry after exchange of labile amide protons with deuterium [27, 28, 29]. For amyloid fibrils or proteins firmly attached to lipid bilayers, solid-state NMR-spectroscopy is an invaluable tool for obtaining structural information on a residue-specific level [30, 31] (Figure 1). If molecular tumbling rates or conformational changes are slower than the spectral time scale (i.e., slower than in the ms range), chemical shift anisotropy and dipolar couplings give rise to well-defined anisotropic resonance broadening which can easily be eliminated by magic angle spinning (MAS) and thus allows for obtaining precise information about secondary structure, residual dynamics and intra-and intermolecular distance restraints. Assemblies of intermediate size with molecular tumbling rates or molecular regions undergoing conformational changes at a rate close to the spectral time scale of NMR give rise to severe homogeneous line broadening and can thus not be detected by NMR-spectroscopy at all. Thus, protein regions with reduced flexibility may not be detected by solution NMR-Spectroscopy [24, 25], whereas semi-flexible regions are often absent from solid-state NMR spectra of fibrils.

An alternative tool to obtain information about intra- or intermolecular distances or dynamics is electron paramagnetic resonance (EPR) spectroscopy. This method requires the introduction of one or more spin labels by site-selective mutation of one or two amino acids into cysteine to which subsequently a suitable stable radical is attached. As the spectral time-scale of EPR-spectroscopy is in the nanosecond to microsecond regime, the line shape of the EPR signal is highly sensitive to overall molecular tumbling as well as segmental flexibility. Dipolar interactions between spin labels are a direct measure for the distance between spin labels, and are best detected in rigid systems like fibrils, lipid bilayers or frozen solutions. Distances below 2 nm can be directly extracted from the line shape of a continuous wave (CW) spectrum, whereas larger distances require distance measurements by pulsed EPR [32]. A linear array of dipolar coupled spins in a fibrillary assembly, on the other hand, leads to exchange narrowing of the signal in the CW spectrum; thus, core regions of fibrils with in register parallel arrangement can be easily identified from line shape analyses of EPR spectra from spin-labeled fibrils, where only labels in the core region yield exchange narrowed lines [33].

A third spectroscopic technique for probing molecular dynamics and structure involving an even shorter time-scale is fluorescence spectroscopy. The fluorescence anisotropy of fluorescing amino acid residues as tryptophan or tyrosine increases with increasing correlation time of the fluorophore. Thus, flexibility of protein regions which are not detectable by NMR-spectroscopy is easily accessible without the need to modify the protein. For distance determination over ranges up to 40 nm, Förster resonance transfer fluorescence (FRET) can be applied. For such measurements, two fluorophores, a donor and an acceptor which different excitation wavelengths have to be introduced into the protein, where the rate of the energy transfer is inversely proportional to the sixth power of the distance [32]. Site-selective labeling of α-synuclein with two fluorophores may be employed for determination of intramolecular distances in conformational ensembles, while intermolecular interactions can easily be identified from a mixture of monomers which are singly labeled with either the acceptor or the donor fluorophore, or by the detection of fluorescence excimers [34].

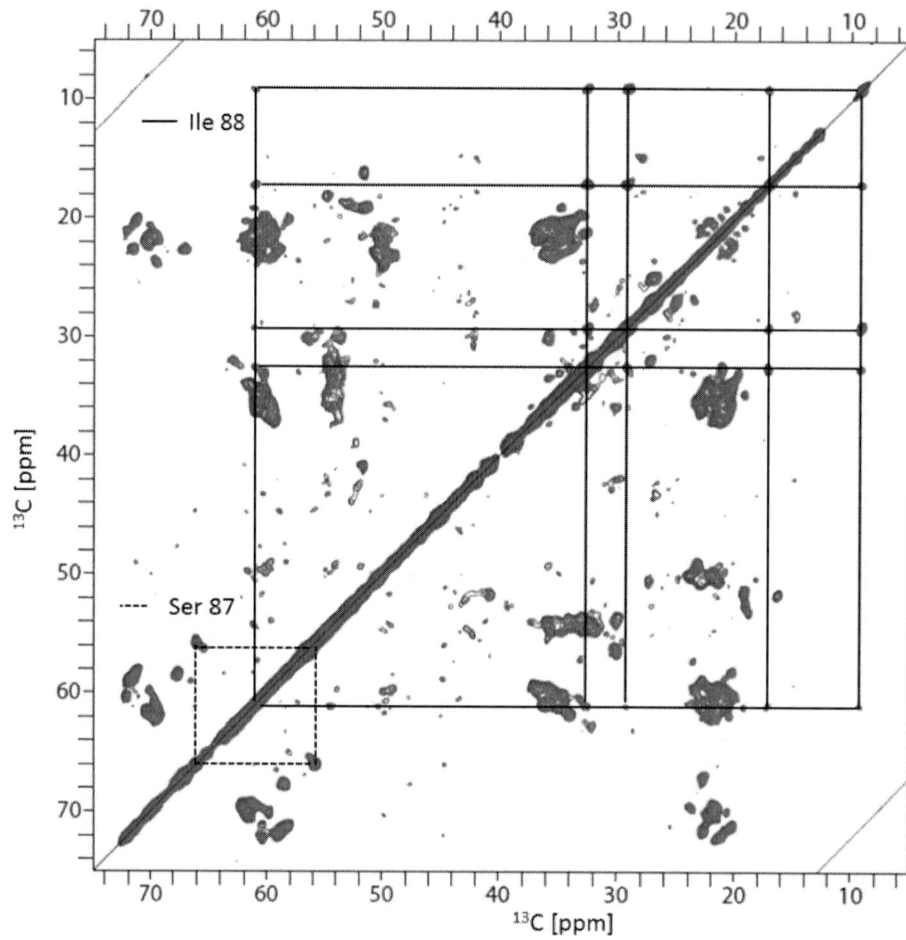

Figure 1. Solid-state NMR-spectrum (obtained by spin diffusion with a mixing time of 20 ms at 14.1 T, spinning speed of 11 kHz) of α-synuclein fibrils in a hitherto unobserved conformation. Spin systems of isoleucine 88 and serine 87 are indicated exemplarily.

MONOMERIC α-SYNUCLEIN

Native Structure of α-synuclein

The structural versatility of α-synuclein is also evident from the uncertainty about its native protein structure. In a first structural study, recombinantly expressed human α-synuclein was purified under non-denaturing conditions as a comparison to the earlier developed purification protocol [35] including a boiling step to precipitate most cellular proteins [16]. No conformational and chemical differences were observed between protein purified under non-denaturing conditions and after heat-treatment, in both cases CD and FTIR spectroscopy identified the protein as natively unfolded with a lack of a hydrophobic core. Early NMR studies on the monomeric protein in solution supported the finding that α-synuclein is predominantly unfolded [36]. However, chemical shifts of Cα atoms of most of the first 100 amino acids in the sequence were slightly shifted to higher resonance frequencies up to 0.5 ppm with respect to the random coil chemical shifts found in completely unfolded peptides [37]. These rather small secondary chemical shifts [38] are indicative of a slight propensity of the peptide chain to populate transient α-helical conformation [13]. Paramagnetic relaxation enhancement data of three site selectively spin labeled mutants of α-synuclein however were indicative of long-range tertiary contacts between the highly negatively charged C-terminus and the N-terminal and middle region [22]. These long-range contacts were reduced under highly denaturing conditions caused by the addition of urea, as well as at temperatures above 40 °C [22]. Further, residual dipolar couplings [39] in a weakly aligning medium were characteristic of some residual degree of order, which again were reduced at elevated temperatures [22]. Upon addition of SDS detergent micelles as lipid-mimetic, a conformational change towards a state with a high degree of α-helicity could be observed. In multidimensional NMR-spectra, in the presence of SDS micelles, significant secondary Cα chemical shifts of up to 2 ppm were observed for the N-terminal region of α-synuclein [13, 40, 41], which confirms its propensity to form amphipathic helices in the presence of lipids [42].

The natively disordered monomeric conformation of α-synuclein, which hitherto had been widely accepted by the scientific community, has recently been challenged by two studies which proposed a helically folded tetrameric structure as the native structure of α-synuclein from red blood cells [17] or a fusion construct with 10 additional N-terminal residues in *E. coli* [19], respectively. Native polyacrylamide gel electrophoresis as well as in cell cross-linking with subsequent SDS PAGE were indicative of a prevailing tetrameric complex, its α-helical configuration was assessed by CD spectroscopy of α-synuclein isolated under non-denaturing conditions. Further, it was proposed that this helical tetramer had a significantly higher membrane binding affinity than the unstructured monomer. The fact that this tetrameric assembly had not been detected previously was ascribed to the rather harsh denaturing purification conditions commonly applied in recombinant expression of α-synuclein [35]. In contrast, NMR-shifts of the putative tetramer *in vitro* did not differ significantly from those of disordered monomeric α-synuclein [19]. Subsequently, attempts from several independent research groups to reproduce these results using α-synuclein expressed recombinantly or from mammalian cells failed, and the outcome of this combined study suggested that native α-synuclein exists predominantly as a disordered monomer [20, 43]. The hypothesis that posttranslational N-acetylation of α-synuclein in eukaryotic cells may stabilize helically folded oligomers was rebutted by a thorough comparison of N-acetylated and non-acetylated α-synuclein both *in vitro* and in intact *E. coli* cells [44]. Irrespective of the N-acetylation, α-synuclein existed predominantly in the monomeric form, and CD spectra did not reveal any predominant secondary structure for both forms. NMR spectra of N-acetylated and unmodified α-synuclein recorded *in vitro* and in intact *E. coli* cells were essentially similar, which ruled out any large scale structural changes of α-synuclein upon N-terminal acetylation [44], as well as a disruption of the tetramer by purification [21]. However, a slight increase in helicity was observed for the first 10 N-terminal residues in the acetylated form, together with an increase in membrane affinity [45]. Furthermore, the existence of highly labile oligomeric forms in equilibrium with the unfolded monomer could not be completely ruled out [46]. Taken together, the recent debate about the native form of soluble α-synuclein seems to converge towards a picture of a highly dynamic and natively unfolded protein which may be able to transiently form multimers, and which may adopt transient α-helical conformation in the N-terminus [12, 47, 48].

Interaction with Lipid Surfaces

The N-terminus of α-synuclein consists of seven imperfect 11-mer repeats which upon formation of an amphipathic helix expose at least 10 positively charged lysine residues to one side, which favors the binding to negatively charged lipid vesicles. While the increase of α-helical conformation upon vesicle binding has been proven by CD spectroscopy and NMR-spectroscopy early on [13, 42], the exact conformation and arrangement of such an amphipathic helix remains as controversial as the monomer conformation. Early solution NMR studies using SDS micelles as a low molecular weight mimetic for phospholipid bilayers suggested that α-synuclein adopts a broken α-helical conformation in the presence of small micelles, with a break between two helical segments around residue 40 [41, 49]. However, regarding the relative arrangement of the two helical segments in the presence of SDS micelles, different results were obtained by two research groups. Site-directed spin labeling with a paramagnetic Mn^{2+} complex in position 87 indicated an antiparallel horseshoe-type arrangement of two α-helices on the micelle surface, whereas studies using a stable nitroxide radical as spin label and detecting paramagnetic relaxation enhancements with spin labels in different positions throughout the first 93 residues, no close interhelical contacts could be detected, thus pointing towards a more extended conformation [50]. However, as solution NMR-spectroscopy is limited by the molecular tumbling rate, well-resolved spectra can only be obtained for α-synuclein in the presence of small detergent micelles; binding to phospholipid bilayers in contrast resulted in a line broadening beyond detection for all residues attached to the membrane surface [13, 41]. Thus, the question whether the antiparallel horseshoe conformation was induced artificially by the small size and the large curvature of the SDS micelles could not be answered by NMR-spectroscopy. Therefore, EPR studies on singly and doubly spin labeled α-synuclein bound to small unilamellar vesicles consisting of lipid bilayers were conducted to shed light onto the helical conformation of membrane bound α-synuclein. First line-shape analysis of labeled α-synuclein singly spin labeled in 40 different sites in combination with paramagnetic quenchers were indicative of an extended α-helix when bound to POPC/POPS vesicles [51], a finding which subsequently could be confirmed by distance measurements in doubly labeled mutants by pulsed EPR [52]. However, for α-synuclein bound to small unilamellar vesicles of POPG, EPR distance measurements were consistent with the horseshoe model [53], whereas later investigations on large unilamellar vesicles from POPG both extended and horseshoe conformation were observed in coexistence [54], a finding which implies that also in its membrane-bound state α-synuclein does not exist in one single conformation but may adapt its shape to its environment. Two recent studies on vesicle-bound α-synuclein by solution-state NMR-spectroscopy, fluorescence anisotropy measurements and solid-state NMR-spectroscopy [24, 25] suggested that α-synuclein can bind to phospholipid vesicles in different competitive binding modes. Irrespective of the lipid to protein ratio, the C-terminal 40 residues were always found flexible enough to give rise to well-resolved resonances in solution NMR-spectra. Attenuation profiles of the N-terminal residues were in agreement with two protein pools where either the first 25 or the first 98 residues were tightly bound to the lipid vesicles, with the ratio between these two protein conformations being dependent on the protein to lipid ratio. Electron microscopy images of lipid vesicles suggested that small unilamellar vesicles largely rearranged upon α-synuclein binding, leading to rod-like structures at higher protein concentrations. However, extended α-helical conformations were ruled out as possible conformations at least for binding to small unilamellar vesicles; instead a multimeric helix bundle with a modest number of phospholipids was proposed [24]. In agreement with these findings, in solid-state NMR spectra of phospholipid bound α-synuclein, resonances from residue 6 to 25 could be unambiguously assigned, indicating that these N-terminal residues are rigid and well-ordered [25]. Taken together, the phospholipid bound state of α-synuclein cannot be described by one defined structure, but rather by equilibrium of different states, which is sensitive to the exact condition in the cell.

Beta-sheets in Monomeric α-synuclein

Although α-synuclein in solution is mainly unfolded and highly flexible, a fact that is manifest in the absence of significant secondary chemical shifts in solution NMR spectra [13, 22], the conformational ensemble of the intrinsically disordered protein may be shifted towards conformations with lower energy by lowering the temperatures. In a super-cooled solution at -15 °C, residual secondary chemical shifts indicative of a slight increase in β-sheet propensity were observed for residues in the central hydrophobic region spanning residues 40 to 94 [55]. Interestingly, the residual secondary chemical shifts obtained in super-cooled solution correlated well with the secondary chemical shifts determined for fibrils by solid-state NMR-spectroscopy [17]. Later, a thorough reinvestigation of intramolecular contacts in monomers from PRE effects also revealed some pairwise tertiary contacts between residues which in the fibrillary state are located in β-sheets. However, those tertiary contacts do not agree with the fibrillary structure [56].

One promising approach to prevent amyloidogenic proteins from aggregating is the sequestration of the most aggregation prone regions with β-sheet binding proteins. Such binding molecules may be selected by phage display technology from combinatorial protein libraries based on small and well-defined protein scaffolds [57, 58]. For Aβ(1-40), the structure of the monomeric peptide stabilized by the homodimeric β-sheet-binding affibody protein $Z_{A\beta3}$ had been determined by solution NMR. Monomeric Aβ(1-40) was stabilized in a β-hairpin conformation [58] with the β-strand regions being identical to β-sheets determined by solid-state NMR in fibrils [59]. Phage display selection from a library based on $Z_{A\beta3}$ towards binding of α-synuclein yielded β-hairpin AS69 which was found to bind α-synuclein with a K_d value of 240 nM [60]. The structure of the complex determined by solution NMR-spectroscopy revealed that α-synuclein(35–56) folds into a β-hairpin comprising residues ^{37}VLYVGSK^{43} (β1) and ^{48}VVHGVAT^{54} (β2). Again these residues have been found in β-sheet conformation also in mature fibrils, however, they comprise only a small fraction of the amyloid core region which extends up to residue ~93 [17, 61, 62]. In particular, the hydrophobic NAC region extending from residue 60 to 95, which has been postulated to be responsible for aggregation, is unaffected by the β-binding protein AS69. These studies show that monomeric α-synuclein may also form β-sheet structures under appropriate conditions or in the presence of adequate interaction partners, which again is a signature of the extreme versatility of this protein.

Structural Studies on α-synuclein Oligomers

The first step towards fibrillation is the formation of oligomeric intermediates or protofibrils. However, the term "oligomer" does not refer to one well-defined species of aggregate but rather covers a plethora of different states comprising early stage fibrillary assemblies as well as off-pathway oligomers, which may be in equilibrium with each other, with the unfolded monomers, or with the mature fibrils. Oligomeric assemblies of amyloidogenic proteins have been proposed to be the toxic agents in degenerative diseases rather than the mature fibrils [12, 63], and their membrane-disrupting effects have been demonstrated [64, 65, 66]. Therefore, the nature of toxic oligomers is of high interest, but, due to the transient nature of oligomeric aggregates and their inherent polydispersity, structural details are even less well defined as for the intrinsically unfolded monomer of α-synuclein. Although it will not be possible to determine one single well-defined structure of α-synuclein in oligomeric form, several attempts have been made to obtain at least some information about the β-strand core region, the amount of secondary structure, site-selective solvent exposure and dynamics, and intra- and intermolecular distance distributions in addition to size distributions in oligomeric α-synuclein preparations. One of the most obvious characteristics of oligomeric assemblies is their size or size distribution, as well as the shape of the aggregate. Time-resolved small angle X-ray scattering experiments following the kinetics of α-synuclein aggregation and fibrillation revealed the existence of an oligomeric intermediate which was hypothesized to be an on-pathway oligomer. This oligomeric species could be isolated from abundant monomers by gel filtration. Subsequently, the ability to permeabilize membranes was proven by incubation with POPC vesicles containing the fluorescent dye calcein above self-quenching concentrations. A rupture of the lipid vesicles leading to calcein release was then observed only after incubation with α-synuclein oligomers but not after incubation with monomers. The SAXS profile of the oligomers was characteristic for an elongated annular shape with a long axis of 18 nm and a short axis of 9 nm [66]. Subsequent studies using size-exclusion chromatography in combination with dynamic light scattering and small angle X-ray scattering revealed the coexistence of two monomer types of different size [67]: small oligomers consisting of roughly 30 monomers with dimensions agreeing to those found in the previous study, and larger oligomers roughly one order of magnitude larger. For both types of oligomers a small but significant amount of antiparallel β-sheets could be detected by Fourier transform infrared spectroscopy. Both types of oligomers were found to disrupt lipid vesicles, but they were not able to incorporate into fibrillary seeds or act as seeds [67]. A preference for oligomers consisting of ~30 monomers had independently been observed by photo bleaching experiments on oligomers containing a defined substoichiometric amount of monomers labeled with one fluorophore [68], whereas the prevalence of distinct antiparallel β-sheet in toxic oligomers had been confirmed by infrared spectroscopy in an independent study [69]. Characterization of a mixture of α-synuclein moieties during the fibrillation process with deuterium exchange followed by mass spectrometry revealed two distinct oligomeric species with different stabilities and distinct core regions. For one type of oligomer, the entire N-terminus up to residue 90 was protected from deuterium exchange; however, this oligomeric species vanished after longer times, whereas for a second oligomer which appeared stable for over 100 minutes, a reduced core region from residue 38 to ~85 was detected [70]. Likewise, solvent protection of distinct sites was probed by site-selective substituting different amino acids with the fluorescent amino acid tryptophan which does not occur in the amino acid sequence of α-synuclein. Fluorescence quenching experiments revealed that the full N-terminus up to residue 90 was solvent protected [71]. Similar results were also obtained by a complementary fluorescence study [34]. Taken together, the oligomerization process of α-synuclein is by no means a linear process, and these studies together confirmed that a mixture of oligomers of different size and ultrastructure may coexist in equilibrium. However, one common motif of all oligomers is the highly flexible and solvent exposed C-terminus from residue ~100 to 140, as well as the antiparallel β-sheet core in early oligomers.

THE MANY STRUCTURES OF α-SYNUCLEIN FIBRILS

Given the enormous structural versatility of α-synuclein monomers and oligomers, it is not surprising that amyloid fibrils of this protein, although intrinsically well-structured, can form not only in one conformation, but many polymorphic fibrillary structures can be adopted, depending on the solution and fibrillation conditions (Figure 2). AFM, EM, and fluorescence microscopy studies on different fibril preparation generated *in vitro* demonstrated that the morphology of synuclein fibrils critically depends on pH, salt concentration, and slight variations in the fibrillation conditions may change the appearance of the aggregates [72]. Early solid-state NMR investigations on fibrils formed at pH 7.4 led to the discovery of two polymorphic fibril types dubbed A and B, which could form at identical *in vitro* conditions [17]. The different molecular conformations in both fibril types were also reflected by different morphological appearance of the fibrils in electron microscopy images, where fibrils of type A were characterized by regular twists, and fibrils of type B were straight and flat. In both fibril types the β-sheet core was found to extend at least from residue 38 to roughly residue 94, whereas the C-terminus from residue ~100 until the end was flexible and unstructured in both variants. While the length of the β-sheet core was nearly identical, the location of sheets and turns varied slightly, as well as the exact chemical shifts which are a signature of the conformation and environment of the corresponding amino acid residue. The N-termini in both fibril types were characterized by a high degree of structural disorder, but were found to appear rigid on the sub-μs time scale. For several amino acids in this region peak doubling indicative of the existence of more than one molecular conformation was observed, and the molecular details were found to vary from preparation to preparation even in fibrils of one morphology. Hydrogen exchange experiments coupled to detection by mass spectrometry confirmed that in fibrillar α-synuclein backbone amide protons of residues 39 to 100 are protected from the solvent due to their incorporation in the β-strand core [27]. A multidisciplinary approach combining solid-state NMR-spectroscopy and hydrogen exchange could reproduce the resonance assignment for conformer B and located the solvent protected core region between residues 35 and 95 [61]. EPR spectra of different fibrils from monomers with site-directed spin labels showed a single exchange-narrowed line characteristic for parallel in-register β-sheets if the spin label was attached to an amino acid residue in the core region between 36 and 98 [33, 73].

Subsequently, further solid-state NMR investigations of α-synuclein fibrils prepared under different conditions revealed at least two or three molecular conformations differing on the molecular level from the first two forms [74, 75, 76]. While the location of the central core region in most studies had been consistent, for one fibril type generated in salt-free solution, denoted as "ribbon" in contrast to the "fibril" conformation, a substantially larger core region spanning the N-terminal 100 residues with only small interruptions was determined [75, 77]. In agreement with these findings, the early-onset mutant A30P, which contains a β-sheet breaking proline substitution outside of the core region found in all fibril conformations readily forms fibrils with a core region largely unaffected by the mutation [28, 78], whereas the formation of ribbons was prevented by this proline substitution [79]. Ribbons and fibrils were also found to propagate their conformation *in vitro* under adequate conditions; however, at salt-free conditions fibrils were unable to propagate their structure. In mammalian neuronal cell cultures, only α-synuclein fibrils could persistently propagate over 95 generations, whereas the phenotype caused by infection with ribbons vanished after 30 days [79]. Different cell assays probing apoptotic markers after incubation with ribbons and fibrils, respectively, indicated a higher toxicity for fibrils than for ribbons, a finding which also correlates well with the differential stabilities of the two isoforms in cellular environment. However, whether these two polymorphic forms can be taken as model systems for prion strains may be debated, as the formation of ribbons requires growth conditions far from physiological cellular environments.

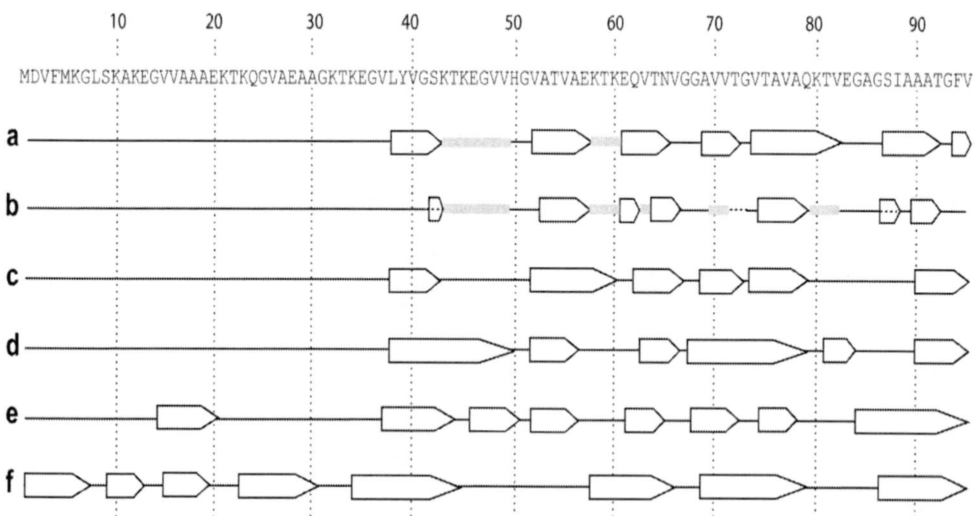

Figure 2. Beta sheet core regions of different fibril polymorphs from wild-type α-synuclein: a,b: form A and B [17], c [61], d [62] e: fibrils [77] f: ribbons [79].

The disease-related mutants A53T [62, 80, 81] and E46K [62, 81] have also been subject to intense solid-state NMR investigations. As for fibrils from wild-type α-synuclein, it can be expected that also α-synuclein bearing several mutations may be able to form different polymorphic forms, thus variations with respect to one single polymorphic form may be interpreted with caution. However, some conclusions by comparing results obtained under identical fibrillation conditions for wild-type and A53T mutants revealed only minor perturbations around the mutation site [81] and a slightly extended β-strand region towards the C-terminus [80], respectively, whereas the E46K mutant led to significant perturbations throughout the β-sheet core, and thus was found to have a more pronounced effect on the fibril structure, a finding which is not surprising as this mutation leads to an inversion of a charge from negative to positive under physiological conditions [62]. Finally, to address the question whether mature fibrils or rather oligomeric or protofibrillar assemblies are the cytotoxic agents in Parkinson's disease, two artificial mutants with diminished aggregation propensities were designed by introducing proline substitutions in β-strand regions. The single proline mutant A56P with one β-sheet breaking proline substituent and the triple mutant A30P/A56P/A76P, where two alanine residues in the core region were substituted by proline in addition to the disease-related A30P point mutation [82]. For both mutants *in vitro* fibrillation as well as aggregation in HEK cells was retarded with respect to wild-type α-synuclein, in particular for the triple mutant. Thus, the hypothetical equilibrium between fibrils and prefibrillar assemblies may be expected to be shifted towards the prefibrillar intermediates. Solid-state NMR spectra of fibrils from the A56P mutant displayed a reduced rigid β-sheet core. In contrast to wild-type fibrils, also some parts of the N-terminus were observed to undergo motions on a sub-μs time scale. For the triple mutant, solid-state NMR spectra displayed only broad and featureless signals indicative of a low degree of order, with secondary chemical shifts characteristic for β-sheets. A higher toxicity for these design mutants on eukaryotic cells was confirmed by overexpression of these mutants in drosophila, *C. elegans* and in cultured mammalian neurons; a finding which supports the hypothesis that oligomers instead of mature fibrils are the toxic agents [82]. In a related study, two artificial mutants with a single lysine to glutamate substitutions in position 35 (i.e., outside of the fibril core region) or 57 (i.e., inside the fibril core) to disrupt possible salt bridges between β-sheets, were found to have a strongly decreased propensity to form fibrils [83]. Instead of mature fibrils or fibrillary structures, electron micrographs revealed annular structures even after long-term incubation. Toxicity towards mammalian neuronal cells was assessed by lentiviral injection of these artificial mutants in addition to two disease related mutants and wild-type α-synuclein into the substantia nigra of rats, and the decrease in dopaminergic cells was monitored. While toxic effects were observed for all of the variants, the two artificial oligomer promoting variants displayed the strongest effect, a further support of the hypothesis that oligomers may be the true toxic agents in neurodegeneration.

Taken together, these studies show that despite the high degree of order which α-synuclein molecules in amyloid fibrils may adopt, there is no such thing as the one and only fibril structure, but rather, a large manifold of structures may be adopted. These properties have thus far also prevented high-resolution 3D structure determination of α-synuclein in fibrils.

CONCLUSION

The title "protein chameleon" which refers to the ability of α-synuclein to adopt its structure to its surrounding, characterizes not only the monomeric or native state, but seems to be the key feature of also oligomeric and fibrillary aggregates of the protein. To date, at least four different fibril types of wild-type α-synuclein have been investigated, and the relation with real disease-related aggregates is still not clarified. Nevertheless, the concerted effort towards structure elucidation in oligomers and fibrils has also yielded some similarities, such as a highly flexible intrinsically disordered C-terminus, a parallel, in register orientation of β-sheets, as well as a minimum central core region spanning residues 38 to 95. Thus, although not completely defined yet, the picture of the multi-faceted protein has gained contours, and may also help to improve the understanding of other amyloid diseases.

REFERENCES

[1] Spillantini MG, Schmidt ML, Lee VM, Trojanowski JQ, Jakes R, et al. (1997) Alpha-synuclein in Lewy bodies. *Nature* 388: 839-840.

[2] Chartier-Harlin MC, Kachergus J, Roumier C, Mouroux V, Douay X, et al. (2004) Alpha-synuclein locus duplication as a cause of familial Parkinson's disease. *Lancet* 364: 1167-1169.

[3] Singleton AB, Farrer M, Johnson J, Singleton A, Hague S, et al. (2003) alpha-Synuclein locus triplication causes Parkinson's disease. *Science* 302: 841.

[4] Polymeropoulos MH, Lavedan C, Leroy E, Ide SE, Dehejia A, et al. (1997) Mutation in the alpha-synuclein gene identified in families with Parkinson's disease. *Science* 276: 2045-2047.

[5] Kruger R, Kuhn W, Muller T, Woitalla D, Graeber M, et al. (1998) Ala30Pro mutation in the gene encoding alpha-synuclein in Parkinson's disease. *Nat Genet* 18: 106-108.

[6] Zarranz JJ, Alegre J, Gomez-Esteban JC, Lezcano E, Ros R, et al. (2004) The new mutation, E46K, of alpha-synuclein causes Parkinson and Lewy body dementia. *Ann Neurol* 55: 164-173.

[7] Lesage S, Anheim M, Letournel F, Bousset L, Honore A, et al. (2013) G51D alpha-synuclein mutation causes a novel parkinsonian-pyramidal syndrome. *Ann Neurol* 73: 459-471.

[8] Kiely AP, Asi YT, Kara E, Limousin P, Ling H, et al. (2013) alpha-Synucleinopathy associated with G51D SNCA mutation: a link between Parkinson's disease and multiple system atrophy? *Acta Neuropathol* 125: 753-769.

[9] Proukakis C, Dudzik CG, Brier T, MacKay DS, Cooper JM, et al. (2013) A novel alpha-synuclein missense mutation in Parkinson disease. *Neurology* 80: 1062-1064.

[10] Appel-Cresswell S, Vilarino-Guell C, Encarnacion M, Sherman H, Yu I, et al. (2013) Alpha-synuclein p.H50Q, a novel pathogenic mutation for Parkinson's disease. *Mov Disord* 28: 811-813.

[11] Pasanen P, Myllykangas L, Siitonen M, Raunio A, Kaakkola S, et al. (2014) Novel alpha-synuclein mutation A53E associated with atypical multiple system atrophy and Parkinson's disease-type pathology. *Neurobiol Aging* 35: 2180 e2181-2185.

[12] Lashuel HA, Overk CR, Oueslati A, Masliah E (2013) The many faces of alpha-synuclein: from structure and toxicity to therapeutic target. *Nat Rev Neurosci* 14: 38-48.

[13] Eliezer D, Kutluay E, Bussell R, Jr., Browne G (2001) Conformational properties of alpha-synuclein in its free and lipid-associated states. *J Mol Biol* 307: 1061-1073.

[14] Auluck PK, Caraveo G, Lindquist S (2010) alpha-Synuclein: membrane interactions and toxicity in Parkinson's disease. *Annu Rev Cell Dev Biol* 26: 211-233.

[15] Uversky VN (2003) A protein-chameleon: conformational plasticity of alpha-synuclein, a disordered protein involved in neurodegenerative disorders. *J Biomol Struct Dyn* 21: 211-234.

[16] Weinreb PH, Zhen W, Poon AW, Conway KA, Lansbury PT, Jr. (1996) NACP, a protein implicated in Alzheimer's disease and learning, is natively unfolded. *Biochemistry* 35: 13709-13715.

[17] Heise H, Hoyer W, Becker S, Andronesi OC, Riedel D, et al. (2005) Molecular-level secondary structure, polymorphism, and dynamics of full-length alpha-synuclein fibrils studied by solid-state NMR. *Proc Natl Acad Sci U S A* 102: 15871-15876.

[18] Bartels T, Choi JG, Selkoe DJ (2011) alpha-Synuclein occurs physiologically as a helically folded tetramer that resists aggregation. *Nature* 477: 107-110.

[19] Wang W, Perovic I, Chittuluru J, Kaganovich A, Nguyen LT, et al. (2011) A soluble alpha-synuclein construct forms a dynamic tetramer. *Proc Natl Acad Sci U S A* 108: 17797-17802.

[20] Fauvet B, Mbefo MK, Fares MB, Desobry C, Michael S, et al. (2012) alpha-Synuclein in central nervous system and from erythrocytes, mammalian cells, and Escherichia coli exists predominantly as disordered monomer. *J Biol Chem* 287: 15345-15364.

[21] Binolfi A, Theillet FX, Selenko P (2012) Bacterial in-cell NMR of human alpha-synuclein: a disordered monomer by nature? *Biochem Soc Trans* 40: 950-954.

[22] Bertoncini CW, Jung YS, Fernandez CO, Hoyer W, Griesinger C, et al. (2005) Release of long-range tertiary interactions potentiates aggregation of natively unstructured alpha-synuclein. *Proc Natl Acad Sci U S A* 102: 1430-1435.

[23] Dedmon MM, Lindorff-Larsen K, Christodoulou J, Vendruscolo M, Dobson CM (2005) Mapping long-range interactions in alpha-synuclein using spin-label NMR and ensemble molecular dynamics simulations. *J Am Chem Soc* 127: 476-477.

[24] Bodner CR, Dobson CM, Bax A (2009) Multiple tight phospholipid-binding modes of alpha-synuclein revealed by solution NMR spectroscopy. *J Mol Biol* 390: 775-790.

[25] Fusco G, De Simone A, Gopinath T, Vostrikov V, Vendruscolo M, et al. (2014) Direct observation of the three regions in alpha-synuclein that determine its membrane-bound behaviour. *Nat Commun* 5: 3827.

[26] Clore GM, Gronenborn AM (1983) Theory of the Time Dependent Transferred Nuclear Overhauser Effect: Applications to Structural Analysis of Ligand-Protein Complexes in Solution. *Journal of Magnetic Resonance* 53: 423-442.

[27] Del Mar C, Greenbaum EA, Mayne L, Englander SW, Woods VL, Jr. (2005) Structure and properties of alpha-synuclein and other amyloids determined at the amino acid level. *Proc Natl Acad Sci U S A* 102: 15477-15482.

[28] Cho MK, Kim HY, Fernandez CO, Becker S, Zweckstetter M (2011) Conserved core of amyloid fibrils of wild type and A30P mutant alpha-synuclein. *Protein Sci* 20: 387-395.

[29] Mysling S, Betzer C, Jensen PH, Jorgensen TJ (2013) Characterizing the dynamics of alpha-synuclein oligomers using hydrogen/deuterium exchange monitored by mass spectrometry. *Biochemistry* 52: 9097-9103.

[30] Hoyer W, Heise H (2013) What Does Solid-State NMR Tell Us about Amyloid Structures? In: Otzen DE, editor. *Amyloid Fibrils and Prefibrillar Aggregates: Molecular and Biological Properties:* John Wiley & Sons, Inc. pp. 39-62.

[31] Tycko R (2011) Solid-state NMR studies of amyloid fibril structure. *Annu Rev Phys Chem* 62: 279-299.

[32] Drescher M, Huber M, Subramaniam V (2012) Hunting the chameleon: structural conformations of the intrinsically disordered protein alpha-synuclein. *Chembiochem* 13: 761-768.

[33] Chen M, Margittai M, Chen J, Langen R (2007) Investigation of alpha-synuclein fibril structure by site-directed spin labeling. *J Biol Chem* 282: 24970-24979.

[34] Gallea JI, Celej MS (2014) Structural insights into amyloid oligomers of the Parkinson disease-related protein alpha-synuclein. *J Biol Chem* 289: 26733-26742.

[35] Jakes R, Spillantini MG, Goedert M (1994) Identification of two distinct synucleins from human brain. *FEBS Lett* 345: 27-32.

[36] Wishart DS, Bigam CG, Holm A, Hodges RS, Sykes BD (1995) 1H, 13C and 15N random coil NMR chemical shifts of the common amino acids. I. Investigations of nearest-neighbor effects. *J Biomol NMR* 5: 67-81.

[37] Schwarzinger S, Kroon GJ, Foss TR, Wright PE, Dyson HJ (2000) Random coil chemical shifts in acidic 8 M urea: implementation of random coil shift data in NMRView. *J Biomol NMR* 18: 43-48.

[38] Wishart DS, Case DA (2002) [1] - *Use of Chemical Shifts in Macromolecular Structure Determination*. In: Thomas L. James VD, Uli S, editors. Methods in Enzymology: Academic Press. pp. 3-34.

[39] Tjandra N, Grzesiek S, Bax A (1996) Magnetic Field Dependence of Nitrogen−Proton J Splittings in 15N-Enriched Human Ubiquitin Resulting from Relaxation Interference and Residual Dipolar Coupling. *Journal of the American Chemical Society* 118: 6264-6272.

[40] Ulmer TS, Bax A, Cole NB, Nussbaum RL (2005) Structure and dynamics of micelle-bound human alpha-synuclein. *J Biol Chem* 280: 9595-9603.

[41] Chandra S, Chen X, Rizo J, Jahn R, Sudhof TC (2003) A broken alpha -helix in folded alpha -Synuclein. *J Biol Chem* 278: 15313-15318.

[42] Davidson WS, Jonas A, Clayton DF, George JM (1998) Stabilization of alpha-synuclein secondary structure upon binding to synthetic membranes. *J Biol Chem* 273: 9443-9449.

[43] Coelho-Cerqueira E, Carmo-Goncalves P, Pinheiro AS, Cortines J, Follmer C (2013) alpha-Synuclein as an intrinsically disordered monomer--fact or artefact? *FEBS J* 280: 4915-4927.

[44] Fauvet B, Fares MB, Samuel F, Dikiy I, Tandon A, et al. (2012) Characterization of semisynthetic and naturally Nalpha-acetylated alpha-synuclein in vitro and in intact cells: implications for aggregation and cellular properties of alpha-synuclein. *J Biol Chem* 287: 28243-28262.

[45] Dikiy I, Eliezer D (2014) N-terminal acetylation stabilizes N-terminal helicity in lipid- and micelle-bound alpha-synuclein and increases its affinity for physiological membranes. *J Biol Chem* 289: 3652-3665.

[46] Luth ES, Bartels T, Dettmer U, Kim NC, Selkoe DJ (2015) Purification of alpha-synuclein from human brain reveals an instability of endogenous multimers as the protein approaches purity. *Biochemistry* 54: 279-292.

[47] Alderson TR, Markley JL (2013) Biophysical characterization of alpha-synuclein and its controversial structure. *Intrinsically Disord Proteins* 1: 18-39.

[48] Gurry T, Ullman O, Fisher CK, Perovic I, Pochapsky T, et al. (2013) The dynamic structure of alpha-synuclein multimers. *J Am Chem Soc* 135: 3865-3872.

[49] Bussell R, Jr., Eliezer D (2003) A structural and functional role for 11-mer repeats in alpha-synuclein and other exchangeable lipid binding proteins. *J Mol Biol* 329: 763-778.

[50] Bussell R, Jr., Ramlall TF, Eliezer D (2005) Helix periodicity, topology, and dynamics of membrane-associated alpha-synuclein. *Protein Sci* 14: 862-872.

[51] Jao CC, Der-Sarkissian A, Chen J, Langen R (2004) Structure of membrane-bound alpha-synuclein studied by site-directed spin labeling. *Proc Natl Acad Sci U S A* 101: 8331-8336.

[52] Jao CC, Hegde BG, Chen J, Haworth IS, Langen R (2008) Structure of membrane-bound alpha-synuclein from site-directed spin labeling and computational refinement. *Proc Natl Acad Sci U S A* 105: 19666-19671.

[53] Drescher M, Veldhuis G, van Rooijen BD, Milikisyants S, Subramaniam V, et al. (2008) Antiparallel arrangement of the helices of vesicle-bound alpha-synuclein. *J Am Chem Soc* 130: 7796-7797.

[54] Robotta M, Braun P, van Rooijen B, Subramaniam V, Huber M, et al. (2011) Direct evidence of coexisting horseshoe and extended helix conformations of membrane-bound alpha-synuclein. *Chemphyschem* 12: 267-269.

[55] Kim HY, Heise H, Fernandez CO, Baldus M, Zweckstetter M (2007) Correlation of amyloid fibril beta-structure with the unfolded state of alpha-synuclein. *Chembiochem* 8: 1671-1674.

[56] Esteban-Martin S, Silvestre-Ryan J, Bertoncini CW, Salvatella X (2013) Identification of fibril-like tertiary contacts in soluble monomeric alpha-synuclein. *Biophys J* 105: 1192-1198.

[57] Gronwall C, Jonsson A, Lindstrom S, Gunneriusson E, Stahl S, et al. (2007) Selection and characterization of Affibody ligands binding to Alzheimer amyloid beta peptides. *J Biotechnol* 128: 162-183.

[58] Hoyer W, Gronwall C, Jonsson A, Stahl S, Hard T (2008) Stabilization of a beta-hairpin in monomeric Alzheimer's amyloid-beta peptide inhibits amyloid formation. *Proc Natl Acad Sci U S A* 105: 5099-5104.

[59] Petkova AT, Ishii Y, Balbach JJ, Antzutkin ON, Leapman RD, et al. (2002) A structural model for Alzheimer's beta -amyloid fibrils based on experimental constraints from solid state NMR. *Proc Natl Acad Sci* U S A 99: 16742-16747.

[60] Mirecka EA, Shaykhalishahi H, Gauhar A, Akgul S, Lecher J, et al. (2014) Sequestration of a beta-hairpin for control of alpha-synuclein aggregation. *Angew Chem Int Ed Engl* 53: 4227-4230.

[61] Vilar M, Chou HT, Luhrs T, Maji SK, Riek-Loher D, et al. (2008) The fold of alpha-synuclein fibrils. *Proc Natl Acad Sci U S A* 105: 8637-8642.

[62] Comellas G, Lemkau LR, Nieuwkoop AJ, Kloepper KD, Ladror DT, et al. (2011) Structured regions of alpha-synuclein fibrils include the early-onset Parkinson's disease mutation sites. *J Mol Biol* 411: 881-895.

[63] Caughey B, Lansbury PT (2003) Protofibrils, pores, fibrils, and neurodegeneration: separating the responsible protein aggregates from the innocent bystanders. *Annu Rev Neurosci* 26: 267-298.

[64] Volles MJ, Lee SJ, Rochet JC, Shtilerman MD, Ding TT, et al. (2001) Vesicle permeabilization by protofibrillar alpha-synuclein: implications for the pathogenesis and treatment of Parkinson's disease. *Biochemistry* 40: 7812-7819.

[65] van Rooijen BD, Claessens MM, Subramaniam V (2009) Lipid bilayer disruption by oligomeric alpha-synuclein depends on bilayer charge and accessibility of the hydrophobic core. *Biochim Biophys Acta* 1788: 1271-1278.

[66] Giehm L, Svergun DI, Otzen DE, Vestergaard B (2011) Low-resolution structure of a vesicle disrupting α-synuclein oligomer that accumulates during fibrillation. *Proc Natl Acad Sci U S A* 108: 3246-3251.

[67] Lorenzen N, Nielsen SB, Buell AK, Kaspersen JD, Arosio P, et al. (2014) The role of stable alpha-synuclein oligomers in the molecular events underlying amyloid formation. *J Am Chem Soc* 136: 3859-3868.

[68] Zijlstra N, Blum C, Segers-Nolten IM, Claessens MM, Subramaniam V (2012) Molecular composition of sub-stoichiometrically labeled alpha-synuclein oligomers determined by single-molecule photobleaching. *Angew Chem Int Ed Engl* 51: 8821-8824.

[69] Celej MS, Sarroukh R, Goormaghtigh E, Fidelio GD, Ruysschaert JM, et al. (2012) Toxic prefibrillar alpha-synuclein amyloid oligomers adopt a distinctive antiparallel beta-sheet structure. *Biochem J* 443: 719-726.

[70] Paslawski W, Mysling S, Thomsen K, Jorgensen TJ, Otzen DE (2014) Co-existence of two different alpha-synuclein oligomers with different core structures determined by hydrogen/deuterium exchange mass spectrometry. *Angew Chem Int Ed Engl* 53: 7560-7563.

[71] van Rooijen BD, van Leijenhorst-Groener KA, Claessens MM, Subramaniam V (2009) Tryptophan fluorescence reveals structural features of alpha-synuclein oligomers. *J Mol Biol* 394: 826-833.

[72] Hoyer W, Antony T, Cherny D, Heim G, Jovin TM, et al. (2002) Dependence of alpha-synuclein aggregate morphology on solution conditions. *J Mol Biol* 322: 383-393.

[73] Der-Sarkissian A, Jao CC, Chen J, Langen R (2003) Structural organization of alpha-synuclein fibrils studied by site-directed spin labeling. *J Biol Chem* 278: 37530-37535.

[74] Kloepper KD, Woods WS, Winter KA, George JM, Rienstra CM (2006) Preparation of alpha-synuclein fibrils for solid-state NMR: expression, purification, and incubation of wild-type and mutant forms. *Protein Expr Purif* 48: 112-117.

[75] Gath J, Habenstein B, Bousset L, Melki R, Meier BH, et al. (2012) Solid-state NMR sequential assignments of alpha-synuclein. *Biomol NMR Assign* 6: 51-55.

[76] Gath J, Bousset L, Habenstein B, Melki R, Meier BH, et al. (2014) Yet another polymorph of alpha-synuclein: solid-state sequential assignments. *Biomol NMR Assign* 8: 395-404.

[77] Gath J, Bousset L, Habenstein B, Melki R, Bockmann A, et al. (2014) Unlike twins: an NMR comparison of two alpha-synuclein polymorphs featuring different toxicity. *PLoS One* 9: e90659.

[78] Lemkau LR, Comellas G, Kloepper KD, Woods WS, George JM, et al. (2012) Mutant protein A30P alpha-synuclein adopts wild-type fibril structure, despite slower fibrillation kinetics. *J Biol Chem* 287: 11526-11532.

[79] Bousset L, Pieri L, Ruiz-Arlandis G, Gath J, Jensen PH, et al. (2013) Structural and functional characterization of two alpha-synuclein strains. *Nat Commun* 4: 2575.

[80] Heise H, Celej MS, Becker S, Riedel D, Pelah A, et al. (2008) Solid-state NMR reveals structural differences between fibrils of wild-type and disease-related A53T mutant alpha-synuclein. *J Mol Biol* 380: 444-450.

[81] Lemkau LR, Comellas G, Lee SW, Rikardsen LK, Woods WS, et al. (2013) Site-specific perturbations of alpha-synuclein fibril structure by the Parkinson's disease associated mutations A53T and E46K. *PLoS One* 8: e49750.

[82] Karpinar DP, Balija MB, Kugler S, Opazo F, Rezaei-Ghaleh N, et al. (2009) Pre-fibrillar alpha-synuclein variants with impaired beta-structure increase neurotoxicity in Parkinson's disease models. *EMBO J* 28: 3256-3268.

[83] Winner B, Jappelli R, Maji SK, Desplats PA, Boyer L, et al. (2011) In vivo demonstration that alpha-synuclein oligomers are toxic. *Proc Natl Acad Sci U S A* 108: 4194-4199.

In: The Prion Phenomena in Neurodegenerative Diseases ISBN: 978-1-63483-399-8
Editors: Giuseppe Legname and Gabriele Giachin

Chapter 7

PRION-LIKE SPREADING OF Aβ AND TAU AGGREGATES AND THEIR RELEVANCE AS DRIVERS OF PATHOLOGY IN ALZHEIMER'S DISEASE

Giuseppe Di Fede, Marcella Catania and Fabrizio Tagliavini*

Fondazione IRCSS "Carlo Besta" Neurological Institute,
Division of Neurology V and Neuropathology, Milan, Italy

ABSTRACT

Misfolding and aggregation of amyloid-β (Aβ) and tau are key events in the pathogenesis of Alzheimer's disease (AD). However, a third essential element is necessary for inducing the full AD pathology, i.e., the intracerebral propagation of abnormal protein aggregates along susceptible neuron networks, which are destroyed by the neurotoxic assemblies. It appears that oligomeric Aβ and phosphorylated-tau "seeds" work together to drive the slow march of AD neuropathology from the vulnerable entorhinal cortex to the upper regions of the cerebral cortex, resulting in the progressive cognitive deterioration observed in AD clinical phenotype. This spreading of pathology is surprisingly similar to what happens in prion diseases where neuropathologic changes are driven by the cell-to-cell propagation of PrP^{Sc} (the abnormal disease-specific conformer of prion protein). Until recently, spreading and transmission of disease by propagation of protein misfolding were thought to be peculiar of prion diseases. However, a series of recent studies provided experimental evidence that 'prion-like' mechanisms underlie the pathological spreading of misfolded proteins in various neurodegenerative diseases, including AD. Furthermore, cell-to-cell transfer appears to be a very early event that gradually induces neurodegenerative pathology, even before the first cell starts to deteriorate. These findings have important implications in the study of molecular mechanisms underlying AD pathogenesis and in the design of strategies to prevent the diffusion of pathology in the brain since the early stages of the disease.

In the present chapter, we will review the evidence supporting the "prion-like" propagation of Aβ and tau seeds in AD, focusing on the missorting and inter-neuronal

* Corresponding Author address: Email: ftagliavini@istituto-besta.it

transfer thereof, the supportive role of cellular dysfunctions that may favor the aggregation and cell-to-cell diffusion of Aβ and tau, the involvement of non-neuronal cells, and the effects of spreading of toxic seeds on synaptic functions. The insights gained from these studies are discussed for their implications in disease progression and their relevance in the development of disease-modifying therapies for AD.

INTRODUCTION

Alzheimer's disease (AD) is neuropathologically characterized by the presence of amyloid plaques and neurofibrillary tangles (NFT) [1, 2]. These neuropathologic hallmarks represent the final result of a series of molecular events that involve misfolding and aggregation of two key proteins: amyloid-β (Aβ) and tau.

Aβ is the cleavage product of a much larger protein, the Amyloid Precursor Protein (APP), by α-, β- and γ-secretases [3]. Aβ deposition in the neuropil leads to the formation of plaques, which are composed of neuronal (neurites and synaptic terminals) and glial (reactive astrocytes and activated microglia) elements, in addition to Aβ aggregates and debris including lipids, zinc/iron/copper ions and various components of the extracellular matrix [4, 5, 6]. The brain topography of Aβ deposition depends on the stage of the disease. According to Braak's schema, it is possible to detect three stages of disease progression: stage A characterized by the presence of amyloid deposits in the ''basal portions'' of the frontal, temporal, and occipital lobes; stage B involving all of the isocortex except the primary cortices, and mildly affecting the hippocampus; and stage C, which is associated with deposits in all areas of the isocortex including the sensory and motor cortices [7]. Thal and others proposed a refinement of this staging system and identified a sequence of involvement that begins with the neocortex and ends with the cerebellum [8].

NFTs are intracellular aggregates of abnormal phosphorylated tau protein that form cytoplasmic fibrils [9]. The first sign of tau pathology in a neuron is the presence of abnormally phosphorylated tau-protein in the axon, soma, and dendrites. At this stage, the neurons are still morphologically normal. Subsequently, fibrillar tau-containing material emerges in the cytoplasm, gradually expanding within the cell soma until the cell dies. After neuronal death occurred, the NFTs appear as extracellular "ghost-tangles" [10]. In addition to NFTs, tau aggregates also occur as neuropil threads within dendrites and as dystrophic neurites in neuritic plaques [11]. NFT pathology consisting of fibrillary tau aggregates initially develop within pyramidal neurons of the transentorhinal region (Braak-NFT-stage I), and expand in a hierarchical sequence to other brain regions [7], the distribution of abnormally phosphorylated tau protein preceding that of NFTs [12].

There is a wide consensus on the close correlation between clinical alterations in AD patients and tau-related rather than amyloid-related pathology. The temporal evolution of the topographic distribution of plaques and NFTs parallels the onset and progression of the neuropsychological deficits [13].

Cerebral amyloid angiopathy (CAA) is the third pathologic feature of AD. It is a disorder affecting leptomeningeal, cortical, and subcortical vessels by the deposition of Aβ within their wall. The distribution of CAA throughout the brain is similar to that of Aβ plaques [12].

The propagation of the neuropathology in AD is generated and sustained by misfolding and spreading of the two main molecular actors involved in the pathogenesis of the disease: Aβ and tau.

While mechanisms underlying the initial misfolding that leads to Aβ and tau aggregation have been deeply investigated, much less is known on the molecular events determining the spreading of misfolded and/or aggregated Aβ and tau and the propagation of their related pathology along the pathways discovered by neuropathological studies. The spreading of AD pathology is very similar to the propagation of brain alterations and dysfunctions occurring in prion diseases where the pathologic changes are driven by the cell-to-cell propagation of PrP^{Sc} (the abnormal disease-specific conformer of prion protein) [14, 15, 16]. These observations support the view that spreading and transmission of disease by propagation of protein misfolding aren't peculiar of prion diseases [17, 18, 19, 20]. Similar prion-like propagation capacities have been suggested also for other neurodegenerative proteins, such as α-synuclein [21, 22].

Here we will focus on the missorting and inter-neuronal transfer of Aβ and tau seeds, the effects of cellular dysfunctions on aggregation and cell-to-cell diffusion of Aβ and tau, the involvement of non-neuronal cells, and the outcome of the intracerebral diffusion of toxic seeds on synaptic functions. These events, occurring very early in the pathogenesis of the disease, provide evidence in favor of a prion-like "nature" of the AD "proteopathic" seeds and have important implications in the identification of targets for disease-modifying therapies against AD.

PROPAGATION OF Aβ- RELATED PATHOLOGY

To be considered as prion-like seeds, misfolded protein aggregates should fulfill at least two conditions: (i) they act as a seed to initiate aggregation by recruiting unfolded or oligomeric species of the same protein in a prion-like mechanism and (ii) they propagate from one cell to another [23].

A "prion-like" mechanism of Aβ pathology propagation is supported by several studies on transgenic mice and primate models showing the induction of Aβ aggregation and the propagation of AD pathology from both injected AD brain extracts [24, 25] and synthetic Aβ [17, 26]. In Tg2576 APP mice (overexpressing human APP carrying the double "Swedish" mutation), which develop amyloid deposits at the age of 9 months, the injection of brain extracts from AD patients, causes an earlier development of Aβ deposits that are around 10-fold more numerous on the injected site [27]. Using injection of different types of brain extracts into various lines of transgenic mice, Meyer-Luehmann et al., could show that the type of deposits that were observed depended both on the agent (that initiated the amyloidogenic process) and the host (that determined the nature of the induced Aβ-deposition), in a manner reminiscent of prion strains [24]. Injection of Aβ-containing brain extracts in the peritoneum also induced amyloid deposition [28]. Intraperitoneal injection required a prolonged incubation time and a larger Aβ inoculum compared with direct intracerebral injection [28]. These observations are evocative of the replication of peripherally applied prions (e.g., following ingestion of contaminated food) and of their propagation within the nervous system. They also infer the ability of Aβ seeds (like infectious prions) to "travel" between different cell types [23]. However, not all these studies have been able to show the induction of propagation by synthetic Aβ [24]. Fibrils formed by synthetic Aβ rarely show seeding capacity [29]. Nevertheless, these data suggest that the ability of transmitting the disease to animals and propagating Aβ-related pathology to adjacent brain areas is different for distinct seeds and may depend on the type of starting seed as well as on the environmental conditions where the spreading of pathology occurs.

Indeed, the molecular mechanisms involved in the transmission of Aβ amyloidosis of Aβ-related pathology among interconnected neurons are poorly known. The neuronal dysfunction induced by Aβ appears to progress trans-synaptically from the neurons in the entorhinal cortex that selectively overexpress APP at the terminal end of the dentate gyrus [30].

Mounting evidence established that formation of Aβ toxic aggregates and deposition of Aβ peptides play key roles in AD pathology [31], and that soluble forms of Aβ oligomers - both extracellular [32] and intracellular [33, 34]- correlate with cognitive impairment and synaptic dysfunction better than insoluble deposits [35, 36]. Intracellular accumulation of soluble Aβ oligomers could come from either Aβ produced intracellularly [37] or Aβ internalized from the extracellular space [38]. Aβ accumulated intracellularly can be transferred from one cell to other connected neurons and may lead to the slow pathological progression that typically occurs in AD [38]. Moreover, even the extracellular Aβ deposits should not be considered as lifeless scars but rather as composite lesions made of a core of Aβ peptides surrounded by a corona of degenerating axons, some of which can be still active. These partially vital axons may contain synaptic vesicles and exhibit cholinesterase activity. The senile plaques, through these axons and synapses, are connected with the contiguous nervous tissue and appear literally innervated [39], hence potentially mediating the transfer of both tau and amyloid pathology to neighbor cells. Their contribution to the propagation of the disease may be favored by dysfunctions in axonal transports, vesicle trafficking and metabolism that are associated with the degenerative process.

The mechanisms involved in this transfer are not yet fully understood. However, previous studies on cell-to-cell transmission with different aggregates suggest that the endosomal–lysosomal pathway or the lysosomal exocytosis process may be involved [40]. It is also known that aging, that is widely recognized as the main risk factor for the development of AD, induces a gradual failure of the degradation systems, thus causing the accumulation of various proteinaceous aggregates [41].

Impairment of proteosomal degradation has also been associated with AD progression because it may lead to intraneuronal accumulations of Aβ aggregates [42, 43, 44]. Additionally, defective Aβ-degrading enzymes and aberrant clearance processes of lipoproteins, ApoE, and low-density lipoprotein receptors play crucial roles in the AD etiology [45]. These findings suggest that the decreased degradation and/or clearance of Aβ are involved in its toxic accumulation and cytotoxic effects [40].

These phenomena could explain how seeds for AD pathology could pass on to new brain areas and gradually induce the AD pathology before cells start to die. This hypothesis is supported by studies demonstrating that oligomers composed of different Aβ-isoforms (including Aβ1-42; Aβ1-40; Aβ 3pyroglutamate-42 and Aβ11-42) can move from cell to cell, and this transfer is conditioned by differential ability to clear and/or degrade distinct oligomeric species. The inadequate clearance of some oligomeric isoforms, such as those mainly composed of Aβ1-42, may lead to larger net accumulations that could promote the cell-to-cell transfer. Interestingly, this transfer is an early event that is seemingly independent of later cellular toxicity, confirming the view that the propagation of amyloid pathology precedes and triggers Aβ-dependent neurotoxicity in AD [40].

It seems that the large prevalence of the Aβ that is gathered intracellularly and is transferred from one cell to another is composed of oligomers mainly accumulating inside the late-endosomes/lysosomes immediately after internalization [40, 46, 47, 48]. Moreover, the intra-lysosomal accumulation of the Aβ species resistant to degradation alters the morphology of lysosomal vesicles and seems to induce cellular starvation and stress that are not paralleled, at least initially, by mitochondrial associated toxicity [40, 49]. However, longer periods of Aβ transfer have been shown to cause endosomal leakage and cytoskeletal damage [38]. These data suggest that cellular transfer might be an early stress response by cells to get rid of intracellular, non-degradable deposition and that only when the intercellular trafficking of Aβ becomes persistent it leads to neurotoxic events.

In general, the potential ability of Aβ species to induce accumulation and transfer to the connected acceptor cells depends on their susceptibility to clearance and/or degradation by cells. Similarly to larger assemblies, the isolated Aβ monomers, dimers and oligomers also participate in cell-to-cell transfer according to their lysosomal accumulations. Purified monomers and dimers are highly unstable and can propagate further to form higher oligomers [50]. However, the lag phase for the aggregation process should be longer for monomers [51], and the monomeric Aβ will be more susceptible to degradation compared to the dimers and oligomers and, as a result, less prone to accumulation and cell-to-cell transfer. In line with these findings, other more degradable isoforms, including oligomers formed by Aβ1–40 or Aβ11–42 have a lower net transfer, and the formation of extra-large lysosomal vesicles is significantly slower [40]. Since only the remaining Aβ aggregates can cause seeding and pathology in the acceptor cells, these results may explain the higher toxic properties of the aggregation-prone and less degradable Aβ1–42.

It is finally conceivable that Aβ intracellular accumulations and their progression from small amounts of non-degradable seeds may take years before causing pathology, supporting the insidious clinical onset and the typical slow progression of AD.

Once a rid of intracellular oligomeric Aβ has been formed, the spread of AD pathology is initiated by a direct transfer of oligomeric Aβ *via* neuron-to-neuron transmission [29, 30, 38] through neuritic contacts between neuronal cells [52]. Transmission of aggregation-prone proteins, including prions, has been suggested to take place in the ER–Golgi pathway and exosomes, but other unconventional secretory pathways may also be involved, including lipid raft/caveolae-mediated endocytic pathway dependent on dynamin or GM1 internalization and, more recently, tunneling nanotubes (TNTs) (for details see in this review the paragraph on common mechanisms of Aβ and tau transfer) [53, 54, 55, 56].

Aβ peptides are generated within neurons through ER–Golgi processing of the APP [57], have been shown to be secreted by neurons upon synaptic stimulation [58, 59, 60] and to be released by cells in association with exosomes [54,61]. Remarkably, exosomal proteins such as Alix [ALG-2 (apoptosis-linked gene 2)-interacting protein X] and flotillin-1 have been found to accumulate in amyloid plaques in the brains of AD patients suggesting that exosomes might play a role in the trafficking of Aβ peptides *in vivo* [54].

Furthermore, oligomeric Aβ was located in vesicles labeled with endosomal and lysosomal markers, suggesting that the transmission of intracellularly aggregated Aβ involves a mechanism of endo- and exocytosis [52, 62]. Macroautophagy is also a possible mechanism for Aβ transfer [44].

Exogenous Aβ42 has also been shown to be internalized in mouse cortical neurons and human neuroblastoma cells (SH-SY5Y cells) and to be delivered to the late endosomes/lysosomal compartment [46]. This process play a role in the intracellular formation of amyloidogenic Aβ aggregates (that could be further delivered to the extracellular space) both by concentrating the internalized peptides in the vesicular lumen and by exposing them to an acidic environment that would facilitate their misfolding and aggregation, leading to lysosome disruption [46, 63]. Moreover, Aβ42 co-localizes with caveolin-1, which is closely associated with lipid rafts and serves as a scaffold protein to coordinate membrane proteins and to regulate cell signaling and caveolae-mediated endocytosis. Altogether these observations suggest that Aβ42 is internalized in neuronal cells endocytic pathway [63].

Interestingly, prion-containing endolysosomal compartments have been shown to fuse with multivesicular bodies, which results in the extracellular release of exosomes containing prions [56, 64]. So, another commonality with prions could be the transfer of Aβ through exocytosis. A very similar mechanism has been proposed also for other misfolded proteins [21, 65, 66], suggesting a common pathway for the spreading of pathology in neurodegenerative disorders.

Other reports have proposed that endocytosis of Aβ42 may be facilitated by the expression on the neuronal cell membranes of different receptors, such as α7 nicotinic acetylcholine receptor [67], N-methyl-D-aspartate (NMDA) receptor [68], low density lipoprotein receptor-related protein 1 (LRP1)/APOE [69] and sortilin, a p75NTR (p75 neurotrophin receptor) co-receptor who shuttles other proteins within the cells [70]. Aβ has been suggested to bind to the cellular prion protein (PrP^C) [71, 72, 73, 74]. It is therefore possible that such binding could trigger Aβ invagination and uptake [52]. The role and relevance of the receptors that have been suggested to bind to Aβ [71, 72, 73, 74] is far to be clear. Since the application of known inhibitors of voltage-gated sodium channels, PrP^C receptors, nAChRs, NMDA or AMPA receptors, did not have significant effects on oligomeric Aβ transmission in highly differentiated neuroblastoma co-cultures, additional studies are required to establish the exact mechanisms of transfer [38].

Overall *in vitro* and *in vivo* evidence suggest that Aβ (especially in the form of oligomers) can drive disease progression, even if the extracellular plaque load is poorly correlated with the degree of cognitive decline [23].

PROPAGATION OF TAU-RELATED PATHOLOGY

In physiological conditions, tau is mainly an axonal protein. In AD and other tauopathies, tau sorting mechanisms fail and tau becomes missorted into the somatodendritic compartment [75]. In AD, aberrant production of amyloid-β might trigger tau missorting [76].

The intraneuronal missorting of tau from axons to the somatodendritic compartment is sustained by progressive abnormal phosphorylation, and by prion-like mechanisms involving folding, and aggregation [77], which are suggested by studies showing that the expression of aggregation-prone mutants of tau can undergo self-assembly and nucleate the co-assembly of endogenous *wild-type* (wt) tau [78]. Given that a polarized tau distribution is important for tau function, several mechanisms have been proposed as key determinants in intracellular tau missorting. They include compartment-specific transport or differential degradation (proteasomal, lysosomal, cytosolic proteases) [79, 80, 81], and they may be protein-based or RNA-based (mRNA transport, translation) [82, 83]. To date, the relevance of such mechanisms is still under debate.

Tau can then spread outside cells and interneuronally. Putative mechanisms include release from one neuron and uptake into another, involving transfer by exo/endocytosis or exosomes [84, 85], but the spreading may also occur by release into the interstitial fluid and subsequent diffusion [86].

If the transferred tau carries a pathological aggregation-prone conformation (for example as an oligomer with β-structure), this may cause the nucleation and aggregation of tau in the receiving neurons [77]. This process clearly infers the concept of a 'prion-like' propagation of tau pathology.

Internalization of tau exosomes in recipient cells has still to be demonstrated. However, tau aggregates have been shown to be internalized *via* fluid-phase internalization. The endocytic process seems to be dynamin-dependent and to involve small oligomers, but not long fibrils or monomers. It is not possible to exclude a role for other endocytic pathways, e.g., receptor-mediated, clathrin-dependent and caveolae-mediated endocytosis in different cell types. Once internalized, tau localizes along the endocytic pathway from which it must escape in order to gain access to the cytosol, but the molecular bases of such passage are unknown [23].

Most scientific data show that the neurofibrillary pathology progresses with time as does the amyloid pathology, through interneuronal connections but only through specific systems of connections [1]. At the early phase of Alzheimer's pathology, the neurofibrillary lesions are exquisitely limited to the enthorinal region and the axons constituting the crown of the senile plaque are necessarily issued from an enthorinal cell body, which has a high probability of bearing a neurofibrillary tangle. Later, the number of senile plaques located in that specific area decreases, leaving way to vacuoles of spongiosis, while new plaques are found in cerebral regions directly connected with the previous ones, suggesting a stepwise spreading of amyloid and tau pathologies where amyloid lesions precede and support the further diffusion of tau-related lesions [1, 2, 39]. Over the past years, this hypothesis have been supported by *in vivo* and *in vitro* studies showing the cell-to-cell propagation of tau filaments [65, 87], induction of NFT-like tau inclusions by injection into the brains of mutant tau transgenic mice of both pure synthetic tau fibrils and tau oligomers isolated from AD brains [88, 89].

Moreover, injection of P301S mouse brain homogenates containing numerous tau filaments into the hippocampus and the overlying cerebral cortex of ALZ17 mice (expressing the longest normal human tau isoform), that never develop tau deposits, induces the assembly of wt human tau of ALZ17 mice into filaments in the form of NFT and oligodendroglial coiled bodies. Induced tau aggregates are not restricted to the injection sites but progress over time to anatomically connected brain regions [87, 90, 91].

Interestingly, the intracerebral injection of different types of tau seeds into ALZ17 mice resulted in the induction of tau-related pathology recapitulating the features of the original source [92]. So, injection of Progressive Supranuclear Palsy (PSP) brain homogenates resulted in the formation of silver-positive astrocytic aggregates that resembled tufted astrocytes (the hallmark lesions of PSP) [93, 94]; injection of Corticobasal Degeneration (CBD) homogenates gave rise to the formation of silver-positive structures reminiscent of the astrocytic plaques found in CBD [95]; injection of Argyrophilic Grain Disease (AGD) homogenates resulted in the formation of silver-negative astrocytic tau pathology as observed in human AGD [96]. Similar inclusions also formed after intracerebral injection of brain homogenates from human tauopathies into non-transgenic mice [92]. These findings confirm that the specific features of different tauopathies, including AD, are consistent with the existence of tau strains [97, 98, 99], likewise classical prion diseases [92]. This series of experiments also suggests that the wt protein of the host may take an abnormal conformation, at the contact of the injected misfolded protein – the process described by Prusiner as characteristic of prion diseases [100, 101].

To stay within the AD field, Lasagna-Reeves and others have demonstrated that soluble tau oligomers extracted from AD brains and injected into the hippocampi of three month-old wt C57BL/6 mice could disseminate the neuropathology from endogenously produced taues [88]. Thus, tau oligomers seem to act *via* a prion-like mechanism, which is strikingly pertinent to AD.

Furthermore, a seed-dependent polymerization of tau has been demonstrated in studies showing that intracellular tau misfolds after contact with extracellular tau aggregates, is able to seed further aggregation and can move between co-cultured cells [65, 102]. Moreover, filaments made of either wt or mutant tau adopt distinct conformations that are maintained *via* a templated conformational change [103], and that tau filament formation occurs through a nucleation-dependent polymerization mechanism evocative of prion diseases [104]. As for transfer of Aβ assemblies, the intracellular entry of tau filaments seems to occur through endocytosis [105]. Altogether, these data support the view that movement of misfolded tau between cells is responsible for disease propagation [96].

COMMON MECHANISMS IN THE PROPAGATION OF Aβ- AND TAU-RELATED PATHOLOGIES

The causal relationship between Aβ and tau pathology in AD is still widely questioned [106, 107] and a review of the data on this scientific debate goes beyond the intention of this chapter. However, in this context it is intriguing that both misfolded proteins may follow common pathological pathways, some of which strongly evoke prion-like mechanisms, and may act in concert to propagate neurodegeneration and to cause synaptic pathology in AD [108].

Strikingly, in neuronal cell cultures, tau missorting and synapse loss is readily reversed (within 12 h) once the toxic stimuli (which may include Aβ oligomers) disappear [109]. This implies that the progression of tau pathology can be halted or even reversed, but the conditions for achieving this desirable result for the human disease are still largely unknown [77].

Among mechanisms involved in cell-to-cell transfer of both Aβ and tau aggregates, a particular relevance has been ascribed to TNTs. TNTs were discovered only a few years ago as a novel form of cell-to-cell communication [110]. They have been found in many cell types, from neuronal cells and primary cells to immune and epithelial cells in culture, acting as conduits for the exchange of cytosolic and membrane-bound molecules and organelles, as well as for the spreading of pathogens. In particular, they have been shown to transfer viruses and bacteria as well as proteinaceous aggregates linked to several neurodegenerative diseases [111, 112]. Both inside transit of vesicles and organelles (endosomes, lysosomes, mitochondria, Golgi and ER), as well as surfing of cargoes on the extracellular TNT membrane or in the intracellular leaflet have been reported [112], suggesting a key role of these structures in cell-to-cell transfer and communication [23].

Aβ and tau are packaged into endocytic vesicles upon internalization in receiving cells. However, in order to exert their seeding activity a mechanism that allows them to gain access to the cytosol is required. As for α-synuclein, studies conducted on phospholipid bilayers demonstrated the ability of Aβ40 and Aβ42 to intercalate into the phospholipid bilayer of the plasma membrane mainly by establishing electrostatic interactions between charged peptide residues and lipid head groups [113, 114]. Interestingly, a study by Nath et al., has shown the importance of direct cell–cell contact in the transmission of Aβ soluble oligomeric species in an *in vitro* co-culture of primary rat hippocampal neurons and human neuroblastoma cells, which resulted in progressive cytotoxicity of the acceptor cells after 3 days of co-culture with the cell population producing Aβ [38]. Furthermore, Wang et al., [62] have shown that extracellular Aβ, once internalized in primary astrocytes, is found in TNTs established with co-cultured neurons. TNTs are thin actin-rich membrane bridges connecting the cytoplasm of distant cells [110], thereby allowing intercellular exchange of cell components, but also of pathogens [111, 112]. Their involvement in the intercellular spreading of prions has already been shown [55, 115]. Therefore it is possible that TNTs act as transport conduits for other prion-like protein aggregates and their toxic signals [23].

How Aβ aggregates are transported along TNTs is not clear. Following uptake, endocytic vesicles containing Aβ might shuttle within TNT structures. Alternatively, Aβ oligomers could surf along TNTs upon insertion in the lipid bilayer. Further study is required to specifically address this question. Remarkably, even tau short fibrils have been detected within TNTs between neuronal suggesting a more general role for TNTs in the spreading of protein aggregates [23].

Involvement of Non-Neuronal Cells

It has been assumed that only neurons make and spread Aβ and tau seeds as toxic drivers of AD pathology, whereas their associated astrocytes are considered just bystanders/scavengers. But this view is likely to radically change by increasing findings revealing the existence of a vital neuron-astrocyte teamwork that can become dangerously disruptive. In this view, when Aβ42 production in neurons exceeds the safe limit, toxic Aβ42 oligomers may spill out of the neuronal cells and onto their enveloping astrocytes and/or may disperse in the extracellular milieu. This diffusion is favored by the fact that both cell types are endowed with an intricate fence of Aβ42 oligomer-binding receptors [116]. Talantova et al., demonstrated that Aβ oligomers released by neurons can directly bind to the α-7nAChRs of their partner astrocytes [117]. As a result, the signals from these receptors induce the astrocytes to exocytose the glutamate they have swept up from the neuronal synapses [117]. The discharged glutamate activates the extrasynaptic NMDARs of the astrocytes' partner neurons. The resulting signals alter Ca^{2+} homeostasis evoking a cascade of events, including dysfunctional mitochondria pumping out ROS, which cause oxidative damage destroying neuronal synapses and severing communications within the astrocyte's neurons client group and beyond [118]. These data suggest that the spreading of Aβ-dependent pathology in AD is the result of a neuron-astrocyte collaboration [116], rather than a suicidal act of neurons that progressively accumulate misfolded/aggregated Aβ peptides and transfer them to the connected cells [119].

Furthermore, in this intricate teamwork connecting neurons and astrocytes, a relevant role is attributed even to surrounding vascular cells [120]. Indeed, one foremost anatomical feature unique to the cerebral microvasculature is its extensive and intimate network of interactions with neurons and glia [121, 122, 123, 124]. Perivascular neurons, glia (astrocytes, microglia, and oligodendrocytes), and vascular cells (endothelial cells, smooth muscle cells, and pericytes) are structurally juxtaposed, capable of secreting multiple neuroactive and vasoactive substances, functionally interconnected, forming the basis for cerebral homeostasis and the regulation of the cerebral micro-environment [125, 126]. Therefore, the term "neurovascular unit" highlights the integrated structural and functional relationship among these cell types [120].

Normally functioning neurons, glia, and endothelial cells of the neurovascular unit each secrete a complex array of peptides and bioactive factors that when misregulated may contribute to alter homeostasis in adjacent cells. By recognizing these cellular subtypes together as an integrated functional unit, we may better understand the initiation and "spreading" mechanisms common to many neurological disorders, such as AD, and other related neurodegenerative diseases with cerebral vascular involvement. To this regard, it's interesting to remember here the role of activated glial cells in the pathogenesis of AD. Microglia, functioning as cerebral macrophages, can recruit and stimulate astrocytes; however, unlike astrocytes, microglia are more likely to be activated by fibrillary Aβ peptides and the "mature" forms of Aβ peptides associated with senile plaques [120]. Activated microglia also produce toxins and pro-inflammatory cytokines such as IL-1β, IL-6, and TNF-α; the chemokine IL-8, macrophage inflammatory proteins; MCP-1; growth factor macrophage-colony stimulating factor; and pentraxins [127, 128]. These toxins and inflammatory factors, secreted by both astrocytes and microglia, further trigger inflammatory cascades, thereby exacerbating conditions in AD brain that may be either pathogenic or beneficial [128].

Interestingly, both astrocytes and microglia function in an attempt to remove Aβ deposits through either phagocytosis or enzymatic degradation [129, 130]. Moreover, after exposure of cerebral vasculature to Aβ peptides, endothelial angiogenic processes appear to be targeted, and soluble Aβ peptides also induce significant production of ROS in endothelial cells, generating oxidative stress within the cerebral vascular lining [131, 132].

Overall these factors may result in dysfunction of cell membrane permeability, cell-to-cell transfer mechanisms and clearance of misfolded/aggregated peptides, leading to a "pain chain" that can amplifies the effects of Aβ and tau spreading pathologies. Indeed, the set of inflammatory mediators and toxins produced within the neurovascular network may collectively support a neuroinflammatory cascade that can kill neurons and further damage the integrity of the neurovascular unit, which in turn induces progressive release of toxic products, potentially enabling "spreading effects" among susceptible cell types [120, 133].

Similar conclusions could be applied to the spreading of tau-related pathology in AD. As discussed above, the concept of trans-synaptically transmittable, prion-like, oligomeric tau "seeds" has been claimed during the last few years by several groups [87, 134, 135, 136]. However, the results of other studies point to rule out that hyperphosphorylated tau proteins can cross synaptic terminals as do prions [137].

On the other hand, recent studies have reported that human tau can be secreted by neurons but also non-neuronal cells when it was overexpressed indicating that tau secretion could contribute to the spreading of tau pathology in the brain and could lead to its accumulation in the CSF [138]. These data suggest that, similarly to Aβ, cells other than neurons may participate in the spreading of tau pathology through secretory rather than trans-synaptic pathways, the last anyway representing the "highway" of tau pathology propagation.

The majority of tau aggregates in AD brains are made by tau holoproteins [139]. They also contain a minority of tau species cleaved by an activated caspase-3/7 and by calpain in neurons exposed to Aβ and to various proinflammatory cytokines released by astrocytes and microglia [140]. The same cytokines also intensify the Aβ-triggered pathological phosphorylation of tau [141]. Being more aggregation-prone than full-length tau, these truncated phosphotau forms likely accelerate the generation of NFTs [142, 143] and/or are released extracellularly where they are taken up by neurons [144]. They can be internalized by massive endocytosis into the somatodentritic compartment or the axon terminals and thenceforth be carried by the anterograde or retrograde transports.

In summary, toxic tau "seeds" or their derivatives can be spread from degenerated neurons to normal neurons *via* exosomes or axonal varicosities or synapses or maybe other means. Nevertheless, the hyperphosphorylated tau buildup triggered in a neuron by the accumulating Aβ oligomers may induce an Aβ-independent spreading wave of "contagious" exosomes or other vectors loaded with toxic phosphotau proteins [145].

In other words, the two neurotoxic "seeds" can at some point go their own toxic ways in an AD brain, through diffusion in the astrocyte-neuron network, following both interneuronal transynaptic pathways and neuron-glial transfer. A recent study by Dal Prà and others [116] supported this hypothesis by demonstrating that normal human astrocytes freshly isolated from adult cerebral cortex can be induced by exogenous Aβ25-35, an Aβ42 proxy, to make and secrete increased amounts of endogenous Aβ42.

Role of Cellular Dysfunctions and Environmental Modifications in the Propagation of Aβ and Tau Seeds

The propagation of toxic seeds of Aβ and tau to connected cells and their catalyzing effect to induce further aggregates, in a prion-like "fashion," is receiving increasing consensus [26, 146]. However, the prion theory for pathology propagation ignores many other influencing factors in the AD etiology [147]. Many of these factors, including dietary cholesterol, metabolic disorders, ApoE lipoprotein, low-density lipoprotein receptors and insufficient lysosomal-proteosomal and insulin-degrading enzymes [148], influence cellular clearance or degradation systems and have a relevant impact on AD pathology. The role of such factors not necessarily is independent and unrelated with prion-like mechanisms. On the contrary, most of these factors can create the conditions that favor misfolding, missorting, aggregation of Aβ and tau, and cell-to-cell propagation of their seeds.

The inability to clear and/or degrade more resistant isoforms, such as oligomeric Aβ and tau, leads to larger net accumulations that could promote the cell-to-cell transfer [40].

The involvement of lysosomal system in the seeding and spreading of Aβ and tau has been discussed in the previous sections of this chapter.

Evidence from multiple neurodegenerative disease models indicated proteasome dysfunction as a key molecular event in the neurotoxicity mediated by protein aggregates. Tau assemblies as well as Aβ oligomers can functionally impact cell homeostasis by forming proteasome-blocking complexes [149]. Activation of the immunoproteasome together with variable alterations of the different protease activities of the ubiquitin-proteasome system can be induced by modifications in the production of β-amyloid and have important implications in the pathogenesis of AD [150, 151, 152].

Neurons, glia, and endothelial cells secrete various peptides and bio-active factors that may alter the homeostatic function in adjacent brain cell types *via* paracrine effects and under non-homeostatic conditions, one brain cell type has considerable potential to contribute to coordinated dysfunction of the neurovascular unit.

Indeed, if exposed to brief periods of hypoxia, human brain microvessel endothelial cells (hBMECs) have been shown to induce rapid and dramatic changes in homeostatic gene expression patterns in human primary neural cells *in vitro* [153, 154]. Moreover, hypoxia-stressed hBMECs were found to secrete significantly more IL-1β than age-matched controls [155, 156]. In turn, IL-1β secreted at physiological concentrations from hBMECs was found to induce Aβ42 peptide secretion when added at the same concentrations to HN cells [120].

These data strengthen the concept that non-homeostatic paracrine interactions among neurons, glia, and endothelial cells may contribute to Aβ42-mediated pathogenic processes, and these may be important in interneural cell signaling and cell-to-cell "spreading effects" characteristic of chronic, inflammatory, and degenerative brain disease [157], including AD [158].

Strikingly, a recent study showed the existence of individually distinct Aβ fibril conformations in AD patients, depending on the type of AD pathology found [159]. These results, together with data from other studies [160], suggest the existence of distinct types of Aβ seeds and imply that the stochastically induced multiple nucleated Aβ seeds *in vivo* could have been eliminated by amyloid clearance mechanisms. However, individuals with decreased clearance efficiency could have failed to degrade a particular type of seed leading to propagation of pathology with distinct Aβ fibril conformations [40, 159]. In this perspective, degradation and clearance of toxic products such as non-degradable Aβ and tau seeds may represent mechanisms that can even determine the type of seed that will spread to neighbor cells.

In this view, that still needs supportive experimental data, the strain-like features of AD-related proteins could be the results of:

1. an interaction between intrinsic prion-like Aβ and tau misfolding properties, and
2. specific micro-environmental conditions, which can act by selecting a particular seed among those stochastically generated by protein misfolding.

This still hypothetical process is at least in part reminiscent of what happens for prion strains [100, 161].

EFFECTS OF Aβ AND TAU TOXIC SEEDS ON SYNAPTIC FUNCTIONS

The spread of neurodegenerative diseases through protein misfolding appears to be a truly generic phenomenon. However, spreading of misfolded protein is not evidence of neurodegeneration, and this raises critical questions about the link between transmission of pathological proteins and their neurotoxic effects [162]. Indeed, the existence of a direct relationship between propagation of protein aggregates and neurotoxicity remains elusive [23]. In most neurodegenerative diseases protein deposition does not appear to be associated with neuronal dysfunction and degeneration [163, 164]. On the other hand, several studies suggest that the formation of large protein aggregates is beneficial for cell survival [23]. Recent studies have even revealed that amyloids may also play beneficial roles in cells [165]. Cellular processes that could be regulated by amyloids are diverse and include translational regulation, programmed cell death and protein storage. These data put forward the intriguing hypothesis that distinct types of amyloid, including the one formed by prions, are used by cells for physiological processes [165, 166, 167, 168, 169, 170].

However, there is a huge of data in favor of a relevant role of Aβ and tau aggregates in neurotoxicity associated with AD. In particular, there is increasing evidence of correlations between intraneuronal oligomeric Aβ1–42 and synaptic dysfunction, subcellular pathology, and cell death before the development of extracellular amyloid deposits [33, 34, 171].

Aβ oligomers might lead to synaptic damage by forming pore-like structures with channel activity; alterations in glutamate receptors; circuitry hyper-excitability; mitochondrial dysfunction; lysosomal failure and alterations in signaling pathways related to synaptic plasticity, neuronal cell and neurogenesis. A number of signaling proteins, including fyn kinase; glycogen synthase kinase-3beta (GSK3beta) and cyclin-dependent kinase-5 (CDK5), are involved in the neurodegenerative progression of AD and are linked with Aβ [172] and tau [173, 174].

It is intriguing that both Aβ and tau share with prions most of their neurotoxic mechanisms [175]. A sudden, abrupt reduction in the number of synaptic proteins has been found correlated with increasing prion replication and rising levels of misfolded PrP in animal models [162]. This critical reduction in both synapse number and neurotransmission results in cognitive decline and is closely followed by neuronal loss [176]. The reduction in synaptic protein levels was also correlated with dysfunction of the ubiquitin-proteasome pathway causing a reduction, in protein degradation [177]. The involvement of the unfolded protein response (UPR) has been recognized as a relevant mechanism in the pathogenesis of prion diseases [162]. The UPR is a protective cellular mechanism that is induced during periods of cellular and endoplasmic reticulum stress, which aims to maintain protein-folding homeostasis. UPR is activated in prion disease, inhibiting protein translation and leading to a reduction in the levels of synaptic proteins. Interestingly, increased levels of UPR activation have been described in the brains of Alzheimer disease, Parkinson disease, and prion disease patients [140].

A recent study highlighted the relevance of Aβ1–42 transfer in neurodegeneration observed in AD that is not observed in cells without Aβ1–42 oligomers. The intracellular accumulation of oligomeric Aβ, as an effect of cell-to-cell transfer, results in progressive tubulin beading, a sign of axonal damage [38, 178]. Prion-like intercellular spread and amplification of protein misfolding may be triggered by internalized Aβ and tau oligomers that can increase the accumulation of newly synthesized Aβ [179, 180] and act as seeds for aggregation of endogenous proteins [140]. Thus, it is possible that Aβ transfer could not only cause additional seeding of Aβ oligomerization but might also result in subsequent tau pathology, thereby spreading neurodegeneration to anatomically connected brain areas [38].

Indeed, Aβ accumulation (most likely the intracellular soluble oligomeric form) has been indicated as the *primum movens* that precedes tau-related neurotoxicity [31], triggers tau-dependent pathology and then cooperates with tau in driving the disease [33, 34, 145, 171]. The propagation of AD pathology along the vulnerable brain networks results in reduction of the number of spines and inhibition of synaptic plasticity in neurons [71]. Neuronal dysfunctions induced by Aβ can progress trans-synaptically from the neurons in the entorhinal cortex that selectively overexpress APP at the terminal end of the dentate gyrus [30], suggesting a selective vulnerability of these neuronal network whose molecular bases are far to be elucidated [137], and increasing the overlaps between the pathogenic mechanisms common to prions and AD-related proteins [181].

With regard to these commonalities and the presence of a cross-talking between PrP and Aβ in the pathogenesis of AD, several authors showed that: *(i)* pathologic effects of Aβ can be mediated by binding to PrP^C [140]; *(ii)* the positioning of endoproteolytic processing events of APP by pathologic (β-cleavage + γ-cleavage) and non-pathologic (α-cleavage + γ-cleavage) secretase pathways is paralleled by analogous α- and β-like cleavage of PrP^C [182], *(iii)* PrP^C and APP processing machinery occur in similar lipid raft environments [183, 184]; *(iv)* there are overlaps in repertoire of the PrP^C and APP protein "interactors" [185, 186]. Extracellular applications of aggregated forms of both PrP and Aβ have been shown to induce electrophysiological changes in neuronal cells that could result in a disruption of ionic homeostasis, cell dysfunction and eventual cell death [187, 188, 189]. Of particular relevance to AD, an identical suite of ionic channels in cholinergic basal forebrain neurons are modulated by both an internal (106–126) PrP peptide and soluble oligomeric Aβ1–42 [190, 191].

Furthermore, the effects of Aβ1–42 in depressing potassium conductances in such neurons are absent in animals that do not express PrP^C and the PrP-Aβ interactions in neurons from wt mice can be blocked by a PrP antibody [192]. Freir et al., [193] reported that standardized Aβ-derived diffusible ligand (ADDL) preparations disrupt hippocampal synaptic plasticity in a PrP-dependent manner and that Aβ obtained from *ex vivo* human material does the same. Furthermore, using monoclonal antibodies directed at two different PrP^C epitopes, these and other authors successfully blocked the Aβ-mediated disruption of synaptic plasticity [182, 194].

According to the results from several studies [88,195,196], tau oligomers may be the most toxic form and the species responsible for the synaptopathy in AD. In line with this view, it has been reported that specific targeting of tau oligomers in animal models can prevent cognitive impairment and tau toxicity induced by injection with tau oligomeric seeds [197]. In AD, tau becomes hyperphosphorylated and misfolded at both presynaptic and postsynaptic terminals. Synaptic tau seems to be hyperphosphorylated and ubiquitinated, and forms stable oligomers resistant to SDS denaturation. The accumulation of hyperphosphorylated tau oligomers at human AD synapses is associated with increased ubiquitinated substrates and increased proteasome components, consistent with dysfunction of the ubiquitin-proteasome system, leading to disruption of synapses [198]. Oligomers of recombinant full-length human tau protein have been shown to be neurotoxic *in vivo* after subcortical stereotaxic injection into mice. Tau oligomers impair memory consolidation, whereas tau fibrils and monomers do not. Additionally, tau oligomers induce synaptic dysfunction by reducing the levels of synaptic vesicle-associated proteins synaptophysin and septin-11. Furthermore, tau oligomers produce mitochondrial dysfunction by interfering with electron transport chain complex I and caspase-9 [199].

It seems that Aβ and tau, especially their oligomeric forms, work together to decrease the density of dendritic spines and alter their morphology in AD. These changes appear to be reversible by a large variety of treatments or simply by the removal of Aβ [78, 200]. Since it is clear that interventions that restore spine density and morphology to normal levels also cause behavioral and electrophysiological alterations to return to normal levels, it would be conceivable that treatments than can maintain spine density and integrity might slow the intellectual alterations seen in AD.

Conclusion

The mechanisms of how misfolded seeds spread in the brain are not clear and are probably different depending on whether aggregates accumulate intra- or extra-cellularly [201]. In one hand, Aβ and prion aggregates are mostly located outside the cell, so a strong extracellular component present in their spread is suggested. On the other hand, tau aggregates accumulate inside the cytoplasm and thus transference likely requires some type of cell contacts, such as through synapses or TNTs [140]. Indeed, trans-cellular spread has been described for these proteins, which may explain why pathological changes progress in a hierarchical manner during the disease [7]. However, these intracellular aggregates can also be secreted alone or within exosomes, thus an extracellular factor for the dispersion of these molecules cannot be discarded.

No human epidemiological studies support the idea of inter-individual transmission of Aβ and tau pathologies, and a recent report provided evidence against this possibility [202]. However, it is important to highlight that epidemiological tracking of an infectious origin for these diseases would be complicated by the multifactorial nature of these illnesses, the many risk factors and co-morbidities and the likely variable and extended time between exposure to the infectious agent and the onset of clinical symptoms [203]. Actually, in the case of typical human TSEs this interval can be decades [204]. Further research involving detailed and carefully controlled epidemiological studies and more specific experiments in animal models should clarify whether inter-individual transmission may occur in humans, or is restricted to artificial experimental conditions.

It appears that oligomeric Aβ42 and phospho-tau "seeds" tandemly drive the long lasting slow march of sporadic AD neuropathology from the vulnerable entorhinal layer II neurons [205] to upper cognitive regions of the cerebral cortex. The initiators of this spreading pathology are "contagious" Aβ42 oligomers temporally followed by accumulated phospho-tau oligomers [116]. Both kinds of "seeds" are then widely spread along the entorhinal-dentate gyral perforant pathway and beyond by the oligomer making and oligomer exchanging, closely inter-digitating members of neuron-astrocyte networks. A huge of data indicate that both Aβ and tau oligomers are localized at synaptic level where they exert their main toxic effects. Hence, the most urgent task is finding a way to stop or prevent the endocerebral diffusion of both kinds of oligomers, particularly of the initiating Aβ42 oligomers [116].

In the same line, the prion-like replication of misfolding proteins in AD suggest that strategies aimed at trapping and inactivating oligomers could be useful to stop the progression of pathological features. Additionally, the recent results showing that peripheral administration of seeds are able to induce brain pathology [28, 92] support the idea that an active cross-talk between the brain and the periphery occurs in AD. In this sense, modifications of current therapeutic strategies, such as vaccinations and peripheral sink approaches could be and should be importantly improved [203].

Interestingly, data from several studies placed Aβ upstream of tau in AD pathogenesis and indicated tau as an essential protein in development of the disease [206, 207, 208]. Traditionally, these Aβ-tau connections are supposed to be indirect, but there is also evidence for a direct pathogenic connection between the two proteins. Indeed, Aβ can bind to tau [209] and tau monomers can be induced to oligomerize *in vitro* after exposure to low substoichiometric levels of Aβ oligomers [210]. Hence, the intriguing possibility that, *in vivo*, Aβ oligomers seed the initial formation of tau oligomers, which can then self-propagate in the absence of additional input from Aβ [175]. This hypothesis might explain the failure of the Aβ targeting clinical trials whose experimental treatments start long after tau pathology is already well underway, Aβ-independent and self-sustaining [175].

In conclusion, the increasing knowledge collected for prions can be constructively applied to Aβ and tau, which share similar mechanisms of conformational changes and pathology propagation, in order to identify the best molecular targets for therapeutic interventions and prevention strategies in AD.

REFERENCES

[1] Duyckaerts C, Delatour B, Potier MC (2009) Classification and basic pathology of Alzheimer disease. *Acta Neuropathol* 118: 5-36.

[2] Hyman BT, Phelps CH, Beach TG, Bigio EH, Cairns NJ, et al. (2012) National Institute on Aging-Alzheimer's Association guidelines for the neuropathologic assessment of Alzheimer's disease. *Alzheimers Dement* 8: 1-13.

[3] Selkoe DJ (2001) Presenilin, Notch, and the genesis and treatment of Alzheimer's disease. *Proc Natl Acad Sci USA* 98: 11039-11041.

[4] Dickson DW, Crystal HA, Bevona C, Honer W, Vincent I, et al. (1995) Correlations of synaptic and pathological markers with cognition of the elderly. *Neurobiol Aging* 16: 285-298; discussion 298-304.

[5] Metsaars WP, Hauw JJ, van Welsem ME, Duyckaerts C (2003) A grading system of Alzheimer disease lesions in neocortical areas. *Neurobiol Aging* 24: 563-572.

[6] Di Fede G, Giaccone G, Tagliavini F (2013) Hereditary and sporadic beta-amyloidoses. *Front Biosci* (Landmark Ed) 18: 1202-1226.

[7] Braak H, Braak E (1991) Neuropathological stageing of Alzheimer-related changes. *Acta Neuropathol* 82: 239-259.

[8] Thal DR, Rüb U, Orantes M, Braak H (2002) Phases of A beta-deposition in the human brain and its relevance for the development of AD. *Neurology* 58: 1791-1800.

[9] Braak E, Braak H, Mandelkow EM (1994) A sequence of cytoskeleton changes related to the formation of neurofibrillary tangles and neuropil threads. *Acta Neuropathol* 87: 554-567.

[10] Bancher C, Brunner C, Lassmann H, Budka H, Jellinger K, et al. (1989) Accumulation of abnormally phosphorylated tau precedes the formation of neurofibrillary tangles in Alzheimer's disease. *Brain Res* 477: 90-99.

[11] Braak H, Braak E (1988) Neuropil threads occur in dendrites of tangle-bearing nerve cells. *Neuropathol Appl Neurobiol* 14: 39-44.

[12] Thal DR, Attems J, Ewers M (2014) Spreading of amyloid, tau, and microvascular pathology in Alzheimer's disease: findings from neuropathological and neuroimaging studies. *J Alzheimers Dis 42 Suppl* 4: S421-429.

[13] Storey E, Slavin MJ, Kinsella GJ (2002) Patterns of cognitive impairment in Alzheimer's disease: assessment and differential diagnosis. *Front Biosci* 7: e155-184.

[14] Prusiner SB (1982) Novel proteinaceous infectious particles cause scrapie. *Science* 216: 136-144.

[15] Selvaggini C, De Gioia L, Cantù L, Ghibaudi E, Diomede L, et al. (1993) Molecular characteristics of a protease-resistant, amyloidogenic and neurotoxic peptide homologous to residues 106-126 of the prion protein. *Biochem Biophys Res Commun* 194: 1380-1386.

[16] Capobianco R, Casalone C, Suardi S, Mangieri M, Miccolo C, et al. (2007) Conversion of the BASE prion strain into the BSE strain: the origin of BSE? *PLoS Pathog* 3: e31.

[17] Jucker M, Walker LC (2013) Self-propagation of pathogenic protein aggregates in neurodegenerative diseases. *Nature* 501: 45-51.

[18] Guo JL, Lee VM (2014) Cell-to-cell transmission of pathogenic proteins in neurodegenerative diseases. *Nat Med* 20: 130-138.

[19] Fraser PE (2014) Prions and prion-like proteins. *J Biol Chem* 289: 19839-19840.

[20] Aguzzi A, Rajendran L (2009) The transcellular spread of cytosolic amyloids, prions, and prionoids. *Neuron* 64: 783-790.

[21] Desplats P, Lee HJ, Bae EJ, Patrick C, Rockenstein E, et al. (2009) Inclusion formation and neuronal cell death through neuron-to-neuron transmission of alpha-synuclein. *Proc Natl Acad Sci USA* 106: 13010-13015.

[22] Oueslati A, Ximerakis M, Vekrellis K (2014) Protein Transmission, Seeding and Degradation: Key Steps for α-Synuclein Prion-Like Propagation. *Exp Neurobiol* 23: 324-336.

[23] Costanzo M, Zurzolo C (2013) The cell biology of prion-like spread of protein aggregates: mechanisms and implication in neurodegeneration. *Biochem J* 452: 1-17.

[24] Meyer-Luehmann M, Coomaraswamy J, Bolmont T, Kaeser S, Schaefer C, et al. (2006) Exogenous induction of cerebral beta-amyloidogenesis is governed by agent and host. *Science* 313: 1781-1784.

[25] Ridley RM, Baker HF, Windle CP, Cummings RM (2006) Very long term studies of the seeding of beta-amyloidosis in primates. *J Neural Transm* 113: 1243-1251.

[26] Stöhr J, Watts JC, Mensinger ZL, Oehler A, Grillo SK, et al. (2012) Purified and synthetic Alzheimer's amyloid beta (Aβ) prions. *Proc Natl Acad Sci USA* 109: 11025-11030.

[27] Kane MD, Lipinski WJ, Callahan MJ, Bian F, Durham RA, et al. (2000) Evidence for seeding of beta -amyloid by intracerebral infusion of Alzheimer brain extracts in beta - amyloid precursor protein-transgenic mice. *J Neurosci* 20: 3606-3611.

[28] Eisele YS, Obermüller U, Heilbronner G, Baumann F, Kaeser SA, et al. (2010) Peripherally applied Abeta-containing inoculates induce cerebral beta-amyloidosis. *Science* 330: 980-982.

[29] Langer F, Eisele YS, Fritschi SK, Staufenbiel M, Walker LC, et al. (2011) Soluble Aβ seeds are potent inducers of cerebral β-amyloid deposition. *J Neurosci* 31: 14488-14495.

[30] Harris JA, Devidze N, Verret L, Ho K, Halabisky B, et al. (2010) Transsynaptic progression of amyloid-β-induced neuronal dysfunction within the entorhinal-hippocampal network. *Neuron* 68: 428-441.

[31] Hardy J, Selkoe DJ (2002) The amyloid hypothesis of Alzheimer's disease: progress and problems on the road to therapeutics. *Science* 297: 353-356.

[32] Benilova I, Karran E, De Strooper B (2012) The toxic Aβ oligomer and Alzheimer's disease: an emperor in need of clothes. *Nat Neurosci* 15: 349-357.

[33] Gouras GK, Willén K, Tampellini D (2012) Critical role of intraneuronal Aβ in Alzheimer's disease: technical challenges in studying intracellular Aβ. *Life Sci* 91: 1153-1158.

[34] LaFerla FM, Green KN, Oddo S (2007) Intracellular amyloid-beta in Alzheimer's disease. *Nat Rev Neurosci* 8: 499-509.

[35] Brouillette J, Caillierez R, Zommer N, Alves-Pires C, Benilova I, et al. (2012) Neurotoxicity and memory deficits induced by soluble low-molecular-weight amyloid-β1-42 oligomers are revealed in vivo by using a novel animal model. *J Neurosci* 32: 7852-7861.

[36] Selkoe DJ (2008) Soluble oligomers of the amyloid beta-protein impair synaptic plasticity and behavior. *Behav Brain Res* 192: 106-113.

[37] Wirths O, Multhaup G, Czech C, Blanchard V, Moussaoui S, et al. (2001) Intraneuronal Abeta accumulation precedes plaque formation in beta-amyloid precursor protein and presenilin-1 double-transgenic mice. *Neurosci Lett* 306: 116-120.

[38] Nath S, Agholme L, Kurudenkandy FR, Granseth B, Marcusson J, et al. (2012) Spreading of neurodegenerative pathology via neuron-to-neuron transmission of β-amyloid. *J Neurosci* 32: 8767-8777.

[39] Duyckaerts C (2013) Neurodegenerative lesions: seeding and spreading. *Rev Neurol* (Paris) 169: 825-833.

[40] Domert J, Rao SB, Agholme L, Brorsson AC, Marcusson J, et al. (2014) Spreading of amyloid-β peptides via neuritic cell-to-cell transfer is dependent on insufficient cellular clearance. *Neurobiol Dis* 65: 82-92.

[41] Villeda SA, Luo J, Mosher KI, Zou B, Britschgi M, et al. (2011) The ageing systemic milieu negatively regulates neurogenesis and cognitive function. *Nature* 477: 90-94.

[42] Agholme L, Hallbeck M, Benedikz E, Marcusson J, Kågedal K (2012) Amyloid-β secretion, generation, and lysosomal sequestration in response to proteasome inhibition: involvement of autophagy. *J Alzheimers Dis* 31: 343-358.

[43] Nixon RA, Yang DS, Lee JH (2008) Neurodegenerative lysosomal disorders: a continuum from development to late age. *Autophagy* 4: 590-599.

[44] Zheng L, Terman A, Hallbeck M, Dehvari N, Cowburn RF, et al. (2011) Macroautophagy-generated increase of lysosomal amyloid β-protein mediates oxidant-induced apoptosis of cultured neuroblastoma cells. *Autophagy* 7: 1528-1545.
[45] Deane R, Sagare A, Hamm K, Parisi M, Lane S, et al. (2008) apoE isoform-specific disruption of amyloid beta peptide clearance from mouse brain. *J Clin Invest* 118: 4002-4013.
[46] Hu X, Crick SL, Bu G, Frieden C, Pappu RV, et al. (2009) Amyloid seeds formed by cellular uptake, concentration, and aggregation of the amyloid-beta peptide. *Proc Natl Acad Sci USA* 106: 20324-20329.
[47] Umeda T, Tomiyama T, Sakama N, Tanaka S, Lambert MP, et al. (2011) Intraneuronal amyloid β oligomers cause cell death via endoplasmic reticulum stress, endosomal/lysosomal leakage, and mitochondrial dysfunction in vivo. *J Neurosci Res* 89: 1031-1042.
[48] Ahmed M, Davis J, Aucoin D, Sato T, Ahuja S, et al. (2010) Structural conversion of neurotoxic amyloid-beta(1-42) oligomers to fibrils. *Nat Struct Mol Biol* 17: 561-567.
[49] Lee S, Sato Y, Nixon RA (2011) Lysosomal proteolysis inhibition selectively disrupts axonal transport of degradative organelles and causes an Alzheimer's-like axonal dystrophy. *J Neurosci* 31: 7817-7830.
[50] Shankar GM, Li S, Mehta TH, Garcia-Munoz A, Shepardson NE, et al. (2008) Amyloid-beta protein dimers isolated directly from Alzheimer's brains impair synaptic plasticity and memory. *Nat Med* 14: 837-842.
[51] Nag S, Sarkar B, Bandyopadhyay A, Sahoo B, Sreenivasan VK, et al. (2011) Nature of the amyloid-beta monomer and the monomer-oligomer equilibrium. *J Biol Chem* 286: 13827-13833.
[52] Agholme L, Hallbeck M (2014) Getting rid of intracellular Aβ- loss of cellular degradation leads to transfer between connected neurons. *Curr Pharm Des* 20: 2458-2468.
[53] Alvarez-Erviti L, Seow Y, Schapira AH, Gardiner C, Sargent IL, et al. (2011) Lysosomal dysfunction increases exosome-mediated alpha-synuclein release and transmission. *Neurobiol Dis* 42: 360-367.
[54] Rajendran L, Honsho M, Zahn TR, Keller P, Geiger KD, et al. (2006) Alzheimer's disease beta-amyloid peptides are released in association with exosomes. *Proc Natl Acad Sci USA* 103: 11172-11177.
[55] Gousset K, Schiff E, Langevin C, Marijanovic Z, Caputo A, et al. (2009) Prions hijack tunnelling nanotubes for intercellular spread. *Nat Cell Biol* 11: 328-336.
[56] Fevrier B, Vilette D, Archer F, Loew D, Faigle W, et al. (2004) Cells release prions in association with exosomes. *Proc Natl Acad Sci USA* 101: 9683-9688.
[57] Teich AF, Arancio O (2012) Is the amyloid hypothesis of Alzheimer's disease therapeutically relevant? *Biochem J* 446: 165-177.
[58] Cirrito JR, Kang JE, Lee J, Stewart FR, Verges DK, et al. (2008) Endocytosis is required for synaptic activity-dependent release of amyloid-beta in vivo. *Neuron* 58: 42-51.
[59] Cirrito JR, Yamada KA, Finn MB, Sloviter RS, Bales KR, et al. (2005) Synaptic activity regulates interstitial fluid amyloid-beta levels in vivo. *Neuron* 48: 913-922.
[60] Kamenetz F, Tomita T, Hsieh H, Seabrook G, Borchelt D, et al. (2003) APP processing and synaptic function. *Neuron* 37: 925-937.

[61] Sharples RA, Vella LJ, Nisbet RM, Naylor R, Perez K, et al. (2008) Inhibition of gamma-secretase causes increased secretion of amyloid precursor protein C-terminal fragments in association with exosomes. *FASEB J* 22: 1469-1478.
[62] Wang Y, Cui J, Sun X, Zhang Y (2011) Tunneling-nanotube development in astrocytes depends on p53 activation. *Cell Death Differ* 18: 732-742.
[63] Omtri RS, Davidson MW, Arumugam B, Poduslo JF, Kandimalla KK (2012) Differences in the cellular uptake and intracellular itineraries of amyloid beta proteins 40 and 42: ramifications for the Alzheimer's drug discovery. *Mol Pharm* 9: 1887-1897.
[64] Medina DL, Fraldi A, Bouche V, Annunziata F, Mansueto G, et al. (2011) Transcriptional activation of lysosomal exocytosis promotes cellular clearance. *Dev Cell* 21: 421-430.
[65] Frost B, Jacks RL, Diamond MI (2009) Propagation of tau misfolding from the outside to the inside of a cell. *J Biol Chem* 284: 12845-12852.
[66] Hansen C, Angot E, Bergström AL, Steiner JA, Pieri L, et al. (2011) α-Synuclein propagates from mouse brain to grafted dopaminergic neurons and seeds aggregation in cultured human cells. *J Clin Invest* 121: 715-725.
[67] Clifford PM, Siu G, Kosciuk M, Levin EC, Venkataraman V, et al. (2008) Alpha7 nicotinic acetylcholine receptor expression by vascular smooth muscle cells facilitates the deposition of Abeta peptides and promotes cerebrovascular amyloid angiopathy. *Brain Res* 1234: 158-171.
[68] Bi X, Gall CM, Zhou J, Lynch G (2002) Uptake and pathogenic effects of amyloid beta peptide 1-42 are enhanced by integrin antagonists and blocked by NMDA receptor antagonists. *Neuroscienc*e 112: 827-840.
[69] Zerbinatti CV, Wahrle SE, Kim H, Cam JA, Bales K, et al. (2006) Apolipoprotein E and low density lipoprotein receptor-related protein facilitate intraneuronal Abeta42 accumulation in amyloid model mice. *J Biol Chem* 281: 36180-36186.
[70] Takamura A, Sato Y, Watabe D, Okamoto Y, Nakata T, et al. (2012) Sortilin is required for toxic action of Aβ oligomers (AβOs): extracellular AβOs trigger apoptosis, and intraneuronal AβOs impair degradation pathways. *Life Sci* 91: 1177-1186.
[71] Wei W, Nguyen LN, Kessels HW, Hagiwara H, Sisodia S, et al. (2010) Amyloid beta from axons and dendrites reduces local spine number and plasticity. *Nat Neurosci* 13: 190-196.
[72] Ganzinger KA, Narayan P, Qamar SS, Weimann L, Ranasinghe RT, et al. (2014) Single-molecule imaging reveals that small amyloid-β1-42 oligomers interact with the cellular prion protein (PrP(C)). *Chembiochem* 15: 2515-2521.
[73] Kessels HW, Nguyen LN, Nabavi S, Malinow R (2010) The prion protein as a receptor for amyloid-beta. *Nature* 466: E3-4; discussion E4-5.
[74] Laurén J, Gimbel DA, Nygaard HB, Gilbert JW, Strittmatter SM (2009) Cellular prion protein mediates impairment of synaptic plasticity by amyloid-beta oligomers. *Nature* 457: 1128-1132.
[75] Cochran JN, Hall AM, Roberson ED (2014) The dendritic hypothesis for Alzheimer's disease pathophysiology. *Brain Res Bull* 103: 18-28.
[76] Zempel H, Thies E, Mandelkow E, Mandelkow EM (2010) Abeta oligomers cause localized Ca(2+) elevation, missorting of endogenous Tau into dendrites, Tau phosphorylation, and destruction of microtubules and spines. *J Neurosci* 30: 11938-11950.

[77] Zempel H, Mandelkow E (2014) Lost after translation: missorting of Tau protein and consequences for Alzheimer disease. *Trends Neurosci* 37: 721-732.

[78] Sydow A, Van der Jeugd A, Zheng F, Ahmed T, Balschun D, et al. (2011) Tau-induced defects in synaptic plasticity, learning, and memory are reversible in transgenic mice after switching off the toxic Tau mutant. *J Neurosci* 31: 2511-2525.

[79] Hirokawa N, Funakoshi T, Sato-Harada R, Kanai Y (1996) Selective stabilization of tau in axons and microtubule-associated protein 2C in cell bodies and dendrites contributes to polarized localization of cytoskeletal proteins in mature neurons. *J Cell Biol* 132: 667-679.

[80] Lee MJ, Lee JH, Rubinsztein DC (2013) Tau degradation: the ubiquitin-proteasome system versus the autophagy-lysosome system. *Prog Neurobiol* 105: 49-59.

[81] Wang Y, Mandelkow E (2012) Degradation of tau protein by autophagy and proteasomal pathways. *Biochem Soc Trans* 40: 644-652.

[82] Aronov S, Aranda G, Behar L, Ginzburg I (2001) Axonal tau mRNA localization coincides with tau protein in living neuronal cells and depends on axonal targeting signal. *J Neurosci* 21: 6577-6587.

[83] Morita T, Sobue K (2009) Specification of neuronal polarity regulated by local translation of CRMP2 and Tau via the mTOR-p70S6K pathway. *J Biol Chem* 284: 27734-27745.

[84] Frost B, Diamond MI (2010) Prion-like mechanisms in neurodegenerative diseases. *Nat Rev Neurosci* 11: 155-159.

[85] Walker LC, Diamond MI, Duff KE, Hyman BT (2013) Mechanisms of protein seeding in neurodegenerative diseases. *JAMA Neurol* 70: 304-310.

[86] Yamada K, Cirrito JR, Stewart FR, Jiang H, Finn MB, et al. (2011) In vivo microdialysis reveals age-dependent decrease of brain interstitial fluid tau levels in P301S human tau transgenic mice. *J Neurosci* 31: 13110-13117.

[87] Clavaguera F, Bolmont T, Crowther RA, Abramowski D, Frank S, et al. (2009) Transmission and spreading of tauopathy in transgenic mouse brain. *Nat Cell Biol* 11: 909-913.

[88] Lasagna-Reeves CA, Castillo-Carranza DL, Sengupta U, Guerrero-Munoz MJ, Kiritoshi T, et al. (2012) Alzheimer brain-derived tau oligomers propagate pathology from endogenous tau. *Sci Rep* 2: 700.

[89] Iba M, Guo JL, McBride JD, Zhang B, Trojanowski JQ, et al. (2013) Synthetic tau fibrils mediate transmission of neurofibrillary tangles in a transgenic mouse model of Alzheimer's-like tauopathy. *J Neurosci* 33: 1024-1037.

[90] Allen B, Ingram E, Takao M, Smith MJ, Jakes R, et al. (2002) Abundant tau filaments and nonapoptotic neurodegeneration in transgenic mice expressing human P301S tau protein. *J Neurosci* 22: 9340-9351.

[91] Probst A, Götz J, Wiederhold KH, Tolnay M, Mistl C, et al. (2000) Axonopathy and amyotrophy in mice transgenic for human four-repeat tau protein. *Acta Neuropathol* 99: 469-481.

[92] Clavaguera F, Grueninger F, Tolnay M (2014) Intercellular transfer of tau aggregates and spreading of tau pathology: Implications for therapeutic strategies. *Neuropharmacology* 76 Pt A: 9-15.

[93] Nishimura M, Namba Y, Ikeda K, Oda M (1992) Glial fibrillary tangles with straight tubules in the brains of patients with progressive supranuclear palsy. *Neurosci Lett* 143: 35-38.

[94] Yamada T, McGeer PL, McGeer EG (1992) Appearance of paired nucleated, Tau-positive glia in patients with progressive supranuclear palsy brain tissue. *Neurosci Lett* 135: 99-102.

[95] Komori T (1999) Tau-positive glial inclusions in progressive supranuclear palsy, corticobasal degeneration and Pick's disease. *Brain Pathol* 9: 663-679.

[96] Tolnay M, Clavaguera F (2004) Argyrophilic grain disease: a late-onset dementia with distinctive features among tauopathies. *Neuropathology* 24: 269-283.

[97] Hyman BT (2014) Tau propagation, different tau phenotypes, and prion-like properties of tau. *Neuron* 82: 1189-1190.

[98] Sanders DW, Kaufman SK, DeVos SL, Sharma AM, Mirbaha H, et al. (2014) Distinct tau prion strains propagate in cells and mice and define different tauopathies. *Neuron* 82: 1271-1288.

[99] Clavaguera F, Hench J, Goedert M, Tolnay M (2015) Invited review: Prion-like transmission and spreading of tau pathology. *Neuropathol Appl Neurobiol* 41: 47-58.

[100] Prusiner SB (1998) Prions. *Proc Natl Acad Sci USA* 95: 13363-13383.

[101] Morinet F (2014) Prions: a model of conformational disease? *Pathol Biol* (Paris) 62: 96-99.

[102] Nonaka T, Watanabe ST, Iwatsubo T, Hasegawa M (2010) Seeded aggregation and toxicity of {alpha}-synuclein and tau: cellular models of neurodegenerative diseases. *J Biol Chem* 285: 34885-34898.

[103] Frost B, Ollesch J, Wille H, Diamond MI (2009) Conformational diversity of wild-type Tau fibrils specified by templated conformation change. *J Biol Chem* 284: 3546-3551.

[104] Friedhoff P, von Bergen M, Mandelkow EM, Davies P, Mandelkow E (1998) A nucleated assembly mechanism of Alzheimer paired helical filaments. *Proc Natl Acad Sci USA* 95: 15712-15717.

[105] Guo JL, Lee VM (2011) Seeding of normal Tau by pathological Tau conformers drives pathogenesis of Alzheimer-like tangles. *J Biol Chem* 286: 15317-15331.

[106] Armstrong RA (2014) A critical analysis of the 'amyloid cascade hypothesis'. *Folia Neuropathol* 52: 211-225.

[107] Bolmont T, Clavaguera F, Meyer-Luehmann M, Herzig MC, Radde R, et al. (2007) Induction of tau pathology by intracerebral infusion of amyloid-beta -containing brain extract and by amyloid-beta deposition in APP x Tau transgenic mice. *Am J Pathol* 171: 2012-2020.

[108] Crimins JL, Pooler A, Polydoro M, Luebke JI, Spires-Jones TL (2013) The intersection of amyloid β and tau in glutamatergic synaptic dysfunction and collapse in Alzheimer's disease. *Ageing Res Rev* 12: 757-763.

[109] Zempel H, Luedtke J, Kumar Y, Biernat J, Dawson H, et al. (2013) Amyloid-β oligomers induce synaptic damage via Tau-dependent microtubule severing by TTLL6 and spastin. *EMBO J* 32: 2920-2937.

[110] Rustom A, Saffrich R, Markovic I, Walther P, Gerdes HH (2004) Nanotubular highways for intercellular organelle transport. *Science* 303: 1007-1010.

[111] Abounit S, Zurzolo C (2012) Wiring through tunneling nanotubes--from electrical signals to organelle transfer. *J Cell Sci* 125: 1089-1098.

[112] Marzo L, Gousset K, Zurzolo C (2012) Multifaceted roles of tunneling nanotubes in intercellular communication. *Front Physiol* 3: 72.

[113] Williams TL, Serpell LC (2011) Membrane and surface interactions of Alzheimer's Aβ peptide--insights into the mechanism of cytotoxicity. *FEBS J* 278: 3905-3917.

[114] Tofoleanu F, Buchete NV (2012) Alzheimer Aβ peptide interactions with lipid membranes: fibrils, oligomers and polymorphic amyloid channels. *Prion* 6: 339-345.

[115] Rustom A (2009) Hen or egg?: some thoughts on tunneling nanotubes. *Ann N Y Acad Sci* 1178: 129-136.

[116] Dal Prà I, Chiarini A, Gui L, Chakravarthy B, Pacchiana R, et al. (2015) Do astrocytes collaborate with neurons in spreading the "infectious" aβ and tau drivers of Alzheimer's disease? *Neuroscientist* 21: 9-29.

[117] Talantova M, Sanz-Blasco S, Zhang X, Xia P, Akhtar MW, et al. (2013) Aβ induces astrocytic glutamate release, extrasynaptic NMDA receptor activation, and synaptic loss. *Proc Natl Acad Sci USA* 110: E2518-2527.

[118] Klein WL (2013) Synaptotoxic amyloid-β oligomers: a molecular basis for the cause, diagnosis, and treatment of Alzheimer's disease? *J Alzheimers Dis* 33 Suppl 1: S49-65.

[119] Bero AW, Yan P, Roh JH, Cirrito JR, Stewart FR, et al. (2011) Neuronal activity regulates the regional vulnerability to amyloid-β deposition. *Nat Neurosci* 14: 750-756.

[120] Zhao Y, Cui JG, Lukiw WJ (2006) Natural secretory products of human neural and microvessel endothelial cells: Implications in pathogenic "spreading" and Alzheimer's disease. *Mol Neurobiol* 34: 181-192.

[121] Iadecola C (2004) Neurovascular regulation in the normal brain and in Alzheimer's disease. *Nat Rev Neurosci* 5: 347-360.

[122] Hawkins BT, Davis TP (2005) The blood-brain barrier/neurovascular unit in health and disease. *Pharmacol Rev* 57: 173-185.

[123] Zlokovic BV (2005) Neurovascular mechanisms of Alzheimer's neurodegeneration. *Trends Neurosci* 28: 202-208.

[124] Kandimalla KK, Scott OG, Fulzele S, Davidson MW, Poduslo JF (2009) Mechanism of neuronal versus endothelial cell uptake of Alzheimer's disease amyloid beta protein. *PLoS One* 4: e4627.

[125] Benarroch EE (2005) Neuron-astrocyte interactions: partnership for normal function and disease in the central nervous system. *Mayo Clin Proc* 80: 1326-1338.

[126] Ward NL, Lamanna JC (2004) The neurovascular unit and its growth factors: coordinated response in the vascular and nervous systems. *Neurol Res* 26: 870-883.

[127] McGeer PL, McGeer EG (2002) Local neuroinflammation and the progression of Alzheimer's disease. *J Neurovirol* 8: 529-538.

[128] Rogers J, Strohmeyer R, Kovelowski CJ, Li R (2002) Microglia and inflammatory mechanisms in the clearance of amyloid beta peptide. *Glia* 40: 260-269.

[129] Bard F, Cannon C, Barbour R, Burke RL, Games D, et al. (2000) Peripherally administered antibodies against amyloid beta-peptide enter the central nervous system and reduce pathology in a mouse model of Alzheimer disease. *Nat Med* 6: 916-919.

[130] Nagele RG, Wegiel J, Venkataraman V, Imaki H, Wang KC (2004) Contribution of glial cells to the development of amyloid plaques in Alzheimer's disease. *Neurobiol Aging* 25: 663-674.

[131] Grammas P, Ovase R (2001) Inflammatory factors are elevated in brain microvessels in Alzheimer's disease. *Neurobiol Aging* 22: 837-842.

[132] Bailey TL, Rivara CB, Rocher AB, Hof PR (2004) The nature and effects of cortical microvascular pathology in aging and Alzheimer's disease. *Neurol Res* 26: 573-578.

[133] Christov A, Ottman JT, Grammas P (2004) Vascular inflammatory, oxidative and protease-based processes: implications for neuronal cell death in Alzheimer's disease. *Neurol Res* 26: 540-546.

[134] Clavaguera F, Akatsu H, Fraser G, Crowther RA, Frank S, et al. (2013) Brain homogenates from human tauopathies induce tau inclusions in mouse brain. *Proc Natl Acad Sci USA* 110: 9535-9540.

[135] Clavaguera F, Lavenir I, Falcon B, Frank S, Goedert M, et al. (2013) "Prion-like" templated misfolding in tauopathies. *Brain Pathol* 23: 342-349.

[136] Gerson JE, Kayed R (2013) Formation and propagation of tau oligomeric seeds. *Front Neurol* 4: 93.

[137] Stranahan AM, Mattson MP (2010) Selective vulnerability of neurons in layer II of the entorhinal cortex during aging and Alzheimer's disease. *Neural Plast* 2010: 108190.

[138] Plouffe V, Mohamed NV, Rivest-McGraw J, Bertrand J, Lauzon M, et al. (2012) Hyperphosphorylation and cleavage at D421 enhance tau secretion. *PLoS One* 7: e36873.

[139] Wray S, Saxton M, Anderton BH, Hanger DP (2008) Direct analysis of tau from PSP brain identifies new phosphorylation sites and a major fragment of N-terminally cleaved tau containing four microtubule-binding repeats. *J Neurochem* 105: 2343-2352.

[140] (!!! INVALID CITATION !!!).

[141] Garwood CJ, Pooler AM, Atherton J, Hanger DP, Noble W (2011) Astrocytes are important mediators of Aβ-induced neurotoxicity and tau phosphorylation in primary culture. *Cell Death Dis* 2: e167.

[142] Avila J (2010) Alzheimer disease: caspases first. *Nat Rev Neurol* 6: 587-588.

[143] Gamblin TC, Chen F, Zambrano A, Abraha A, Lagalwar S, et al. (2003) Caspase cleavage of tau: linking amyloid and neurofibrillary tangles in Alzheimer's disease. *Proc Natl Acad Sci USA* 100: 10032-10037.

[144] Wu JW, Herman M, Liu L, Simoes S, Acker CM, et al. (2013) Small misfolded Tau species are internalized via bulk endocytosis and anterogradely and retrogradely transported in neurons. *J Biol Chem* 288: 1856-1870.

[145] Medeiros R, Chabrier MA, LaFerla FM (2013) Elucidating the triggers, progression, and effects of Alzheimer's disease. *J Alzheimers Dis* 33 Suppl 1: S195-210.

[146] Nussbaum JM, Schilling S, Cynis H, Silva A, Swanson E, et al. (2012) Prion-like behaviour and tau-dependent cytotoxicity of pyroglutamylated amyloid-β. *Nature* 485: 651-655.

[147] Lahiri DK (2012) Prions: a piece of the puzzle? *Science* 337: 1172.

[148] Selkoe DJ (1997) Alzheimer's disease: genotypes, phenotypes, and treatments. *Science* 275: 630-631.

[149] Ayyadevara S, Balasubramaniam M, Gao Y, Yu LR, Alla R, et al. (2015) Proteins in aggregates functionally impact multiple neurodegenerative disease models by forming proteasome-blocking complexes. *Aging Cell* 14: 35-48.

[150] Aso E, Lomoio S, López-González I, Joda L, Carmona M, et al. (2012) Amyloid generation and dysfunctional immunoproteasome activation with disease progression in animal model of familial Alzheimer's disease. *Brain Pathol* 22: 636-653.

[151] Sulistio YA, Heese K (2015) The Ubiquitin-Proteasome System and Molecular Chaperone Deregulation in Alzheimer's Disease. *Mol Neurobiol.*

[152] Cárdenas-Aguayo MeC, Gómez-Virgilio L, DeRosa S, Meraz-Ríos MA (2014) The role of tau oligomers in the onset of Alzheimer's disease neuropathology. *ACS Chem Neurosci* 5: 1178-1191.

[153] Cui JG, Kuroda H, Chandrasekharan NV, Pelaez RP, Simmons DL, et al. (2004) Cyclooxygenase-3 gene expression in Alzheimer hippocampus and in stressed human neural cells. *Neurochem Res* 29: 1731-1737.

[154] Bazan NG, Lukiw WJ (2002) Cyclooxygenase-2 and presenilin-1 gene expression induced by interleukin-1beta and amyloid beta 42 peptide is potentiated by hypoxia in primary human neural cells. *J Biol Chem* 277: 30359-30367.

[155] Blasko I, Stampfer-Kountchev M, Robatscher P, Veerhuis R, Eikelenboom P, et al. (2004) How chronic inflammation can affect the brain and support the development of Alzheimer's disease in old age: the role of microglia and astrocytes. *Aging Cell* 3: 169-176.

[156] Liao YF, Wang BJ, Cheng HT, Kuo LH, Wolfe MS (2004) Tumor necrosis factor-alpha, interleukin-1beta, and interferon-gamma stimulate gamma-secretase-mediated cleavage of amyloid precursor protein through a JNK-dependent MAPK pathway. *J Biol Chem* 279: 49523-49532.

[157] Griffin WS (2006) Inflammation and neurodegenerative diseases. *Am J Clin Nutr* 83: 470S-474S.

[158] Borenstein AR, Copenhaver CI, Mortimer JA (2006) Early-life risk factors for Alzheimer disease. *Alzheimer Dis Assoc Disord* 20: 63-72.

[159] Lu JX, Qiang W, Yau WM, Schwieters CD, Meredith SC, et al. (2013) Molecular structure of β-amyloid fibrils in Alzheimer's disease brain tissue. *Cell* 154: 1257-1268.

[160] Stöhr J, Condello C, Watts JC, Bloch L, Oehler A, et al. (2014) Distinct synthetic Aβ prion strains producing different amyloid deposits in bigenic mice. *Proc Natl Acad Sci USA* 111: 10329-10334.

[161] Colby DW, Prusiner SB (2011) Prions. *Cold Spring Harb Perspect Biol* 3: a006833.

[162] Halliday M, Radford H, Mallucci GR (2014) Prions: generation and spread versus neurotoxicity. *J Biol Chem* 289: 19862-19868.

[163] Cicchetti F, Saporta S, Hauser RA, Parent M, Saint-Pierre M, et al. (2009) Neural transplants in patients with Huntington's disease undergo disease-like neuronal degeneration. *Proc Natl Acad Sci USA* 106: 12483-12488.

[164] Mendez I, Viñuela A, Astradsson A, Mukhida K, Hallett P, et al. (2008) Dopamine neurons implanted into people with Parkinson's disease survive without pathology for 14 years. *Nat Med* 14: 507-509.

[165] Sugiyama S, Tanaka M (2014) Self-propagating amyloid as a critical regulator for diverse cellular functions. *J Biochem* 155: 345-351.

[166] Holmes DL, Lancaster AK, Lindquist S, Halfmann R (2013) Heritable remodeling of yeast multicellularity by an environmentally responsive prion. *Cell* 153: 153-165.

[167] Suzuki G, Tanaka M (2013) Active conversion to the prion state as a molecular switch for cellular adaptation to environmental stress. *Bioessays* 35: 12-16.

[168] Carrillo-Mora P, Luna R, Colín-Barenque L (2014) Amyloid beta: multiple mechanisms of toxicity and only some protective effects? *Oxid Med Cell Longev* 2014: 795375.

[169] Castellani RJ, Lee HG, Siedlak SL, Nunomura A, Hayashi T, et al. (2009) Reexamining Alzheimer's disease: evidence for a protective role for amyloid-beta protein precursor and amyloid-beta. J Alzheimers Dis 18: 447-452.

[170] Cowan CM, Quraishe S, Mudher A (2012) What is the pathological significance of tau oligomers? *Biochem Soc Trans* 40: 693-697.

[171] Gouras GK, Willén K, Faideau M (2014) The inside-out amyloid hypothesis and synapse pathology in Alzheimer's disease. *Neurodegener* Dis 13: 142-146.

[172] Crews L, Masliah E (2010) Molecular mechanisms of neurodegeneration in Alzheimer's disease. *Hum Mol Genet* 19: R12-20.

[173] Liao D, Miller EC, Teravskis PJ (2014) Tau acts as a mediator for Alzheimer's disease-related synaptic deficits. *Eur J Neurosci* 39: 1202-1213.

[174] Terwel D, Dewachter I, Van Leuven F (2002) Axonal transport, tau protein, and neurodegeneration in Alzheimer's disease. *Neuromolecular Med* 2: 151-165.

[175] Nussbaum JM, Seward ME, Bloom GS (2013) Alzheimer disease: a tale of two prions. *Prion* 7: 14-19.

[176] Moreno JA, Radford H, Peretti D, Steinert JR, Verity N, et al. (2012) Sustained translational repression by eIF2α-P mediates prion neurodegeneration. *Nature* 485: 507-511.

[177] Andre R, Tabrizi SJ (2012) Misfolded PrP and a novel mechanism of proteasome inhibition. *Prion* 6: 32-36.

[178] Shah SB, Nolan R, Davis E, Stokin GB, Niesman I, et al. (2009) Examination of potential mechanisms of amyloid-induced defects in neuronal transport. *Neurobiol Dis* 36: 11-25.

[179] Bahr BA, Hoffman KB, Yang AJ, Hess US, Glabe CG, et al. (1998) Amyloid beta protein is internalized selectively by hippocampal field CA1 and causes neurons to accumulate amyloidogenic carboxyterminal fragments of the amyloid precursor protein. *J Comp Neurol* 397: 139-147.

[180] Glabe C (2001) Intracellular mechanisms of amyloid accumulation and pathogenesis in Alzheimer's disease. *J Mol Neurosci* 17: 137-145.

[181] Jackson WS (2014) Selective vulnerability to neurodegenerative disease: the curious case of Prion Protein. *Dis Model Mech* 7: 21-29.

[182] Westaway D, Jhamandas JH (2012) The P's and Q's of cellular PrP-Aβ interactions. *Prion* 6: 359-363.

[183] Walmsley AR, Zeng F, Hooper NM (2003) The N-terminal region of the prion protein ectodomain contains a lipid raft targeting determinant. *J Biol Chem* 278: 37241-37248.

[184] Vetrivel KS, Cheng H, Lin W, Sakurai T, Li T, et al. (2004) Association of gamma-secretase with lipid rafts in post-Golgi and endosome membranes. *J Biol Chem* 279: 44945-44954.

[185] Bai Y, Markham K, Chen F, Weerasekera R, Watts J, et al. (2008) The in vivo brain interactome of the amyloid precursor protein. *Mol Cell Proteomics* 7: 15-34.

[186] Watts JC, Huo H, Bai Y, Ehsani S, Jeon AH, et al. (2009) Interactome analyses identify ties of PrP and its mammalian paralogs to oligomannosidic N-glycans and endoplasmic reticulum-derived chaperones. *PLoS Pathog* 5: e1000608.

[187] Kourie JI, Culverson A (2000) Prion peptide fragment PrP[106-126] forms distinct cation channel types. *J Neurosci Res* 62: 120-133.

[188] Lin MC, Mirzabekov T, Kagan BL (1997) Channel formation by a neurotoxic prion protein fragment. *J Biol Chem* 272: 44-47.

[189] Calella AM, Farinelli M, Nuvolone M, Mirante O, Moos R, et al. (2010) Prion protein and Abeta-related synaptic toxicity impairment. *EMBO Mol Med* 2: 306-314.

[190] Jhamandas JH, Cho C, Jassar B, Harris K, MacTavish D, et al. (2001) Cellular mechanisms for amyloid beta-protein activation of rat cholinergic basal forebrain neurons. *J Neurophysiol* 86: 1312-1320.

[191] Alier K, Li Z, Mactavish D, Westaway D, Jhamandas JH (2010) Ionic mechanisms of action of prion protein fragment PrP(106-126) in rat basal forebrain neurons. *J Neurosci Res* 88: 2217-2227.

[192] Alier K, Ma L, Yang J, Westaway D, Jhamandas JH (2011) Aβ inhibition of ionic conductance in mouse basal forebrain neurons is dependent upon the cellular prion protein PrPC. *J Neurosci* 31: 16292-16297.

[193] Freir DB, Nicoll AJ, Klyubin I, Panico S, Mc Donald JM, et al. (2011) Interaction between prion protein and toxic amyloid β assemblies can be therapeutically targeted at multiple sites. *Nat Commun* 2: 336.

[194] Barry AE, Klyubin I, Mc Donald JM, Mably AJ, Farrell MA, et al. (2011) Alzheimer's disease brain-derived amyloid-β-mediated inhibition of LTP in vivo is prevented by immunotargeting cellular prion protein. *J Neurosci* 31: 7259-7263.

[195] Lasagna-Reeves CA, Castillo-Carranza DL, Sengupta U, Sarmiento J, Troncoso J, et al. (2012) Identification of oligomers at early stages of tau aggregation in Alzheimer's disease. *FASEB J* 26: 1946-1959.

[196] Patterson KR, Remmers C, Fu Y, Brooker S, Kanaan NM, et al. (2011) Characterization of prefibrillar Tau oligomers in vitro and in Alzheimer disease. *J Biol Chem* 286: 23063-23076.

[197] Castillo-Carranza DL, Gerson JE, Sengupta U, Guerrero-Muñoz MJ, Lasagna-Reeves CA, et al. (2014) Specific targeting of tau oligomers in Htau mice prevents cognitive impairment and tau toxicity following injection with brain-derived tau oligomeric seeds. *J Alzheimers Dis* 40 Suppl 1: S97-S111.

[198] Tai HC, Serrano-Pozo A, Hashimoto T, Frosch MP, Spires-Jones TL, et al. (2012) The synaptic accumulation of hyperphosphorylated tau oligomers in Alzheimer disease is associated with dysfunction of the ubiquitin-proteasome system. *Am J Pathol* 181: 1426-1435.

[199] Lasagna-Reeves CA, Castillo-Carranza DL, Sengupta U, Clos AL, Jackson GR, et al. (2011) Tau oligomers impair memory and induce synaptic and mitochondrial dysfunction in wild-type mice. *Mol Neurodegener* 6: 39.

[200] Pozueta J, Lefort R, Shelanski ML (2013) Synaptic changes in Alzheimer's disease and its models. *Neuroscience* 251: 51-65.

[201] Moreno-Gonzalez I, Soto C (2011) Misfolded protein aggregates: mechanisms, structures and potential for disease transmission. *Semin Cell Dev Biol* 22: 482-487.

[202] Irwin DJ, Abrams JY, Schonberger LB, Leschek EW, Mills JL, et al. (2013) Evaluation of potential infectivity of Alzheimer and Parkinson disease proteins in recipients of cadaver-derived human growth hormone. *JAMA Neurol* 70: 462-468.

[203] Morales R, Callegari K, Soto C (2015) Prion-like features of misfolded Aβ and tau aggregates. *Virus Res.*

[204] Will RG (2003) Acquired prion disease: iatrogenic CJD, variant CJD, kuru. *Br Med Bull* 66: 255-265.
[205] Gallagher M, Koh MT (2011) Episodic memory on the path to Alzheimer's disease. *Curr Opin Neurobiol* 21: 929-934.
[206] Seward ME, Swanson E, Norambuena A, Reimann A, Cochran JN, et al. (2013) Amyloid-β signals through tau to drive ectopic neuronal cell cycle re-entry in Alzheimer's disease. *J Cell Sci* 126: 1278-1286.
[207] Götz J, Chen F, van Dorpe J, Nitsch RM (2001) Formation of neurofibrillary tangles in P301l tau transgenic mice induced by Abeta 42 fibrils. *Science* 293: 1491-1495.
[208] Rapoport M, Dawson HN, Binder LI, Vitek MP, Ferreira A (2002) Tau is essential to beta -amyloid-induced neurotoxicity. *Proc Natl Acad Sci USA* 99: 6364-6369.
[209] Guo JP, Arai T, Miklossy J, McGeer PL (2006) Abeta and tau form soluble complexes that may promote self aggregation of both into the insoluble forms observed in Alzheimer's disease. *Proc Natl Acad Sci USA* 103: 1953-1958.
[210] Lasagna-Reeves CA, Castillo-Carranza DL, Guerrero-Muoz MJ, Jackson GR, Kayed R (2010) Preparation and characterization of neurotoxic tau oligomers. *Biochemistry* 49: 10039-10041.

In: The Prion Phenomena in Neurodegenerative Diseases ISBN: 978-1-63483-399-8
Editors: Giuseppe Legname and Gabriele Giachin

Chapter 8

TAU STRAINS AND THEIR PROPAGATION IN EXPERIMENTAL DISEASE MODELS

Kyle P. McHugh, Olga A. Morozova and David W. Colby*

Department of Chemical and Biomolecular Engineering,
University of Delaware, Newark, Delaware, US

ABSTRACT

Tauopathies encompass a broad family of neurodegenerative diseases, including Alzheimer's disease, which are characterized by the fibrillization of the microtubule-associated tau protein. The normal function of tau is to stabilize and promote the assembly of microtubules in neuronal axons. Sequestration of tau into amyloid fibrils results in destabilization of the microtubule network and may contribute to disease progression. As tau is an intracellular protein and proteins do not passively cross cell membranes, tau fibril formation has been assumed to occur spontaneously within individual cells. However, recent evidence suggests that tau shares several characteristics with prions, which propagate through the brain by protein-protein interactions in the interstitial space; these characteristics include conformational templating of native tau into disease-associated fibrils and intercellular fibril propagation. Tau adopts diverse fibril structures, or strains, which have been shown to self-propagate in the presence of monomeric recombinant tau protein. Exogenous tau fibrils induce misfolding of native tau in both cell culture and animal models, causing strain-dependent cellular dysfunction and differential patterns of neuropathology. Tau fibers have also been found recently in patient samples or models of several diseases not formerly identified as tauopathies, including chronic traumatic encephalopathy, Parkinson's disease, and Huntington's disease, suggesting a common underlying mechanism for neurodegenerative diseases. The possibility that tauopathies and other neurodegenerative diseases involve prion-like mechanisms has implications for studies designed to understand disease pathogenesis and for the development of therapies, which may be devised to impede tau strain propagation and intercellular transmission, allowing clearance of tau fibrils and potentially halting or reversing disease progression.

---

* E-mail address: colby@udel.edu

INTRODUCTION

Misfolding of the microtubule-associated protein tau into deposits of neurofibrillary tangles is a distinguishing feature of a group of neurodegenerative diseases collectively referred to as tauopathies. Tauopathies are movement disorders and dementias that result in a progressive loss of neurons and cognitive impairment and include Alzheimer's disease (AD), Pick's disease, corticobasal degeneration, progressive supranuclear palsy, agyrophilic grain disease, chronic traumatic encephalopathy, and tangle-only dementia, among others [1]. The fibrillization and accumulation of tau is common among these diseases; however, the histopathological progression and clinical presentation differs between them [2], suggesting the possibility of distinct strains of tau fibrils with unique properties that would account for their stereotypic characteristics. Currently there are no reliable methods to diagnose patients with many of these diseases [3] and no therapeutics available to halt or even slow disease progression.

Native tau mainly functions by binding to and stabilizing neuronal microtubules to facilitate cellular structure and intracellular transport of biomolecules [4, 5] though tau may also play a role in many cellular pathways [6, 7]. In the unbound state, tau is an inherently disordered, highly soluble protein [8, 9]. The microtubule-binding region near the C-terminus reversibly associates with axonal microtubules in a phosphorylation-dependent manner [10]. There are 6 different splice variants or isoforms of tau (Figure 1) that are expressed in humans and their relative proportions in neurofibrillary tangles often varies among different tauopathies [11].

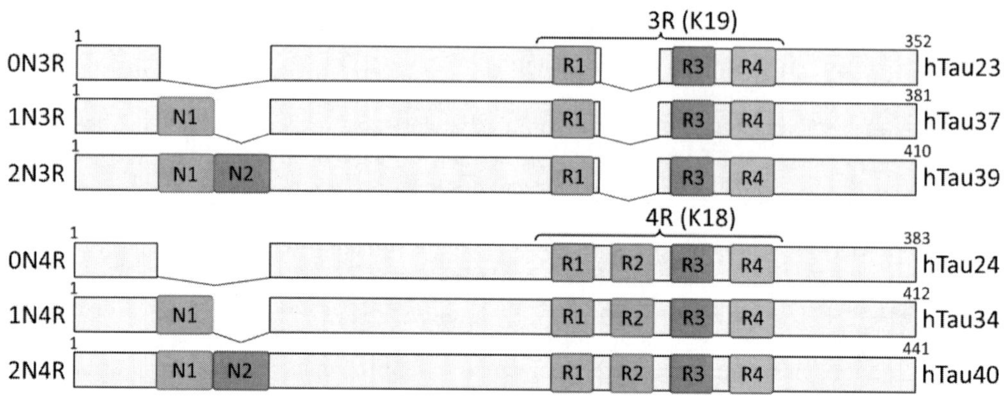

Figure 1. Splice variant isoforms of tau. The six different isoforms of tau generated by alternative splicing of exons 2 and 3 for the N-terminal region, which encode the N1 and N2 segments of the protein (labeled here in orange and red, respectively), and of exon 10 in the microtubule binding region, which encodes the second repeat sequence (R2, shown in green) [20]. Terminology used for describing the isoforms varies among researchers; the more descriptive names listed to the left of each isoform are used throughout this chapter. Historical names are listed to the right, along with the number of residues present in each isoform. The microtubule binding domain is composed of 3 or 4 repeat sequences (blue and green), which have significant homology but are not identical. These domains form the core of tau fibrils, and when expressed recombinantly as truncated protein products, they are referred to as 3R and 4R; alternately they are sometime identified as K19 and K18, respectively.

Alternative splicing produces an N-terminal region that may have zero, one, or two variable polypeptide segments while the microtubule-binding region may contain either three or four repeat sequences with moderate homology. Roughly equal amounts of 3R and 4R isoforms are found in fibrils isolated from the brains of patients with AD [12], chronic traumatic encephalopathy [13], and tangle-only dementia [14]. The 4R isoforms are predominant in fibrils found in progressive supranuclear palsy [15], corticobasal degeneration [16], and agyrophilic grain disease brain tissue [17, 18], while Pick's disease inclusions are predominantly composed of 3R isoforms [19].

Prions are infectious agents composed of alternatively folded protein with the ability to transmit disease through recruitment and conversion of normally folded protein into the alternatively folded conformation [21]; additionally, structurally distinct prion strains, composed of protein with identical polypeptide sequences, induce distinct phenotypic changes in host animals [22, 23]. The mechanism by which initial spontaneous misfolding of tau occurs is still not fully understood; however, increasing evidence suggests that propagation of fibrillar tau may be "prion-like" in its progression not only at the molecular level, but at the cellular level as well (Figure 2) [24, 25, 26, 27]. Neurodegenerative diseases in general appear to follow a pattern of neuronal connectivity in their progression [28, 29, 30] which may signify the propagation of a pathogenic species. Thus, the prion-like propagation of tau strains may provide an opportunity for developing therapeutics to prevent their intercellular spread.

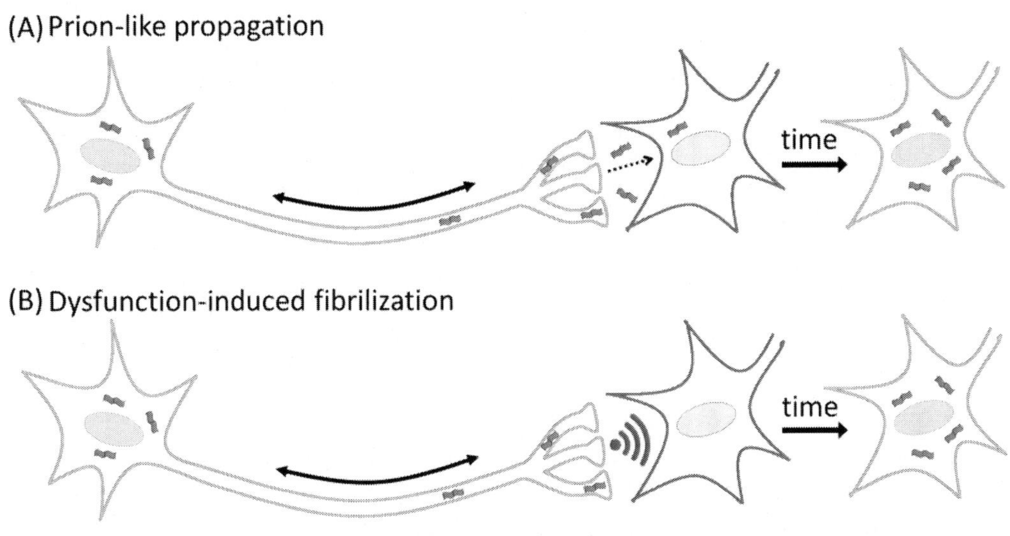

Figure 2. Competing hypotheses for the causative mechanism of disease pathogenesis. (A) The "prion-like" hypothesis of tauopathies suggests that strains of tau fibrils pass from dysfunctioning neurons (green) into healthy neurons (blue) and recruit native tau, resulting in dysfunction of the healthy neuron over time. (B) An alternate hypothesis is that dysfunctioning neurons induce a state of stress in healthy neurons through signaling, causing tau fibrillization as a downstream effect, e.g., through disruption of protein homeostasis or induction of apoptosis [31]; this hypothesis is akin to the amyloid cascade hypothesis in AD. The observation that tau strains are conserved throughout the brain as they spread supports the first hypothesis.

PRION-LIKE PHENOMENON IN TAUOPATHIES

Shortly after the discovery of prions, the most common tauopathy, Alzheimer's disease, was hypothesized to share a common underlying mechanism for pathogenesis [32]. While most tauopathies are sporadic in etiology [33], genetic forms of these diseases caused by destabilizing point mutations have been discovered (Figure 3). The fact that such mutations are sufficient to initiate neurodegeneration suggests that tau fibrillization can initiate disease pathogenesis [34, 35, 36].

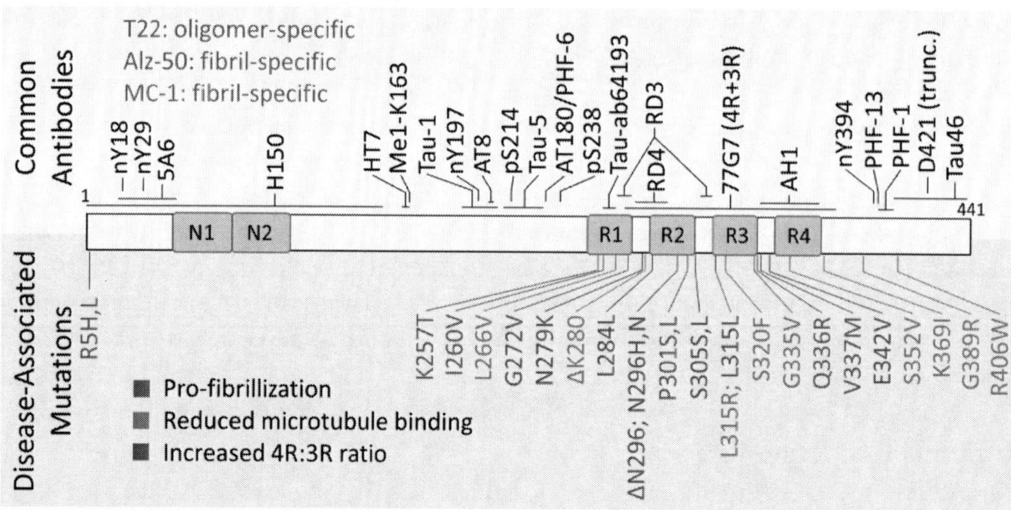

Figure 3. Commonly used tau antibodies and disease-associated mutations. (Top) Antibodies are mapped to the locations of antigens used to raise them, or to their epitopes if known. Antibodies T22, Alz-50, and MC1 are conformation-specific as indicated. The antibodies RD3 and RD4 are specific to the isoforms after which they are named. Several antibodies are specific for post-translational modification, including phosphorylation, nitration, and methylation. (Bottom) Disease-associated mutations are mapped to their locations on the gene. Mutations are associated with increasing fibril formation (blue), reducing the binding affinity for microtubule binding affinity (green), or increasing the 4R:3R splicing ratio (red). Some mutations such as L315L are silent gene mutations that effect tau mRNA splicing (Bottom updated and adapted from [36]).

The first extensive classification of the histopathological stages of AD demonstrated a distinct pattern of the spread of tau tangles in the brain along neuroanatomical connections [37], suggesting either protein-based disease progression or progressive cellular dysfunction in series of neurons (Figure 2). The hierarchical spread of tau pathology has also been documented in other tauopathies [38]. Templated conformational propagation of recombinant tau into structurally distinct strains [39, 40], transynaptic spread of tau fibrils and pathology in mice [41, 42], and the spread of tau fibrils following inoculation of exogenous fibrils [43, 44] all provide supporting evidence for the prion-like spread of tauopathies (Table 1). Serial propagation of strains has also been demonstrated in mice [45, 46] analogous to that of prion inoculation [47].

One distinguishing feature of *bona fide* prions is their transmissibility from one individual to another. An epidemiological study of the prevalence of several neurological diseases associated with protein misfolding in patients receiving injections of human growth hormone isolated from cadaver pituitary glands concluded that, with the exception of prion diseases, such diseases are not iatrogenically transmitted between patients in this fashion [48]. However, intraperitoneal injection of tau fibrils induced tauopathy in the brains of mice in another study [49]. Regardless of whether tauopathies are transmissible, such diseases do share key characteristics with prions at the molecular and cellular level.

Table 1. Summary of evidence for prion-like properties of tau strains

Model System	Evidence of strain-like behavior	References
Biochemical	Synthetic tau strains faithfully propagate using recombinant protein	[39]
	Conformational properties of both mouse and human brain-derived fibrils faithfully propagate using recombinant protein	[40, 77]
Cell Culture	Synthetic strains form unique puncta morphologies and retain biochemical properties	[46]
	Human brain-derived fibrils form unique puncta morphologies	[46]
Transgenic mice	Strains have differential patterns of neuropathology, including brain regions and cell types affected	[45, 46, 93]
	Tauopathy-derived strains exhibit histopathological features of their human counterparts when passaged to mice	[45, 93]
	Fibrils maintaine structural and biochemical features during three serial passages in mice	[46]

FORMATION OF SYNTHETIC TAU STRAINS FROM RECOMBINANT PROTEIN

Analogous to the diversity of conformational strains found in prion disease [22, 23, 50, 51, 52, 53], fibrils isolated from brains of patients diagnosed with different tauopathies also exhibit a range of conformations (Figure 4a) [54, 55, 56, 57]. Tau protein natively exists as an inherently disorganized structure consisting mostly of random coil, adopting a range of monomeric structures over a broad energy potential landscape [5, 58]. The energy potential landscapes of amyloidogenic proteins contain intermediate states which bind to amyloids, leading to elongation of fibrils [59, 60, 61]. This conversion is accompanied by a loss of random coil content and an increase in beta-sheet content [9, 60, 61].

Full-length tau produced recombinantly forms synthetic fibrils [62, 63], a process which is induced by polyanionic cofactors including sulfated glucosaminoglycans (e.g., heparin), RNA, or free fatty acids [64, 65, 66, 67]. Investigation of the protein regions responsible for driving synthetic fibril formation indicated that the third repeat domain and adjacent sequences are sufficient to form fibrils [68]. In the presence of polyanionic inducers, the mechanism of fibril formation follows nucleated monomer-addition kinetics [69, 70, 71, 72]. Such studies have provided insight into the molecular mechanism leading to spontaneous formation and stabilization of fibrils in the early pathogenesis of tauopathies.

Distinct fibril strains have been shown to propagate by sequestering the same recombinant tau substrate. Two different fibril conformations formed from wild-type and mutant tau in the presence of an inducer were subsequently used to seed monomeric wild-type tau; the tau structures formed maintained the structural characteristics of the original seeds [39]. Other studies have shown that two different induced fibrils from 4R tau isoforms had distinct properties, and only one of the conformations was able to seed a 3R tau substrate [73, 74]. In addition to potential roles played by genetic polymorphisms and splice variants, thiol-disulfide interactions may contribute to fibril diversity [75].

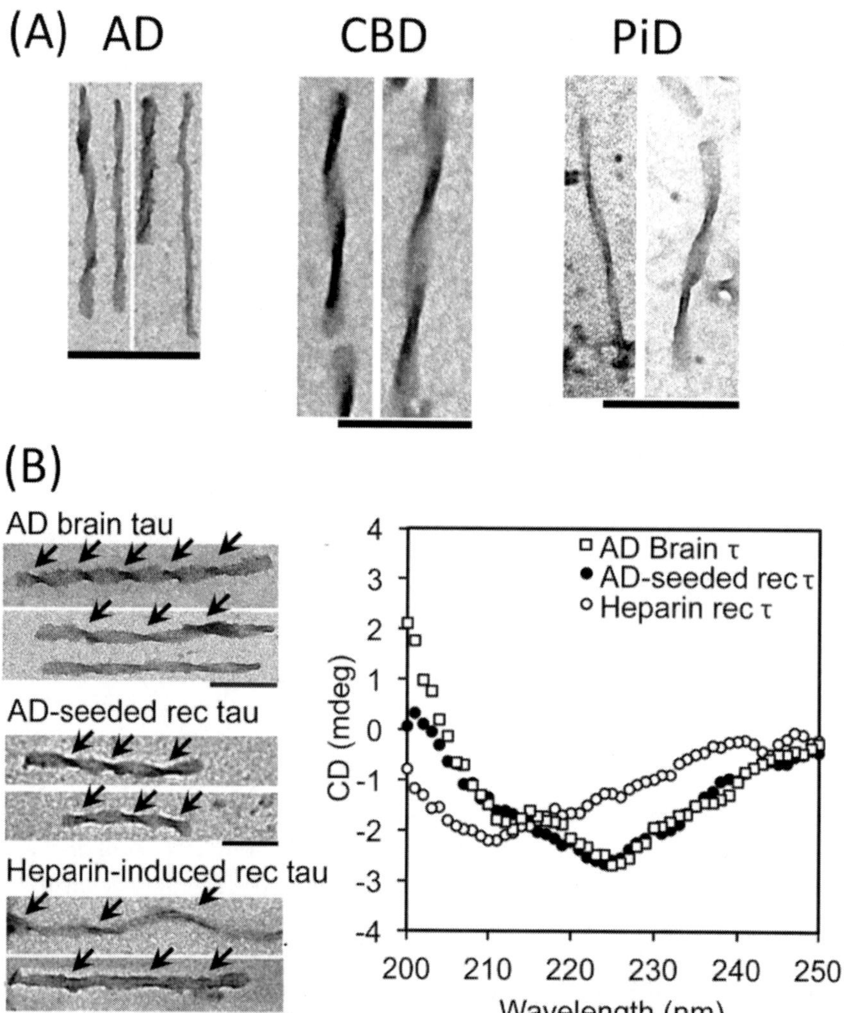

Figure 4. Tau strains and their propagation in cell-free systems without post-translational modification or cofactors. (A) Electron micrographs of the distinct structures of tau fibrils isolated from AD, corticobasal degeneration (CBD), and Pick's disease (PiD) brain homogenates. (B) Monomeric recombinant protein seeded with tau fibrils isolated from AD brain homogenates retains the structural features of the parental seed as assessed by electron microscopy and circular dichroism. For comparison, recombinant tau protein induced to form fibrils by heparin have distinct features. Scale bars represent 200 nm in (A) and 100 nm in (B); arrows indicate period of twist; images in (B) reprinted with permission from [40], copyright 2013 American Chemical Society.

SEEDED AMPLIFICATION OF BRAIN-DERIVED TAU STRAINS

While polyanionic fibril induction has enabled insights into disease processes using recombinant protein, the underlying mechanism of fibril formation in the presence of such inducers appears to follow a different fibrillization mechanism than most amyloidogenic proteins [76], and the fibril strains formed are both structurally and biochemically different from their brain-derived counterparts (Figure 4b) [40, 77]. In contrast to these synthetic tau strains, full-length wild-type tau seeded by fibrils isolated from AD brain without heparin faithfully inherited the seed properties including fibril dimensions and secondary structure, independent of phosphorylation (Figure 4b) [40]. Hyper-phosphorylated tau has a reduced ability to stabilize microtubules so it has been implicated in tauopathy pathogenesis, though its role in fibril formation is a subject of debate [40, 78, 79, 80].

Additionally, recombinant tau seeded by P301S mouse brain-derived fibrils had the seeding potency and biochemical characteristics of the parent brain-derived seeds with and without hyper-phosphorylation [77] confirming the potential for tau strains to template conformational change independently of post-translational modifications [40].

TAU FIBRIL UPTAKE AND STRAIN PROPAGATION IN CELL CULTURE

Cell culture models have been used to study the mechanisms by which tau fibrils become internalized, propagate, and transfer between cells. Synthetic tau fibrils, formed by misfolding tau in the presence of polyanionic cofactors, can be directly taken up by cells, seeding fibrillization of endogenous tau [81, 82, 83]. AD brain-derived tau also seeded intracellular fibrillization in HEK cells and SH-SY5Y cells [84]. Tau fibrils enter primary mouse neurons without lipid-based protein delivery reagents and stimulate conversion of endogenously expressed tau [26, 85, 86, 87].

Tau fibril strains also propagate in cell culture. Fibrils of 4R tau induced several biochemically and morphologically distinct synthetic tau strains in HEK cells [46]. These synthetic strains propagate in HEK cells as the cells divide and infect naïve HEK cells while maintaining the cellular and molecular properties characteristic of each strain. Tau fibrils purified from AD, agyrophilic grain disease, corticobasal degeneration, Pick's disease, and progressive supranuclear palsy brains elicited morphologically distinct patterns of aggregation in HEK cells [46]. Finally, tau fibers purified from end-stage P301S mouse brain seed conversion of tau in HEK293 cells about fifty times more efficiently than biochemically distinct, synthetic fibrils composed of recombinant tau with the same sequence [77].

TRANSMISSION OF TAUOPATHIES IN MICE

The tendency of tau fibrils to be taken up by neurons and recruit endogenous tau into newly formed fibrils has also been demonstrated in mouse models of tauopathies. One mouse model expresses P301S mutant full-length human tau and begins to spontaneously develop tau tangles and neurodegeneration [88]. Intracerebral injection of P301S mouse brain homogenate into ALZ17 mice, a mouse model expressing a wild-type human tau [89], seeded fibrillization of tau in ALZ17 mouse brains [43]. Since the ALZ17 mice do not develop tauopathy in their lifetime, the P301S mouse brain homogenate was inferred to have contained a transmissible species. Likewise, an injection of end-stage P301S brain homogenate into presymptomatic P301S mice accelerated fibrillization before the P301S mice normally develop tauopathy [90].

The induction of tau pathology in mice by synthetic fibrils made from recombinantly expressed tau [44] further supports the protein-only hypothesis. A larger dose of synthetic fibrils made from P301L 4R tau seeded tau fibrillization in mice expressing full-length P301L tau and additionally demonstrated selective neuronal loss in the hippocampus relative to wild-type mice injected with the same quantity of induced fibrils [91]. In addition to the structural differences between fibrils from AD brains and synthetic fibrils induced by heparin [40], brain-derived and synthetic fibrils have different seeding potency in mouse models: enhanced seeding of P301S brain homogenate relative to heparin-induced fibrils was observed [77]; likewise, AD brain-derived seeds fibrillized tau in wild-type mouse brains more potently than heparin-induced fibrils [92].

Mice expressing mutant tau only in the entorhinal cortex induced tau fibrillization in distal, but synaptically connected regions of the brain [41, 42]. Exogenously administered fibrils consistently induce a time- and dose-dependent pattern of transynaptic spread in mice [44, 46, 90, 91]. Patient brain-homogenates from six different tauopathies seeded tau pathology similar to their human counterparts in mice expressing wild-type 2N4R human tau [45] except for Pick's disease in which tau fibrils were confined to the injection site. Pick's disease is a predominantly 3R isoform tauopathy, so there may be a seeding barrier between 3R and 4R tau isoforms [74, 82]. Brain homogenate from corticobasal degeneration and AD patients also induced similar histological progression in mice expressing full-length P301S tau; the number of hippocampal neurons decreased significantly in the AD cohort, but not in the corticobasal degeneration mice [93]. Two synthetic strains successfully propagated biochemical features after multiple sequential inoculations in mice [46]. Tau fibrillization was also propagated through serial inoculation of P301S mouse brain homogenates in ALZ17 mice, and brain homogenate from tangle-only dementia and agyrophilic grain disease patients in wild-type mice [45], although it was not clear whether the specific patterns of tau fibrillization were faithfully propagated as well. The intercellular transfer of tau fibrils in the brain and potential alternate routes of administration indicates that antibody therapies or vaccination may be an effective approach to treat or prevent tauopathies [94]; some groups have demonstrated success with antibodies capable of attenuating disease pathology [95, 96, 97].

MECHANISMS IMPLICATED IN CELL-TO-CELL TRANSFER OF TAU FIBRILS

Unlike disease proteins that are trafficked to the cell surface like prions or Aβ, tau is normally located in the cytosol and tau fibrils localize to the perinuclear space or somatodenritic compartment [98]. Monomeric tau is released into the interstitial space related to neuronal activity [99, 100] and is present in CSF [101]. It is unclear whether the release of pathogenic tau from neurons is related to the normal pathway of physiological release or unconventional secretory mechanisms [102, 103].

Experimentally, tau fibrils have been demonstrated to transfer between cells in cell culture [81, 104, 105] and transynaptically *in vivo* [41, 42, 105, 106]. Transynaptic spread in mouse models and both anterograde and retrograde trafficking of misfolded tau in neurons [87] strongly indicates the importance of synaptic connectivity in tauopathy pathogenesis. Alternatively, tau may be released into the interstitial space by the death of neurons containing tau fibrils. However, tau spreads in a hierarchical pattern following synaptic connectivity to distal regions of the brain [37, 41, 42, 43, 44, 45]; moreover tau levels do not appear to correlate with lactate dehydrogenase or tubulin release [107, 108]. Therefore it is unclear whether cell death is a dominant mechanism of intercellular transfer.

The detailed steps by which pathogenic uptake of tau fibrils occurs are also not fully understood, although several potential mechanisms have been identified (Figure 5).

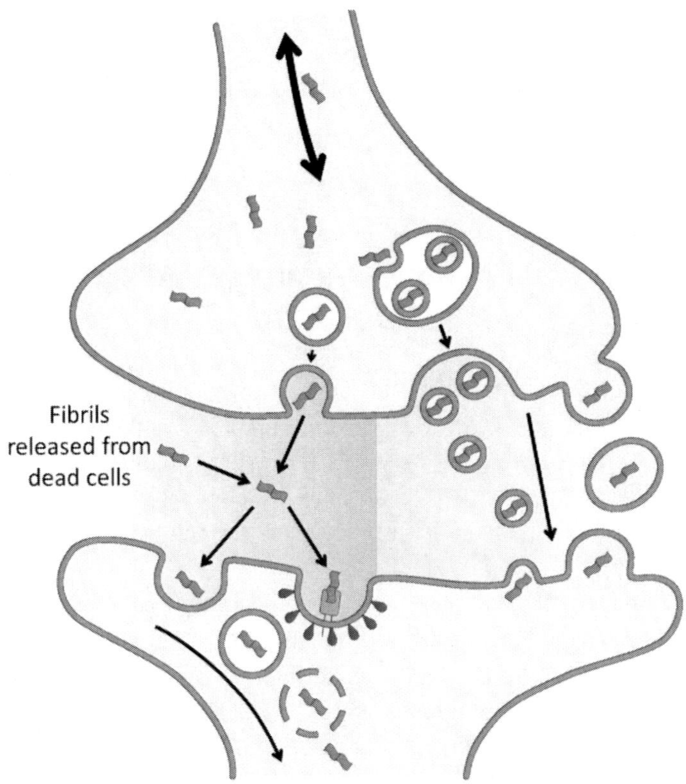

Figure 5. Hypotheses for the intercellular transfer of tau seeding species. Tau fibrils (orange) are transported both retrogradely and anterogradely along axons, as indicated by the large double-headed arrow at top, allowing fibrils to traverse neurons to presynaptic and postsynaptic termini [87]. Fibrillar tau has been observed outside of the cell in free form or in extracellular vesicles [102]. Shown to the left, naked fibrils may enter the extracellular space by release from dying cells or vesicular release by exocytosis potentially related to synaptic activity. Free fibrils may then be taken up by fluid-phase endocytosis or receptor-mediated endocytosis (receptor and vesicular coat proteins indicated in green and purple, respectively). Endosomal tau must then escape into the cytosol before it can recruit native tau into fibrils. Shown to the right, membrane-associated tau originates from exosomal/microvesicular packaging and release [113]. Once the membrane-associated tau reaches a post-synaptic terminal, it may be taken up by exosome/microvesicle fusion with the cell membrane.

Empirically, synthetic and brain-derived tau fibrils enter the cytosol of immortalized cell lines [81, 83, 84] and neurons in culture [85, 87, 109], and in mouse brains [43, 44, 45]; uptake also appears to be related to synaptic connections [37, 41, 42]. Lipid-based transfection reagents are used to promote fibril uptake [82, 83, 109]; however, studies specifically addressing the direct uptake of free tau fibrils in multiple cell types agree that a dominant mechanism is macropinocytosis [84, 86, 87]. Macropinocytosis is an actin-driven endocytic pathway in which the cell membrane encapsulates and pinches off a large intracellular vesicle containing extracellular fluid and local biomolecules [110]. Early work identifying markers of macropinocytosis seemed to suggest non-specific uptake [81, 84, 87]; however, a recent study showed tau fibrils actively stimulate macropinocytosis in a dose-dependent manner [86]. Once internalized into intracellular membrane vesicles, the endosomal escape of tau fibrils must occur before they can interact with endogenous tau. Heparin sulfate proteoglycans have been identified in neuritic plaques [111]; however, it was recently demonstrated that blocking cell surface heparin sulfate proteoglycan interactions strongly inhibits fibril uptake in culture and in mice [86] similar to the heparin-mediated pathways by which some bacteria and viruses enter cells [112]. Exosomal membrane fusion has also been suggested as a possible uptake mechanism [113]. The intercellular transfer of tau may also occur by a combination of these mechanisms [114], although it is not yet clear which is dominant in disease progression.

Role of Tau Fibers in Neuronal Dysfunction and Death

The contribution of the tau fibrillization process to neurodegeneration is unclear, as is that of the fibers themselves [115], with several lines of evidence questioning a direct contribution. Some degree of tau pathology was found in all individuals examined over age 75, increasing steadily with age, in the absence of cognitive impairment (n=26) [116]. Neuronal death in tauopathy patients greatly exceeds the number of neurofibrillary tangles accumulated [117].

Suppression of mutant tau expression, by administration of doxycycline to 'Tet-Off' transgenic mice expressing P301L or ΔK280 mutant human tau and after cognitive deficits and tau pathology have begun to develop, leads to improvement in cognitive function despite the persistence of neurofibrillary tangles [118, 119, 120]. Behavioral impairment and neuronal loss occur in some tauopathy animal models in the absence of detectable insoluble tau [121, 122, 123]. Mice expressing full length mutant tau exhibit neuronal dysfunction before the presence of detectable, mature neurofibrillary tangles [119, 124]; further, fibrils from end-stage P301S mice intracerebrally injected into mice expressing full-length human tau develop clear histological tau pathology without obvious neuronal loss [43, 90]. These findings must be taken into account in dissecting tau's role in neurodegeneration.

The toxicity of tau fibrillization may be directly related to the prefibrillar conversion of tau rather than the presence of mature tau neurofibrillary tangles themselves. It has been hypothesized that destabilization of protein quality control systems by age-related dysfunction or external stress (as in chronic traumatic encephalopathy) by a stressor threshold effect [31] may allow this toxic conversion process to occur more rapidly or accumulate more efficiently, making upregulation of protein chaperones a potential therapeutic target [125, 126, 127]. As tau also has a physiological role in many cellular pathways [6, 7], rapid sequestration of tau by fibril elongation may elicit dysfunction by a sudden loss-of-function of tau [128, 129].

Post-translational modifications including phosphorylation may not be required to template existing strains [40]; however, they may influence the spontaneous origin of strains or affect the interactions of tau in these cellular pathways to cause dysfunction [79, 80]. Tau-induced microglial activation [130] or receptor activation [131, 132] may indirectly cause neuronal dysfunction in surrounding cells (Figure 2b).

Conclusion

The identification of distinct fibril structures and evidence for propagation of strains in tauopathies provides a possible explanation for the divergent histological and clinical characteristics of tauopathies. Although significant progress has been made, additional research is needed to firmly establish the dominant mechanisms of neuronal release and uptake, the role of synaptic connections and activity on cellular transfer, cell type-specific vulnerability, and the conditions or cofactors responsible for the spontaneous origin of tau strains. Accumulating evidence suggests that tau fibrillization progresses within and between cells via templated conversion, similar to prions, Aβ, and other neurodegeneration-associated proteins [133, 134]; however, elucidation of strain-specific contributions to toxicity and cellular dysfunction is complicated by the possibility of mechanisms involving cell-autonomous effects and those arising from interactions with surrounding cells.

There are currently no therapies available to slow or halt the progression of tauopathies. Understanding the mechanisms by which tau strains propagate and cause or contribute to neurodegeneration will likely facilitate the discovery or design of therapies [135, 136, 137] or immunization strategies aimed at particular conformations of tau [138, 139, 140, 141, 142].

Acknowledgments

This chapter was supported by the National Institute of General Medical Sciences of the National Institutes of Health under award number P20GM104316. The content is solely the responsibility of the authors and does not necessarily represent the official views of the National Institutes of Health.

References

[1] Spillantini MG, Goedert M (2013) Tau pathology and neurodegeneration. *The Lancet Neurology* 12: 609-622.

[2] Murray ME, Kouri N, Lin WL, Jack CR, Jr., Dickson DW, et al. (2014) Clinicopathologic assessment and imaging of tauopathies in neurodegenerative dementias. *Alzheimers Res Ther* 6: 1.

[3] Williams DR, Lees AJ (2009) Progressive supranuclear palsy: clinicopathological concepts and diagnostic challenges. *Lancet Neurol.* 8, 270-279.

[4] Weingarten MD, Lockwood AH, Hwo SY, Kirschner MW (1975) A protein factor essential for microtubule assembly. *Proc Natl Acad Sci USA* 72: 1858-1862.

[5] Cleveland DW, Hwo SY, Kirschner MW (1977) Physical and chemical properties of purified tau factor and the role of tau in microtubule assembly. *J Mol Biol* 116: 227-247.

[6] Morris M, Maeda S, Vossel K, Mucke L (2011) The many faces of tau. *Neuron* 70: 410-426.

[7] Hanger DP, Lau DH, Phillips EC, Bondulich MK, Guo T, et al. (2014) Intracellular and extracellular roles for tau in neurodegenerative disease. *J Alzheimers Dis* 40 Suppl 1: S37-45.

[8] Schwalbe M, Ozenne V, Bibow S, Jaremko M, Jaremko L, et al. (2014) Predictive atomic resolution descriptions of intrinsically disordered hTau40 and alpha-synuclein in solution from NMR and small angle scattering. *Structure* 22: 238-249.

[9] von Bergen M, Barghorn S, Biernat J, Mandelkow EM, Mandelkow E (2005) Tau aggregation is driven by a transition from random coil to beta sheet structure. *Biochim Biophys Acta* 1739: 158-166.

[10] Fischer D, Mukrasch MD, Biernat J, Bibow S, Blackledge M, et al. (2009) Conformational changes specific for pseudophosphorylation at serine 262 selectively impair binding of tau to microtubules. *Biochemistry* 48: 10047-10055.

[11] Goedert M, Jakes R (1990) Expression of separate isoforms of human tau protein: correlation with the tau pattern in brain and effects on tubulin polymerization. *EMBO J* 9: 4225-4230.

[12] Goedert M, Spillantini MG, Cairns NJ, Crowther RA (1992) Tau proteins of Alzheimer paired helical filaments: abnormal phosphorylation of all six brain isoforms. *Neuron* 8: 159-168.

[13] Schmidt ML, Zhukareva V, Newell KL, Lee VM, Trojanowski JQ (2001) Tau isoform profile and phosphorylation state in dementia pugilistica recapitulate Alzheimer's disease. *Acta Neuropathol* 101: 518-524.

[14] Noda K, Sasaki K, Fujimi K, Wakisaka Y, Tanizaki Y, et al. (2006) Quantitative analysis of neurofibrillary pathology in a general population to reappraise neuropathological criteria for senile dementia of the neurofibrillary tangle type (tangle-only dementia): the Hisayama Study. *Neuropathology* 26: 508-518.

[15] Flament S, Delacourte A, Verny M, Hauw JJ, Javoy-Agid F (1991) Abnormal Tau proteins in progressive supranuclear palsy. Similarities and differences with the neurofibrillary degeneration of the Alzheimer type. *Acta Neuropathol* 81: 591-596.

[16] Ksiezak-Reding H, Morgan K, Mattiace LA, Davies P, Liu WK, et al. (1994) Ultrastructure and biochemical composition of paired helical filaments in corticobasal degeneration. *Am J Pathol* 145: 1496-1508.

[17] Togo T, Cookson N, Dickson DW (2002) Argyrophilic grain disease: neuropathology, frequency in a dementia brain bank and lack of relationship with apolipoprotein E. *Brain Pathol* 12: 45-52.

[18] Tolnay M, Sergeant N, Ghestem A, Chalbot S, De Vos RA, et al. (2002) Argyrophilic grain disease and Alzheimer's disease are distinguished by their different distribution of tau protein isoforms. *Acta Neuropathol* 104: 425-434.

[19] Delacourte A, Robitaille Y, Sergeant N, Buee L, Hof PR, et al. (1996) Specific pathological Tau protein variants characterize Pick's disease. *J Neuropathol Exp Neurol* 55: 159-168.

[20] Goedert M, Spillantini MG, Jakes R, Rutherford D, Crowther RA (1989) Multiple isoforms of human microtubule-associated protein tau: sequences and localization in neurofibrillary tangles of Alzheimer's disease. *Neuron* 3: 519-526.

[21] Prusiner SB (1982) Novel proteinaceous infectious particles cause scrapie. *Science* 216: 136-144.

[22] Safar J, Cohen FE, Prusiner SB (2000) Quantitative traits of prion strains are enciphered in the conformation of the prion protein. *Arch Virol Suppl*: 227-235.

[23] Legname G, Nguyen HO, Peretz D, Cohen FE, DeArmond SJ, et al. (2006) Continuum of prion protein structures enciphers a multitude of prion isolate-specified phenotypes. *Proc Natl Acad Sci USA* 103: 19105-19110.

[24] Peden AH, Ironside JW (2012) Molecular pathology in neurodegenerative diseases. *Curr Drug Targets* 13: 1548-1559.

[25] Goedert M, Falcon B, Clavaguera F, Tolnay M (2014) Prion-like mechanisms in the pathogenesis of tauopathies and synucleinopathies. *Curr Neurol Neurosci Rep* 14: 495.

[26] Holmes BB, Diamond MI (2014) Prion-like properties of Tau protein: the importance of extracellular Tau as a therapeutic target. *J Biol Chem* 289: 19855-19861.

[27] Clavaguera F, Hench J, Goedert M, Tolnay M (2014) Prion-like transmission and spreading of tau pathology. *Neuropathol Appl* Neurobiol.

[28] Seeley WW, Crawford RK, Zhou J, Miller BL, Greicius MD (2009) Neurodegenerative diseases target large-scale human brain networks. *Neuron* 62: 42-52.

[29] Zhou J, Gennatas ED, Kramer JH, Miller BL, Seeley WW (2012) Predicting regional neurodegeneration from the healthy brain functional connectome. *Neuron* 73: 1216-1227.

[30] Raj A, Kuceyeski A, Weiner M (2012) A network diffusion model of disease progression in dementia. *Neuron* 73: 1204-1215.

[31] Saxena S, Caroni P (2011) Selective neuronal vulnerability in neurodegenerative diseases: from stressor thresholds to degeneration. *Neuron* 71: 35-48.

[32] Prusiner SB (1984) Some speculations about prions, amyloid, and Alzheimer's disease. *N Engl J Med* 310: 661-663.

[33] Lee VM, Goedert M, Trojanowski JQ (2001) Neurodegenerative tauopathies. *Annu Rev Neurosci* 24: 1121-1159.

[34] Hutton M, Lendon CL, Rizzu P, Baker M, Froelich S, et al. (1998) Association of missense and 5'-splice-site mutations in tau with the inherited dementia FTDP-17. *Nature* 393: 702-705.

[35] Wolfe MS (2009) Tau mutations in neurodegenerative diseases. *J Biol Chem* 284: 6021-6025.

[36] Novak P, Prcina M, Kontsekova E (2011) Tauons and prions: infamous cousins? *J Alzheimers Dis* 26: 413-430.

[37] Braak H, Braak E (1991) Neuropathological stageing of Alzheimer-related changes. *Acta Neuropathol* 82: 239-259.

[38] Feany MB, Dickson DW (1996) Neurodegenerative disorders with extensive tau pathology: a comparative study and review. *Ann Neurol* 40: 139-148.

[39] Frost B, Ollesch J, Wille H, Diamond MI (2009) Conformational diversity of wild-type Tau fibrils specified by templated conformation change. *J Biol Chem* 284: 3546-3551.

[40] Morozova OA, March ZM, Robinson AS, Colby DW (2013) Conformational features of tau fibrils from Alzheimer's disease brain are faithfully propagated by unmodified recombinant protein. *Biochemistry* 52: 6960-6967.

[41] Liu L, Drouet V, Wu JW, Witter MP, Small SA, et al. (2012) Trans-synaptic spread of tau pathology in vivo. *PLoS One* 7: e31302.

[42] de Calignon A, Polydoro M, Suarez-Calvet M, William C, Adamowicz DH, et al. (2012) Propagation of tau pathology in a model of early Alzheimer's disease. *Neuron* 73: 685-697.

[43] Clavaguera F, Bolmont T, Crowther RA, Abramowski D, Frank S, et al. (2009) Transmission and spreading of tauopathy in transgenic mouse brain. *Nat Cell Biol* 11: 909-913.

[44] Iba M, Guo JL, McBride JD, Zhang B, Trojanowski JQ, et al. (2013) Synthetic tau fibrils mediate transmission of neurofibrillary tangles in a transgenic mouse model of Alzheimer's-like tauopathy. *J Neurosci* 33: 1024-1037.

[45] Clavaguera F, Akatsu H, Fraser G, Crowther RA, Frank S, et al. (2013) Brain homogenates from human tauopathies induce tau inclusions in mouse brain. *Proc Natl Acad Sci USA* 110: 9535-9540.

[46] Sanders DW, Kaufman SK, DeVos SL, Sharma AM, Mirbaha H, et al. (2014) Distinct tau prion strains propagate in cells and mice and define different tauopathies. *Neuron* 82: 1271-1288.

[47] Collinge J, Clarke AR (2007) A general model of prion strains and their pathogenicity. *Science* 318: 930-936.

[48] Irwin DJ, Abrams JY, Schonberger LB, Leschek EW, Mills JL, et al. (2013) Evaluation of potential infectivity of Alzheimer and Parkinson disease proteins in recipients of cadaver-derived human growth hormone. *JAMA Neurol.* 70(4):462-468.

[49] Clavaguera F, Hench J, Lavenir I, Schweighauser G, Frank S, et al. (2014) Peripheral administration of tau aggregates triggers intracerebral tauopathy in transgenic mice. *Acta Neuropathol* 127: 299-301.

[50] Tanaka M, Chien P, Naber N, Cooke R, Weissman JS (2004) Conformational variations in an infectious protein determine prion strain differences. *Nature* 428: 323-328.

[51] Klimova N, Makarava N, Baskakov IV (2014) The diversity and relationship of prion protein self-replicating states. *Virus Res.*

[52] Kretzschmar H, Tatzelt J (2013) Prion disease: a tale of folds and strains. *Brain Pathol* 23: 321-332.

[53] Sano K, Atarashi R, Ishibashi D, Nakagaki T, Satoh K, et al. (2014) Conformational properties of prion strains can be transmitted to recombinant prion protein fibrils in real-time quaking-induced conversion. *J Virol* 88: 11791-11801.

[54] Kidd M (1963) Paired helical filaments in electron microscopy of Alzheimer's disease. *Nature* 197: 192-193.

[55] Ksiezak-Reding H, Morgan K, Mattiace LA, Davies P, Liu WK, et al. (1994) Ultrastructure and biochemical composition of paired helical filaments in corticobasal degeneration. *Am J Pathol.* 145(6):1496-1508.

[56] Crowther RA, Goedert M (2000) Abnormal tau-containing filaments in neurodegenerative diseases. *J Struct Biol* 130: 271-279.

[57] Zhukareva V, Shah K, Uryu K, Braak H, Del Tredici K, et al. (2002) Biochemical analysis of tau proteins in argyrophilic grain disease, Alzheimer's disease, and Pick's disease : a comparative study. *Am J Pathol* 161: 1135-1141.

[58] Schweers O, Schonbrunn-Hanebeck E, Marx A, Mandelkow E (1994) Structural studies of tau protein and Alzheimer paired helical filaments show no evidence for beta-structure. *J Biol Chem* 269: 24290-24297.

[59] Wolynes PG, Onuchic JN, Thirumalai D (1995) Navigating the folding routes. *Science* 267: 1619-1620.

[60] Dobson CM (2003) Protein folding and misfolding. *Nature* 426: 884-890.

[61] Selkoe DJ (2003) Folding proteins in fatal ways. *Nature* 426: 900-904.

[62] Wille H, Drewes G, Biernat J, Mandelkow EM, Mandelkow E (1992) Alzheimer-like paired helical filaments and antiparallel dimers formed from microtubule-associated protein tau in vitro. *J Cell Biol* 118: 573-584.

[63] Crowther RA, Olesen OF, Smith MJ, Jakes R, Goedert M (1994) Assembly of Alzheimer-like filaments from full-length tau protein. *FEBS Lett* 337: 135-138.

[64] Goedert M, Jakes R, Spillantini MG, Hasegawa M, Smith MJ, et al. (1996) Assembly of microtubule-associated protein tau into Alzheimer-like filaments induced by sulphated glycosaminoglycans. *Nature* 383: 550-553.

[65] Perez M, Valpuesta JM, Medina M, Montejo de Garcini E, Avila J (1996) Polymerization of tau into filaments in the presence of heparin: the minimal sequence required for tau-tau interaction. *J Neurochem* 67: 1183-1190.

[66] Kampers T, Friedhoff P, Biernat J, Mandelkow EM, Mandelkow E (1996) RNA stimulates aggregation of microtubule-associated protein tau into Alzheimer-like paired helical filaments. *FEBS Lett* 399: 344-349.

[67] Wilson DM, Binder LI (1997) Free fatty acids stimulate the polymerization of tau and amyloid beta peptides. In vitro evidence for a common effector of pathogenesis in Alzheimer's disease. *Am J Pathol* 150: 2181-2195.

[68] von Bergen M, Friedhoff P, Biernat J, Heberle J, Mandelkow EM, et al. (2000) Assembly of tau protein into Alzheimer paired helical filaments depends on a local sequence motif ((306)VQIVYK(311)) forming beta structure. *Proc Natl Acad Sci USA* 97: 5129-5134.

[69] Friedhoff P, Schneider A, Mandelkow EM, Mandelkow E (1998) Rapid assembly of Alzheimer-like paired helical filaments from microtubule-associated protein tau monitored by fluorescence in solution. *Biochemistry* 37: 10223-10230.

[70] Barghorn S, Mandelkow E (2002) Toward a unified scheme for the aggregation of tau into Alzheimer paired helical filaments. *Biochemistry* 41: 14885-14896.

[71] Chirita CN, Congdon EE, Yin H, Kuret J (2005) Triggers of full-length tau aggregation: a role for partially folded intermediates. *Biochemistry* 44: 5862-5872.

[72] Ramachandran G, Udgaonkar JB (2011) Understanding the kinetic roles of the inducer heparin and of rod-like protofibrils during amyloid fibril formation by Tau protein. *J Biol Chem* 286: 38948-38959.

[73] Siddiqua A, Luo Y, Meyer V, Swanson MA, Yu X, et al. (2012) Conformational basis for asymmetric seeding barrier in filaments of three- and four-repeat tau. *J Am Chem Soc* 134: 10271-10278.

[74] Dinkel PD, Siddiqua A, Huynh H, Shah M, Margittai M (2011) Variations in filament conformation dictate seeding barrier between three- and four-repeat tau. *Biochemistry* 50: 4330-4336.

[75] Furukawa Y, Kaneko K, Nukina N (2011) Tau protein assembles into isoform- and disulfide-dependent polymorphic fibrils with distinct structural properties. *J Biol Chem* 286: 27236-27246.

[76] Carlson SW, Branden M, Voss K, Sun Q, Rankin CA, et al. (2007) A complex mechanism for inducer mediated tau polymerization. *Biochemistry* 46: 8838-8849.

[77] Falcon B, Cavallini A, Angers R, Glover S, Murray TK, et al. (2015) Conformation determines the seeding potencies of native and recombinant tau aggregates. *J Biol Chem* 290: 1049-1065.

[78] Wischik CM, Harrington CR, Storey JM (2014) Tau-aggregation inhibitor therapy for Alzheimer's disease. *Biochem Pharmacol* 88: 529-539.

[79] Tenreiro S, Eckermann K, Outeiro TF (2014) Protein phosphorylation in neurodegeneration: friend or foe? *Front Mol Neurosci* 7: 42.

[80] Noble W, Hanger DP, Miller CC, Lovestone S (2013) The importance of tau phosphorylation for neurodegenerative diseases. *Front Neurol* 4: 83.

[81] Frost B, Jacks RL, Diamond MI (2009) Propagation of tau misfolding from the outside to the inside of a cell. *J Biol Chem* 284: 12845-12852.

[82] Nonaka T, Watanabe ST, Iwatsubo T, Hasegawa M (2010) Seeded aggregation and toxicity of {alpha}-synuclein and tau: cellular models of neurodegenerative diseases. *J Biol Chem* 285: 34885-34898.

[83] Guo JL, Lee VM (2011) Seeding of normal Tau by pathological Tau conformers drives pathogenesis of Alzheimer-like tangles. *J Biol Chem* 286: 15317-15331.

[84] Santa-Maria I, Varghese M, Ksiezak-Reding H, Dzhun A, Wang J, et al. (2012) Paired helical filaments from Alzheimer disease brain induce intracellular accumulation of Tau protein in aggresomes. *J Biol Chem* 287: 20522-20533.

[85] Guo JL, Lee VM (2013) Neurofibrillary tangle-like tau pathology induced by synthetic tau fibrils in primary neurons over-expressing mutant tau. *FEBS Lett* 587: 717-723.

[86] Holmes BB, DeVos SL, Kfoury N, Li M, Jacks R, et al. (2013) Heparan sulfate proteoglycans mediate internalization and propagation of specific proteopathic seeds. *Proc Natl Acad Sci USA* 110: E3138-3147.

[87] Wu JW, Herman M, Liu L, Simoes S, Acker CM, et al. (2013) Small misfolded Tau species are internalized via bulk endocytosis and anterogradely and retrogradely transported in neurons. *J Biol Chem* 288: 1856-1870.

[88] Allen B, Ingram E, Takao M, Smith MJ, Jakes R, et al. (2002) Abundant tau filaments and nonapoptotic neurodegeneration in transgenic mice expressing human P301S tau protein. *J Neurosci* 22: 9340-9351.

[89] Probst A, Gotz J, Wiederhold KH, Tolnay M, Mistl C, et al. (2000) Axonopathy and amyotrophy in mice transgenic for human four-repeat tau protein. *Acta Neuropathol* 99: 469-481.

[90] Ahmed Z, Cooper J, Murray TK, Garn K, McNaughton E, et al. (2014) A novel in vivo model of tau propagation with rapid and progressive neurofibrillary tangle pathology: the pattern of spread is determined by connectivity, not proximity. *Acta Neuropathol* 127: 667-683.

[91] Peeraer E, Bottelbergs A, Van Kolen K, Stancu IC, Vasconcelos B, et al. (2015) Intracerebral injection of preformed synthetic tau fibrils initiates widespread tauopathy and neuronal loss in the brains of tau transgenic mice. *Neurobiol Dis* 73: 83-95.
[92] Lasagna-Reeves CA, Castillo-Carranza DL, Sengupta U, Guerrero-Munoz MJ, Kiritoshi T, et al. (2012) Alzheimer brain-derived tau oligomers propagate pathology from endogenous tau. *Sci Rep* 2: 700.
[93] Boluda S, Iba M, Zhang B, Raible KM, Lee VM, et al. (2015) Differential induction and spread of tau pathology in young PS19 tau transgenic mice following intracerebral injections of pathological tau from Alzheimer's disease or corticobasal degeneration brains. *Acta Neuropathol* 129: 221-237.
[94] De Genst E, Messer A, Dobson CM (2014) Antibodies and protein misfolding: From structural research tools to therapeutic strategies. *Biochim Biophys Acta* 1844: 1907-1919.
[95] Chai X, Wu S, Murray TK, Kinley R, Cella CV, et al. (2011) Passive immunization with anti-Tau antibodies in two transgenic models: reduction of Tau pathology and delay of disease progression. *J Biol Chem* 286: 34457-34467.
[96] Yanamandra K, Kfoury N, Jiang H, Mahan TE, Ma S, et al. (2013) Anti-tau antibodies that block tau aggregate seeding in vitro markedly decrease pathology and improve cognition in vivo. *Neuron* 80: 402-414.
[97] Yanamandra K, Jiang H, Mahan TE, Maloney SE, Wozniak DF, et al. (2015) Anti-tau antibody reduces insoluble tau and decreases brain atrophy. *Annals of Clinical and Translational Neurology* 2(3):278-288.
[98] Kosik KS, Crandall JE, Mufson EJ, Neve RL (1989) Tau in situ hybridization in normal and Alzheimer brain: localization in the somatodendritic compartment. *Ann Neurol* 26: 352-361.
[99] Pooler AM, Phillips EC, Lau DH, Noble W, Hanger DP (2013) Physiological release of endogenous tau is stimulated by neuronal activity. *EMBO Rep* 14: 389-394.
[100] Yamada K, Holth JK, Liao F, Stewart FR, Mahan TE, et al. (2014) Neuronal activity regulates extracellular tau in vivo. *J Exp Med* 211: 387-393.
[101] Tapiola T, Alafuzoff I, Herukka SK, Parkkinen L, Hartikainen P, et al. (2009) Cerebrospinal Fluid beta-Amyloid 42 and Tau Proteins as Biomarkers of Alzheimer-Type Pathologic Changes in the Brain. *Archives of Neurology* 66: 382-389.
[102] Mohamed NV, Herrou T, Plouffe V, Piperno N, Leclerc N (2013) Spreading of tau pathology in Alzheimer's disease by cell-to-cell transmission. *Eur J Neurosci* 37: 1939-1948.
[103] Nickel W, Rabouille C (2009) Mechanisms of regulated unconventional protein secretion. *Nat Rev Mol Cell Biol* 10: 148-155.
[104] Kfoury N, Holmes BB, Jiang H, Holtzman DM, Diamond MI (2012) Trans-cellular propagation of Tau aggregation by fibrillar species. *J Biol Chem* 287: 19440-19451.
[105] Dujardin S, Lecolle K, Caillierez R, Begard S, Zommer N, et al. (2014) Neuron-to-neuron wild-type Tau protein transfer through a trans-synaptic mechanism: relevance to sporadic tauopathies. *Acta Neuropathol Commun* 2: 14.
[106] Kim W, Lee S, Jung C, Ahmed A, Lee G, et al. (2010) Interneuronal transfer of human tau between Lamprey central neurons in situ. *J Alzheimers Dis* 19: 647-664.

[107] Plouffe V, Mohamed NV, Rivest-McGraw J, Bertrand J, Lauzon M, et al. (2012) Hyperphosphorylation and cleavage at D421 enhance tau secretion. *PLoS One* 7: e36873.

[108] Chai X, Dage JL, Citron M (2012) Constitutive secretion of tau protein by an unconventional mechanism. *Neurobiol Dis* 48: 356-366.

[109] Holmes BB, Furman JL, Mahan TE, Yamasaki TR, Mirbaha H, et al. (2014) Proteopathic tau seeding predicts tauopathy in vivo. *Proc Natl Acad Sci USA* 111: E4376-4385.

[110] Lim JP, Gleeson PA (2011) Macropinocytosis: an endocytic pathway for internalising large gulps. *Immunol Cell Biol* 89: 836-843.

[111] Snow AD, Mar H, Nochlin D, Kimata K, Kato M, et al. (1988) The presence of heparan sulfate proteoglycans in the neuritic plaques and congophilic angiopathy in Alzheimer's disease. *Am J Pathol* 133: 456-463.

[112] Mercer J, Helenius A (2009) Virus entry by macropinocytosis. *Nat Cell Biol* 11: 510-520.

[113] Saman S, Kim W, Raya M, Visnick Y, Miro S, et al. (2012) Exosome-associated tau is secreted in tauopathy models and is selectively phosphorylated in cerebrospinal fluid in early Alzheimer disease. *J Biol Chem* 287: 3842-3849.

[114] Guo JL, Lee VM (2014) Cell-to-cell transmission of pathogenic proteins in neurodegenerative diseases. *Nat Med* 20: 130-138.

[115] Bretteville A, Planel E (2008) Tau aggregates: toxic, inert, or protective species? *J Alzheimers Dis* 14: 431-436.

[116] Price JL, Morris JC (1999) Tangles and plaques in nondemented aging and "preclinical" Alzheimer's disease. *Ann Neurol* 45: 358-368.

[117] Gomez-Isla T, Hollister R, West H, Mui S, Growdon JH, et al. (1997) Neuronal loss correlates with but exceeds neurofibrillary tangles in Alzheimer's disease. *Ann Neurol* 41: 17-24.

[118] Santacruz K, Lewis J, Spires T, Paulson J, Kotilinek L, et al. (2005) Tau suppression in a neurodegenerative mouse model improves memory function. *Science* 309: 476-481.

[119] Spires TL, Orne JD, SantaCruz K, Pitstick R, Carlson GA, et al. (2006) Region-specific dissociation of neuronal loss and neurofibrillary pathology in a mouse model of tauopathy. *Am J Pathol* 168: 1598-1607.

[120] Sydow A, Van der Jeugd A, Zheng F, Ahmed T, Balschun D, et al. (2011) Tau-induced defects in synaptic plasticity, learning, and memory are reversible in transgenic mice after switching off the toxic Tau mutant. *J Neurosci* 31: 2511-2525.

[121] Kimura T, Yamashita S, Fukuda T, Park JM, Murayama M, et al. (2007) Hyperphosphorylated tau in parahippocampal cortex impairs place learning in aged mice expressing wild-type human tau. *EMBO J* 26: 5143-5152.

[122] Taniguchi T, Doe N, Matsuyama S, Kitamura Y, Mori H, et al. (2005) Transgenic mice expressing mutant (N279K) human tau show mutation dependent cognitive deficits without neurofibrillary tangle formation. *FEBS Lett* 579: 5704-5712.

[123] Wittmann CW, Wszolek MF, Shulman JM, Salvaterra PM, Lewis J, et al. (2001) Tauopathy in Drosophila: neurodegeneration without neurofibrillary tangles. *Science* 293: 711-714.

[124] Yoshiyama Y, Higuchi M, Zhang B, Huang SM, Iwata N, et al. (2007) Synapse loss and microglial activation precede tangles in a P301S tauopathy mouse model. *Neuron* 53: 337-351.

[125] Chafekar SM, Wisen S, Thompson AD, Echeverria A, Walter GM, et al. (2012) Pharmacological tuning of heat shock protein 70 modulates polyglutamine toxicity and aggregation. *ACS Chem Biol* 7: 1556-1564.

[126] Stein KC, True HL (2014) Structural variants of yeast prions show conformer-specific requirements for chaperone activity. *Mol Microbiol* 93: 1156-1171.

[127] Sweeny EA, Jackrel ME, Go MS, Sochor MA, Razzo BM, et al. (2015) The Hsp104 N-Terminal Domain Enables Disaggregase Plasticity and Potentiation. *Mol Cell* 57(5):836-849.

[128] Jaworski T, Kugler S, Van Leuven F (2010) Modeling of tau-mediated synaptic and neuronal degeneration in Alzheimer's disease. *Int J Alzheimers Dis* 2010.

[129] Trojanowski JQ, Lee VM (2005) Pathological tau: a loss of normal function or a gain in toxicity? *Nat Neurosci* 8: 1136-1137.

[130] Morales I, Jimenez JM, Mancilla M, Maccioni RB (2013) Tau oligomers and fibrils induce activation of microglial cells. *J Alzheimers Dis* 37: 849-856.

[131] Amadoro G, Ciotti MT, Costanzi M, Cestari V, Calissano P, et al. (2006) NMDA receptor mediates tau-induced neurotoxicity by calpain and ERK/MAPK activation. *Proc Natl Acad Sci USA* 103: 2892-2897.

[132] Gomez-Ramos A, Diaz-Hernandez M, Rubio A, Miras-Portugal MT, Avila J (2008) Extracellular tau promotes intracellular calcium increase through M1 and M3 muscarinic receptors in neuronal cells. *Mol Cell Neurosci* 37: 673-681.

[133] Stohr J, Condello C, Watts JC, Bloch L, Oehler A, et al. (2014) Distinct synthetic Abeta prion strains producing different amyloid deposits in bigenic mice. *Proc Natl Acad Sci USA* 111: 10329-10334.

[134] Arosio P, Cukalevski R, Frohm B, Knowles TP, Linse S (2014) Quantification of the concentration of Abeta42 propagons during the lag phase by an amyloid chain reaction assay. *J Am Chem Soc* 136: 219-225.

[135] Bulic B, Pickhardt M, Mandelkow EM, Mandelkow E (2010) Tau protein and tau aggregation inhibitors. *Neuropharmacolog*y 59: 276-289.

[136] Crowe A, Huang W, Ballatore C, Johnson RL, Hogan AM, et al. (2009) Identification of aminothienopyridazine inhibitors of tau assembly by quantitative high-throughput screening. *Biochemistry* 48: 7732-7745.

[137] Taniguchi S, Suzuki N, Masuda M, Hisanaga S, Iwatsubo T, et al. (2005) Inhibition of heparin-induced tau filament formation by phenothiazines, polyphenols, and porphyrins. *J Biol Chem* 280: 7614-7623.

[138] Brody DL, Holtzman DM (2008) Active and passive immunotherapy for neurodegenerative disorders. *Annu Rev Neurosci* 31: 175-193.

[139] Boutajangout A, Quartermain D, Sigurdsson EM (2010) Immunotherapy targeting pathological tau prevents cognitive decline in a new tangle mouse model. *J Neurosci* 30: 16559-16566.

[140] Bi M, Ittner A, Ke YD, Gotz J, Ittner LM (2011) Tau-targeted immunization impedes progression of neurofibrillary histopathology in aged P301L tau transgenic mice. *PLoS One* 6: e26860.

[141] Sigurdsson EM (2008) Immunotherapy targeting pathological tau protein in Alzheimer's disease and related tauopathies. *J Alzheimers Dis* 15: 157-168.

[142] Kontsekova E, Zilka N, Kovacech B, Novak P, Novak M (2014) First-in-man tau vaccine targeting structural determinants essential for pathological tau-tau interaction reduces tau oligomerisation and neurofibrillary degeneration in an Alzheimer's disease model. *Alzheimers Res Ther* 6: 44.

In: The Prion Phenomena in Neurodegenerative Diseases ISBN: 978-1-63483-399-8
Editors: Giuseppe Legname and Gabriele Giachin

Chapter 9

PRION-LIKE MECHANISMS IN AMYOTROPHIC LATERAL SCLEROSIS

Leslie I. Grad, Edward Pokrishevsky and Neil R. Cashman*

Department of Medicine (Neurology),
Djavad Mowafaghian Centre for Brain Health,
University of British Columbia, Vancouver BC, Canada

ABSTRACT

Prion diseases, such as Creutzfeldt–Jakob disease, are caused by a unique class of proteinaceous infectious agents. Pathologically misfolded prion protein can catalyze the conversion of its natively folded counterpart into a misfolded and toxic form, which serves as a recruiting seed for further rounds of protein misfolding that can spread intercellularly through the nervous system. Amyotrophic lateral sclerosis (ALS), a lethal disease characterized by progressive degeneration of motor neurons is currently understood as a classic proteinopathy, although its etiology remains unclear. The disease is typified by the formation of inclusions consisting of misfolded and/or aggregated protein within motor neurons that contribute to neurotoxicity. Recent work has identified prion-like properties in proteins involved in ALS pathology, including their participation in intracellular recruitment, cell-to-cell transmission and even interorganismal transmission. Along with the transmission of naked protein aggregates, experimental evidence suggests that intercellular spread may be facilitated through the ongoing release and uptake of small membranous extracellular vesicles, containing or decorated with disease-specific misfolded proteins, a mechanism already observed for classical prion diseases. Prion-like propagation and transmission may provide the molecular basis for the clinically observed contiguous spread of the disease through the neuroaxis. The inclusion of ALS as a prion-like disease is a relatively recent development, but the evidence and observations supporting it have come at a furious pace. The goal of this chapter is to summarize the current state of knowledge of prion-like proteins in ALS and their mechanisms of transmission between cells and organisms.

* Corresponding Author address: Email: neil.cashman@vch.ca

INTRODUCTION

Amyotrophic lateral sclerosis (ALS) is a progressive, but ultimately fatal neuromuscular disease characterized by systematic degeneration of the upper and lower motor neurons resulting in weakening and subsequent atrophy of muscles of the limbs, as well as those involved in speech and swallowing [1, 2]. Interestingly, cognitive function is usually spared with only 5% of patients developing frank frontotemporal dementia (FTD) [3]. Clinical onset usually occurs in individuals over 40 and is the most common form of motor neuron disease world-wide with a global incidence of about two in 100,000. Half of affected individuals die within 3 years, and less than 20% survive for more than 5 years [4]. Clinical progression of ALS is relentless and spreads by one of two observable patterns: single focal point initiation, where symptoms appear to begin at a single site and subsequently spreads through adjacent neuroanatomical regions in a spatiotemporal manner [5], or *via* multifocal initiation, where several regions are initially affected, but each focal point serves as the epicenter for contiguous spread of pathology through local propagation [6]. These patterns of disease initiation are highly reminiscent of the spread of prion disease and thus could be explained through the prion-like mechanism of propagated protein misfolding. In addition, prion-like protein misfolding could account for how a mutant or even wild-type protein can dominate pathogenesis of a phenotypically diverse disease such as seen for ALS, akin to when the normal cellular isoform of prion protein (PrP^{C}) is converted to its pathologically dominant form, PrP^{Sc} in prion disease.

The etiology of ALS remains unknown and the mechanisms leading to the selective vulnerability and degeneration of motor neurons in ALS are not well understood; however similar to other neurodegenerative diseases such as Alzheimer disease and Creutzfeldt–Jakob disease (CJD), the disease can be divided into two categories, sporadic and familial (inheritable). 90-95% of ALS cases are sporadic (SALS) where only some predisposing gene mutations have been identified, such as the ataxin-2 intermediate repeat expansions [7]. The remainder of cases are familial (FALS) [8], which are predominantly associated with Mendelian-inherited, primarily autosomal dominant mutations in genes encoding Cu/Zn superoxide dismutase (SOD1), TAR-DNA binding protein 43 (TDP-43), fused in sarcoma/translocated in liposarcoma (FUS/TLS), and C9ORF72, but have been associated with mutations in other genes as well (reviewed in [9]) [10, 11, 12, 13]. ALS-associated mutations involving several of these genes increase the propensity of the respective protein to misfold, aggregate and form fibrils [14]. Although the majority of ALS cases are sporadic with no identifiable mutations, pathological forms of these proteins are often present within proteinaceous inclusions found in a large subset of ALS patients, strongly suggesting that protein misfolding plays a key role in disease pathogenesis and/or pathology [15, 16]. In addition, both categories of disease show very similar clinical presentations, suggesting that a common downstream pathogenic mechanism, regardless of disease origin, may lie at the heart of the disease [17].

The post-mortem pathology of ALS patients typically features loss of motor neurons in the brain stem and ventral horn of the spinal cord, accompanied with signs of inflammation such as astrocyte activation and proliferation of microglia [18]. Spinal cord histology often reveals abnormal accumulations of ubiquitinated proteinaceous inclusions in motor neurons and neural accessory cells, which are thought to be the result of aggregated misfolded protein.

Protein misfolding can be triggered by a multitude of factors, including genetic mutation, aberrant oxidation and post-translational modification, dysfunctional proteostasis and seeded polymerization [19]. For example, in FALS cases where a SOD1 mutation is identified, the primary component of these protein inclusions is SOD1 itself [20]. Curiously, in sporadic cases in which SOD1 mutations have been excluded, there is also evidence supporting the presence of misfolded SOD1 [21, 22, 23, 24], suggesting a more expanded role for SOD1 in ALS pathology, although this observation is not one of consensus [25]. A more universally agreed observation is that ubiquitinated and phosphorylated TDP-43 is a primary component of cytosolic inclusions in the vast majority of SALS, in combination with its depletion from the nucleus, where the majority of native TDP-43 normally resides [26]. The presence of misfolded/aggregated protein in ALS, along with the distinct spatiotemporal spread of pathology though the spinal cord makes it a likely candidate as a disease with prion-like mechanistic properties. This chapter will examine the current state of knowledge regarding the prion-like properties of proteins associated with ALS pathology (summarized in Table 1) as well as their possible mechanisms of transmission within and between cells, as well as transmission between organisms.

Table 1. Summary of known evidence of prion-like phenomena in ALS-associated proteins

Protein	Seeded aggregation/ induction of misfolding *in vitro*	Seeded aggregation in cell culture	Seeded aggregation *in vivo*	Intercellular transmission in cell culture	Interorganismal transmission
SOD1	Yes [27, 28].	Yes [28, 29].	Indirect evidence only [30,31].	Yes [24,29].	Yes, under specific experimental conditions [32].
TDP-43	Yes [144].	Yes [33, 34].	n.d.	Yes [34].	n.d.
FUS	Yes [35].	n.d.	n.d.	n.d.	n.d.
C90RF72	Only self-aggregation of DPRs [36, 37].	n.d.	n.d.	n.d.	n.d.
EWRS1	Only self-aggregation *via* prion-like domain [38].	n.d.	n.d.	n.d.	n.d.
TAT15	Only self-aggregation *via* prion-like domain [38].	n.d.	n.d.	n.d.	n.d.
hnRNPA2B1/A1	Yes [39]	Accelerated recruitment into stress granules [39]	n.d.	n.d.	n.d.

n.d., not determined.

THE ROLE OF SOD1 IN ALS PATHOLOGY

In 1993, Rosen et al., identified the first protein to be implicated in familial ALS: Cu/Zn superoxide dismutase (SOD1), a highly abundant and ubiquitously-expressed cytosolic protein whose function is primarily to serve as a free-radical defense enzyme that converts highly toxic free-radical superoxide produced within the cell to less harmful molecules hydrogen peroxide and water [40, 41]. SOD1 mutations occur in 20% of familial ALS patients and have also been detected in a small subset of sporadic ALS patients [42]. To date, over 180 disease-causing mutations have been identified in the 154 amino-acid long protein [10]. Mutant SOD1 proteins display a number of thermodynamic signatures conducive to misfolding, including decreased thermal stability, increased susceptibility to mechanical deformation, increased propensity to monomerize, decreased affinity for metals, and accelerated unfolding under stress conditions [43, 44]. This can lead to the formation of a pool of misfolded SOD1 protein in the cell, potentially through the depletion of copper or structurally-stabilizing zinc under stress [43, 45]. Ultimately, SOD1 aggregation occurs through a mechanism by which the highly-stable native SOD1 homodimer is disrupted producing misfolded monomer intermediates that can be incorporated into higher-order structures [46, 47, 48]. Genetic mutation is not the only way to destabilize, misfold and aggregate SOD1. Aberrant oxidation or post-translational modification of wild-type (WT) SOD1 has been observed to mimic the aggregation-prone effects of mutant SOD1 *in vitro* [47, 49, 50] in a concentration-dependent manner [47]. There is increasing evidence that all types of ALS, including non-SOD1-linked familial and sporadic cases are associated with SOD1 misfolding, oxidation and subsequent aggregation [51]. Inclusions containing aggregated SOD1 have been detected in spinal cord tissues from both FALS and SALS patients [52, 53, 54] in addition to biochemical, genetic and immunological evidence of misfolded SOD1 in cases of mutant SOD1-excluded SALS [21, 22, 23, 24, 55, 56]. Misfolded SOD1 is therefore a prime candidate as a common molecular determinant for all forms of ALS and may play a key role in disease pathogenesis.

The mechanisms by which misfolded SOD1 causes or contributes to ALS pathology are not yet fully understood. Mutations in SOD1 often impair enzymatic function; however loss of superoxide dismutase function is not the primary cause of disease as *SOD1* knockout mice do not develop an ALS-like motor neuron disease [57], but rather a distinctly different motor axonopathy [58]. Conversely, a mutant *SOD1* transgenic mouse developed a progressive motor neuron disease despite increased SOD1 enzymatic activity over and above the mouse endogenous protein [59]. Instead, aberrant folding and subsequent aggregation of SOD1 conferred by mutation, oxidation or other cell stresses is generally thought to acquire a toxic gain of function [57, 59, 60], although the precise nature of this toxicity and its specificity for motor neurons remain to be elucidated. Experimentally, all transgenic mouse strains expressing ALS-causing SOD1 mutants develop cytosolic inclusions in motor neurons and accessory neural cells that coincide with the onset of motor neuron disease and increase in size and number throughout the course of disease progression [61, 62]. When misfolded, SOD1 can react non-specifically with a variety of substrates, causing it to actually become a net producer of reactive oxygen and nitrogen species [63], as opposed to performing its native function as a free-radical scavenger. Aberrant production of free radicals can lead to damage of cellular protein, lipid, and nucleic acid [64, 65]. Toxicity of misfolded SOD1 has also been attributed to other deleterious cellular effects including: cytoskeletal and mitochondrial disruption, caspase activation, microglial activation, and proteasomal and autophagy pathway disruption [66, 67, 68]. With regard to the latter pathways, pathological SOD1 appears to exert its effects on the protein homeostatic pathways in ALS models even before disease symptoms appear, suggesting other disease functions outside of the inefficient clearance of free radicals within the cell. For example, pathways of the unfolded protein response (UPR) are activated in G93A-SOD1 transgenic mice before the earliest signs of disease are observed [69]. In addition, misfolded mutant SOD1 has been observed to induce dysfunction in both autophagy and the proteasome-dependent degradation pathways [70, 71]. Coincidently, reduced proteasome subunit levels and activity are a common molecular signature in both FALS and SALS patients [72], suggesting deficits in proteasome activity are part of the general molecular disease pathology in humans and may be linked to SOD1 misfolding/aggregation.

Prion-Like Conversion of SOD1

The central dogma of the prion hypothesis, as outlined by Prusiner in 1982 [73], stipulates that protein alone is sufficient to act as an infectious agent. On a molecular level, a prion-like protein is often defined as a pathologically misfolded protein that can impart its misfold onto a neighbouring native protein through physical interaction, thus providing more template for subsequent rounds of conversion. Although the breadth of experimental evidence is not as well-established compared to the prion protein itself, an ever-growing body of evidence in the literature suggests that misfolded SOD1 has the ability to transfer conformational information from one SOD1 molecule to another, meeting at least the intermolecular requirements of prion-like activity [27, 28, 29].

Native functional SOD1 enzyme exists as a soluble ubiquitously-expressed homodimer that makes up 1-2% of the total protein of neurons and other neural accessory cells [74]. Monomers are bound to one another *via* hydrophobic interaction at the dimer interface. Furthermore, each monomer contains an intramolecular disulfide bond, believed to contribute to the high conformational stability and resistance to proteolytic digestion of native dimeric SOD1 [75]. Despite its intrinsic stability, destabilization of the enzyme is apparent when the protein monomers are mutated and/or aberrantly oxidized, making them highly susceptible to misfold and form multimeric species and aggregates. More than 180 *SOD1* mutations have been identified in ALS patients [10] affecting at least 75 of the 154 amino acids of the SOD1 protein [76]. Aggregation of mutant misfolded SOD1 inside the cell may not simply be a random process as ubiquitinated misfolded SOD1 is found to cluster into distinct aggregates *via* the juxtanuclear quality control (JUNQ) pathway as a means of sequestering potentially toxic protein from the rest of the cellular machinery [77]. Under denaturing conditions wild-type and mutant forms of SOD1 can spontaneously form aggregates and fibrils *in vitro* [27], where the relative propensity for aggregation is dependent upon the SOD1 mutant variant [78]. *In vivo* SOD1 fibril formation has been observed in transgenic mice expressing mutant SOD1 [79, 80]; however, the formation of amyloid fibrils does not appear to be a consistent feature of SOD1 in human disease as SOD1-positive inclusions from FALS patients do not stain with amyloid-specific dyes [25].

Observations from *in vivo* studies have provided the first, albeit indirect observations of intramolecular conversion of native SOD1 to a pathological form. Acceleration of motor neuron degeneration in mutant SOD1 mouse models is observed upon co-expression of human WTSOD1 [31, 81], possibly through intermolecular stabilization of mutant species *via* WTSOD1 interactions [82] or *via* formation of non-native disulfide interactions that induce insoluble aggregate formation [83].

In addition, co-aggregation of mutant and WTSOD1 has also been detected in tissue derived from familial ALS patients [30], suggestive of intermolecular conversion occurring in patients. More recently, direct evidence of intermolecular WTSOD1 conversion to a misfolded isoform has been observed in human mesenchymal and neuronal cell lines [23, 28]. Expression of misfolded human SOD1 mutants can convert resident WTSOD1 to a misfolded form that is revealed by conformation-specific antibodies that recognize epitopes only accessible when the protein is in a misfolded disease state. The resultant misfolded WTSOD1 in mutant SOD1-transfected cells is highly protease sensitivity, an indicator of overall structural loosening of the polypeptide backbone. Conversion of WTSOD1 to a misfolded conformer by mutant SOD1 has also been shown to occur in a cell-free system, thus eliminating any extraneous protein, lipid or nucleic acid co-factors from the process [28] and further supporting the 'protein-only' paradigm of prion-like protein misfolding.

Interaction between misfolded SOD1 template and native WTSOD1 substrate is a sequence- and/or structure-dependent process akin to the species barrier observed for classical prion diseases such as chronic wasting disease, a transmissible spongiform encephalopathy that is thus far restricted to certain cervid species [84], as mutant human SOD1 does not convert endogenous WTSOD1 to a misfolded species in mouse cells. WTSOD1 conversion appears dependent upon the presence of a single amino acid residue, tryptophan (Trp) at position 32 [28], indicating a potential point of contact between the converting and the converted species that is separate from the dimer interface region, once thought as a more intuitive point of contact between SOD1 molecules. Trp32 is the only tryptophan residue present in the human WTSOD1 amino acid sequence and has previously been identified as a site prone to oxidative modification and a potentiator of aggregation [85]. For example, oxidation of Trp32 caused by SOD1 bicarbonate-dependent peroxidase activity has been shown to trigger SOD1 aggregation, including covalently cross-linking of monomers through ditryptophan bonds [86].

Substitution of the tryptophan by a serine (present in the mouse SOD1 homolog) in ALS-associated mutants of SOD1 serving as 'seed' for the conversion of WTSOD1 fails to induce WTSOD1 misfolding in human cell lines [28], likely explaining why mutant human SOD1 is inert in converting WTSOD1 in mouse cells. The structure/sequence requirements for intermolecular conversion of SOD1 is also seen *in vivo* as human WTSOD1 does not accelerate motor neuron disease in mice expressing mutant murine SOD1 with a G86R substitution [87], analogous to the human G85R mutation linked to FALS. Furthermore, murine SOD1 is not incorporated into aggregates of human mutant SOD1 [31, 83, 88].

PROPAGATION OF SOD1 MISFOLDING

As presented in the previous section, there is ample evidence supporting the intermolecular conversion of WTSOD1 by mutant SOD1; however the mechanism by which this process occurs remains unclear. For the prion protein, two possible mechanisms of propagation have been proposed: nucleated polymerization and template directed misfolding [89]. Nucleated polymerization occurs when the misfolded protein species is intrinsically less stable as a monomer but becomes more stable than its native counterpart when recruited to a multimeric aggregate. When misfolded monomer encounters a nucleating oligomer, the former is incorporated into the latter and eventually leads to fibril elongation, which may break-up into multiple oligomeric seeds that subsequently become the new recruiters. In template-directed misfolding, the misfolded conformer is more stable than the native form but is kinetically inaccessible without catalysis by an interaction with other misfolded conformers; a misfolded SOD1 oligomer becomes a physical template for the misfolding of the native WTSOD1. Once converted, misfolded SOD1 can further propagate by catalyzing additional rounds of conversion, thus forming aggregates and fibril structures in increasing size and number. Evidence for both propagated protein misfolding mechanisms have been observed for SOD1 and suggests that prion-like propagation of both mutant and WTSOD1 likely spans a continuum between the two models. Aggregation of partially unfolded mutant SOD1 may self-propagate primarily by nucleated polymerization. For example, exogenous soluble mutant SOD1 was observed to incorporate into endogenous mutant SOD1 aggregates inside transfected mouse neuroblastoma cells [29]. On the other hand, conversion of WTSOD1 may require structural loosening induced by contact with a mutant or misfolded wild-type template [47] before recruitment to the misfolded SOD1 seed. In support of this notion is the finding that WTSOD1 can only participate in nucleated polymerization upon exposure to low pH and the chaotrope guanidine *in vitro* [21, 27], conditions that destabilize the native state and favour monomer recruitment into aggregates.

The dynamics of mutant SOD1 propagated misfolding depend on the intrinsic aggregation properties and structural stabilities of the different mutant isoforms, and play an essential role in disease progression and patient survival with SOD1-FALS [90]. Crystal structures from recombinant metal-deficient mutant SOD1 proteins reveal assemblies of aligned beta-sheets forming amyloid-like filaments and water-filled nanotubes that result in enzymatic dysfunction [91] suggesting this conformational rearrangement in the metal-deficient enzyme could contribute to SOD1-linked FALS pathology. Recombinant apo-SOD1 without disulphide bonds, ALS mutant SOD1 protein or insoluble SOD1-containing aggregates isolated from mutant SOD1-expressing transgenic mice have all been shown to possess spontaneous fibrillization and seeding activity *in vitro* under various non-physiological conditions [27, 80]. Recent observations have also shown that protein to protein conversion induced by both mutant [29] and over-expressed WTSOD1 [28] can be self-sustaining. Induced misfolding of WTSOD1 can persist even in the absence of the original mutant SOD1 seed in cell culture, suggesting that the induced misfolded SOD1 can act as template for subsequent cycles of misfolding [24]. Similarly, exogenous fibrils of recombinant mutant human SOD1 can be taken up by mouse neuroblastoma cells expressing the same human SOD1 mutant and trigger intracellular aggregation [92].

In the case of propagating WTSOD1 misfolding, it is unclear what the conformational state of the substrate is in prior to conversion. It would be highly thermodynamically unfavorable for natively-folded WTSOD1, or even an enzymatically functional mutant SOD1 in a near-native state to be susceptible to induced misfolding. In fact, co-expression of WTSOD1 is observed to stabilize mutant misfolded SOD1 [93, 94]. FALS-linked mutant SOD1 species are known to have delayed post-translational folding kinetics, thereby increasing the population of partially folded intermediates [95]. Thus, nascent WTSOD1 polypeptide newly-emerged from the cellular translation machinery may provide a thermodynamically favourable substrate for recruitment (Figure 1). However, WTSOD1 does possess relatively quicker folding kinetics compared to mutant isoforms, thus producing significantly smaller populations of partially-folded intermediates. Other mechanisms may be at work in the ALS disease state that slow post-translational folding of WTSOD1, making it more susceptible to induced misfolding; however, such factors have yet to be identified.

INTERCELLULAR TRANSMISSION OF SOD1 MISFOLDING

The regional spread of protein misfolding and aggregate formation is a prevalent feature of neurodegenerative disease, with the spread of misfolded protein seed playing the critical role of expanding the pathology beyond the site of original protein conversion. A misfolded protein that cannot escape the local cellular environment in which it was formed cannot effectively spread pathology to adjacent anatomical regions. The mechanisms of intercellular transmsision of misfolded protein in ALS have yet to be fully elucidated, but various pieces of experimental evidence have provided some insight thay may explain the spatiotemporal spread of disease pathology. Simple release and uptake of soluble misfolded protein, aggregates or proto-fibrils have been observed experiementally in cell lines. For example, exogenous mutant [24, 29] and WTSOD1 [24] aggregates have been shown to efficiently penetrate the cell membrane of neuron-like cells in a macropinocytosis-dependent mechanism, and become self-perpetuating in recruiting soluble SOD1 into insoluble aggregates. Aggregates of misfolded SOD1 likely represent a conformationally and thermodynamically stable form [96] that can better survive the relative hostilities of the extracellular environment than lower-order soluble forms, possibly becoming available when dying neurons release their contents to the extracellular environment.

Although the presence of large proteinaceous inclusions containing SOD1 is a common pathological characteristic in cases of SOD1-FALS , there is a question as to whether these protein structures represent the actual transmissible neurotoxic form of pathological SOD1. In other neurodegenerative diseases, there is growing evidence pointing to *soluble* misfolded protein as the primary toxic species as opposed to large protein aggregates, inclusions or fibrils, which appear for the most part to be pathologically inert [97]. In Alzheimer's disease, it is smaller oligomeric forms of amyloid-β that impair synaptic function [98, 99], plasticity and memory [100]. Likewise, there is growing evidence that pre-fibrillar oligomers of α-synuclein are responsible for disease progression in Parkinson disease [101, 102] as opposed to the hallmark Lewy bodies, which may serve as benign 'dumps' of aggregated protein. A similar situation may exist for misfolded SOD1 in ALS. For example, misfolded SOD1 is detectable in mutant SOD1-excluded sporadic and familial cases, but not typically in the form of large protein inclusions usually observed in mutant SOD1-associated FALS [21, 22, 24], suggesting that misfolded SOD1 in SALS is likely present in the form of smaller soluble structures that are not readily detectable by gross histochemical staining of tissue sections. Mechanistically, the spread of ALS pathology would likely occur prior to neuronal cell death, *via* a more active cellular process.

There is increasing evidence supporting the role of extracellular vesicles (EVs) in the pathobiology of neurodegenerative disease as a means of transmitting toxic proteins from region to region [103]. EVs are membrane-bounded vesices that range in size from 30-1000 nm and are released by various cell types including motor neurons and neural accessory cells. EVs have been shown to carry an assortment of macromolecular cargo inclduing mRNAs, miRNAs, lipds and proteins [104, 105]. Exosomes represent an EV subtype, ranging in size from 30-80 nm that arise from the inward budding of the late endosome and are held within the cell by mutlivesicular bodies (MVB). MVBs are normally involved in the lysosomal pathway, trafficking proteins to the lysosome for proteolysis. Alternatively, MVBs can fuse with the plasma membrane, leading to the release of its intraluminal vesicles into the extracellular milieu as exosomes [106]. Exosomes have been increasingly implicated in the spread of misfolded or aggregated proteins involved in a number of neurodegenerative proteinopathies, such as Alzheimer's disease [107], Parkinson's disease [108, 109] and the prion diseases [110, 111]. It is thought that as misfolded and aggregated proteins accrue in the intracellular environment, it begins to overwhelm the protein clearance pathway leading the cell to release aggregated protein packaged in EVs. Consequently, other cells take up the secreted EVs with their toxic cargo. Evidence continues to build that an analogous EV-associated mechanism may be involved in the pathobiology of ALS (Figure 1). SOD1 itself is a known resident protein of exosomes from multiple cell types and species [112]. Subsequent studies have identified exosomes as a secretion mechanism for both wild-type and mutant SOD1 in a motor neuron-like cell model [113], potentially mediated by chromogranins [114], acidic components of neurotransmitter-enriched secretory vesicles [115] that could serve as a secretory chaperone. However, expression of mutant SOD1 has also been shown to impair its own secretion, possibly contributing to intraneuronal toxicity [116], thus confounding the precise role of exosomes in mutant SOD1 transmission. Other evidence suggests that mutant SOD1 oligomers accumulate in the endoplasmic reticulum (ER) -Golgi compartments of the endocytic pathway prior to its subsequent secretion [117]. In another case, exogenous mutant and misfolded WT SOD1 taken up by neuronal cells inhibits protein transport between the Golgi and ER, ultimately leading to Golgi fragmentation, ER stress and apoptosis [118]. In addition, Golgi fragmentation is observed as an early event in the pathology of a mutant SOD-ALS mouse model [119], further complicating a potential role of the secretory pathway in pathological SOD1 transmission during disease. Other work has established that both mutant and wild-type misfolded SOD1 can be secreted from neuron-like cells *via* exosomes [120]; these exosomes can be subsequently taken up by fresh cells where the misfolded SOD1 cargo provides a template for subsequent induction of protein misfolding [24]. Exosome-independent uptake of SOD1 is not aggregate-specific as aggregated forms are taken up as efficiently as non-aggregated forms. However, the process does show specificity, as an irrelevant cellular aggregate, such as glutathione S-transferase, is not taken up in the same manner as SOD1, suggesting the possible involvement of receptors in this process. Previous work with mouse microglial cells found that scavenger receptors specifically participate in the uptake of aggregated SOD1 [121], whereas heparin sulfate proteoglycans have been shown to be involved in aggregate uptake of tau, alpha-synuclein, and prion protein [122, 123] in other neurodegenerative diseases. More recently, mouse astrocyte-derived exosomes were observed to efficiently transfer mutant SOD1 to spinal neurons and subsequently cause selective motor neuron death [120], providing further evidence that exosome-mediated transmission of misfolded SOD1 is pathogenic.

INTERORGANISMAL TRANSMISSION OF PATHOLOGICAL SOD1

Misfolded SOD1 appears to satisfy both the intermolecular conversion and intercellular propagation characteristics of prions; however, one could argue that despite fulfilling these biochemical properties, SOD1, and by extension other misfolded proteins involved in neurodegenerative proteinopathies, do not share key traits of the classical prion diseases, namely transmission between organisms [96] and the evidence of strains that vary in their stability, infectivity and toxicity [124]. Moreover, there is little evidence in the literature to date that resolutely confirms the protein-only hypothesis in any of the other neurodegenerative proteinopathies. SOD1 could be considered the lone exception as propagated conversion of WTSOD1 to a misfolded conformer was observed in a completely cell-free environment using purified recombinant protein [28] with the caveat that the solution conditions were only a rough approximation of the intracellular environment. When it comes to organismal infectivity no other misfolded protein comes close to the degree of pathogenicity of PrP^{Sc} in the classical prion diseases. PrP^{Sc} is a highly-stable isoform compared to normal PrP^{C} and represents the epitome of a robust infectious agent that is able to withstand the environmental rigours of animal-to-animal transmission. Conversely, many pathological isoforms of misfolded SOD1 are highly protease-sensitive and unstable [28, 75] making long-term survival outside of an organism or even in the extracellular milieu highly unlikely, although the presence of native wild-type SOD1 has been shown to increase the stability of mutant misfolded SOD1 [125]. The point of entry of prion-like agents is likely another crucial factor for efficient transmission. Interorganismal transmission of propagated SOD1 misfolding would likely need to be directly introduced to the anatomical region of pathology; for ALS this would typically be the spinal cord or brain stem. At the time of writing this chapter only one published account has demonstrated a model for interorganismal transmission of motor neuron disease, which indeed utilizes the aforementioned routes of entry. In this experiment, transgenic mice expressing human mutant G85R-SOD1 fused to a YFP reporter (G85R-SOD1:YFP) at levels too low to induce disease were intracerebro-ventricularly injected with spinal cord homogenate isolated from diseased G93A-SOD1 mice [32]. Recipient mice showed the induction of G85R-SOD1:YFP aggregation and the progressive development of motor neuron disease, demonstrating for the first time interorganismal transmission of motor neuron disease pathology. Furthermore, the study showed that spinal cord homogenate from G37R-SOD1 transgenic mice does not induce disease, suggesting the possibility of strain-like characteristics for different misfolded isoforms of SOD1 [32]. Superficially, key prion characteristics are observed in this study, however the authors are quick to point out that disease transmission was relatively inconsistent and disease pathology varied considerably from animal to animal, indicating partial penetrance of disease. If misfolded SOD1 pathology is indeed transmissible, its virulence is several orders of magnitude lower than PrP^{Sc}, the archetypal proteinaceous infectious particle.

TDP-43 MISFOLDING IN DISEASE

The formation of ubiquitin-positive inclusions is a common feature of many neurodegenerative diseases [126]. Two independent discoveries in 2006 identified pathological TAR-DNA binding protein 43 (TDP-43) as a major protein in ubiquitin-positive, tau- and α-synuclein-negative neuronal and glial inclusions, hallmark structures in certain cases of frontotemporal lobar dementia (FTLD), and in the majority of SALS cases [26, 127], providing a common mechanistic link between the two disorders. Interestingly, TDP-43 immunoreactivity has also been observed in inclusions found in Huntington's disease [128], Parkinson's disease [129], and nearly 20% of Alzheimer's disease cases [130], which implicate TDP-43 in a wide spectrum of neurodegenerative disorders. In addition to its translocation from the nucleus to the cytoplasm and subsequent aggregation, pathological TDP-43 also becomes hyperphosphorylated and ubiquitinated [26, 127]. Mutations in the gene encoding TDP-43, *TARDBP*, were subsequently identified in patients with FALS and SALS, suggesting a direct causal nature between the protein and disease [131, 132, 133, 134, 135, 136]. Intriguingly, almost all of the *TARDBP* mutations identified in ALS are located in exon six encoding the C-terminal domain [132, 133] and result in autosomal dominant inheritance [137]. Originally, TDP-43 was thought to be involved in early embryonic development as disruption of *TARDBP* expression is lethal at the embryonic stage [138, 139]. However, the protein is now known to be involved in gene regulation, and mRNA splicing and localization [140]. Studies have determined that TDP-43 mislocalization and aggregation is directly related to disease pathogenesis as opposed to being an end-stage marker of disease. However, the precise role of TDP-43 in disease presently remains ambiguous; it is unclear whether pathology is caused by a toxic gain-of-function due to cytoplasmic mislocalization, loss-of-function due its resultant nuclear depletion, or a combination thereof.

Functionally, TDP-43 is an important regulatory protein in the nervous system: it binds over 6,000 pre-mRNAs, affects the splicing patterns of 965 mRNAs and affects expression levels of another 600 mRNAs [141]. Due to its substantial role in transcription regulation, some propose that the loss of function of pathological TDP-43 in disease can cause neuronal loss due to altered proteostasis of proteins that rely on TDP-43 for their synthesis [142]. Others believe that cytoplasmic mislocalization of pathological TDP-43 is toxic to neurons, potentially by leading to the formation of cytotoxic misfolded SOD1 protein, which could implicate both proteins in a common pathological pathway in ALS [23, 143]. Structurally, the 414 residue TDP-43 protein belongs to the heterogeneous ribonucleoprotein family. In addition to its nuclear localization and export domains that enable it to shuttle sequences of nucleic acid in and out of the nucleus, TDP-43 also contains two RNA recognition motifs (RRM1 and RRM2), and an arginine/glycine-rich C-terminal domain through which it interacts with other proteins [144, 145]. Screening of the entire database of known human proteins using a hidden Markov Model algorithm designed to detect prion-like sequences in yeast found TDP-43 to be the 69th most likely protein to contain a prion-like domain out of 27,879 [146], where the C-terminal region in particular was predicted to be prone to misfolding [147]. Pathological TDP-43 is abnormally cleaved into the cytotoxic 25- and 35-kDa C-terminal fragments (CTFs) [133], becoming themselves susceptible to hyperphosphorylation, ubiquitination and aggregation [148]. These fragments have been shown to be necessary and sufficient for TDP-43 self-aggregation [140, 149] as even truncation constructs featuring minimal C-terminal portions of the protein are aggregation-competent *in vitro* and in cultured cells [14, 33, 150]. Udan-Johns et al., observed that both endogenous and fluorescent-tagged wild-type human TDP-43 undergo reversible aggregation in the nucleus in response to heat shock [151]. The same study confirms that deletion of the C-terminal prion-like domain markedly reduces aggregation of TDP-43, and that replacement of the prion domain in TDP-43 with a prion domain from TIA-1 recapitulates the heat shock induced aggregation. Yeast models of TDP-43 proteinopathy successfully replicate the cytoplasmic mislocalization and toxicity seen in disease and show that the prion-like domain of TDP-43 is essential for its aggregation and cellular toxicity, demonstrating a proposed role in human disease [149]. Other studies have shown that the prion-like domain is essential for the normal function of the protein as deletion mutants fail to properly splice normal TDP-43 targets while substitution of a yeast prion domain into the C-terminus of TDP-43 successfully rescues function [152].

TDP-43 Shows Prion-Like Phenomena

Evidence is rapidly emerging demonstrating prion-like behavior in TDP-43. It is firmly established that, similar to mutant and/or aberrantly oxidized forms of SOD1, TDP-43 and its derived fragments have a high propensity to aggregate *in vitro* [33, 140] and pathological mutations expressed within the protein can enhance this property [14, 140]. Aggregates of TDP-43 CTFs can form detergent-insoluble fibril-like structures [127, 153] localized to the cytoplasm. Synthetic CTFs were able to also form detergent and heat resistant high molecular weight multimers as well as partially protease-resistant low molecular weight species in primary neurons [14]. Interestingly, the low molecular weight TDP-43 species were able to form neurotoxic β-sheet amyloid fibrils, reminiscent of amyloid-like TDP-43-positive inclusions found in post-mortem ALS spinal cord samples [154], although TDP-43 can also be generally found in non-amyloid forms as well [155]. Investigations into the process by which TDP-43 aggregates and fibrils are formed have revealed prion-like characteristics that contribute to its pathology. TDP-43 can be cross-seeded in cultured cells by poly-Q aggregates , a process dependent upon the protein's glutamine/asparagine (Q/N)-rich prion-like domain [156], resulting in TDP-43 nuclear depletion and accumulation into misfolded aggregates in the cytoplasm. Work by Furukawa et al., has demonstrated that exogenously applied detergent-insoluble aggregates of full-length TDP-43 generated *in vitro* can be taken up by human embryonic kidney cells, and act as seed for the aggregation of endogenous TDP-43 [33]. These induced aggregates are themselves detergent-insoluble and ubiquitinated, similar to that observed for pathological TDP-43 in ALS patients, but are not hyperphosphorylated. Despite this, the results clearly implicate the process of seeded aggregation in TDP-43 pathology. Comparable mechanisms have been implicated in several other notable neurodegenerative proteinopathies, including the prion diseases [157], Alzheimer's disease [158, 159] and Parkinson's disease [160].

Even more convincing self-templating properties have been observed for TDP-43 in a recent study by Nonaka et al., Aggregated TDP-43 isolated from the brains of ALS and frontotemporal lobar degeneration patients exogenously applied to cultured human neuroblastoma cells can serve as seed for the self-propagation of additional ubiquitinated and phosphorylated TDP-43 aggregates [34], with the aggregation of full length TDP-43 preceding the C-terminal cleavage of the protein by caspases [161]. Interestingly, treatment of detergent-insoluble TDP-43 with protease, which degrades the protein to <20 kDa fragments, does not diminish its seeding ability, further suggesting that full-length TDP-43 is not necessary for disease pathogenesis [34]. In addition, Nonaka et al., found that the seeding ability of tissue-derived aggregated TDP-43 is resistant to heat, protease digestion and formic acid, similar to that found for pathological prion protein. Furthermore, TDP-43 aggregates could propagate between cells through several passages, suggesting propagated misfolding may persist even in the absence of the original templating seed, indicative of an authentic prion-like self-propagating mechanism. It was further observed that accumulation of pathological TDP-43 in a self-templating manner leads to proteasomal dysfunction, possibly driving further cytoplasmic accumulation of TDP-43 aggregates in a positive-feedback manner [34,162] thus establishing a solid link between propagated TDP-43 misfolding and disease pathology. The proposed prion-like activities of TDP-43 are summarized in Figure 1.

A key characteristic of infectious prions is the existence of distinct strains, a property that has confounded researchers for decades. Despite the gene encoding PrP having no identifiable genetic mutations, different strains of infectious PrP^{Sc} have been identified possessing stable and distinct incubation periods, patterns of pathology, and disease severity [163].

Although not as firmly established as PrP^{Sc} in the various forms of transmissible spongiform encephalopathies, there is emerging evidence suggesting different strains of TDP-43 may be responsible for distinct pathological subtypes of fronto-temporal lobar degeneration with TDP-43 pathology (FTLD-TDP) based on the type of TDP-43-positive inclusions observed [164]. Furthermore, different structural conformations of sarkosyl insoluble TDP-43 from cortex and spinal cord from ALS and FTLD patients produced distinct phosphorylated TDP-43 fragments *via* protease digestion [165]. The distinct patterns of fragments produced by protease digestion were specific for different TDP-43 proteinopathy subtypes [164], suggesting that different conformational changes to TDP-43 cause different patterns of pathology and disease phenotypes, highly reminiscent of distinct strains of infectious prion protein.

Experimental evidence for the intercellular transmission of pathological TDP-43 [34] could also help to explain the prion-like spatiotemporal spread that is clinically observed in ALS [5]. In support of this, TDP-43 pathology is observed to spread in a four-stage process starting from the agranular frontal neocortex and somatomotor neurons of the spinal cord and brain stem, followed by subsequent spreading to the medial temporal lobe and hippocampus by the last stage [166], a pathological progression highly reminiscent of prion-like spread. Although the mechanism of pathological TDP-43 transmission and propagation has yet to be identified, it has been speculated that pathological TDP-43 could spread transynaptically *via* corticofugal axonal projections using anterograde axonal transport [167]. In addition, exosomes may play a role in the intercellular transmission of pathological TDP-43, similar to that observed for misfolded SOD1, as full-length TDP-43 is enriched in exosome fractions isolated from human neuroblastoma cells treated with seed from ALS patient extract [34], although other mechanisms of transmissions could also be at play, such as direct uptake of aggregates by the plasma membrane as seen for aggregates of SOD1 [24] (Figure 1).

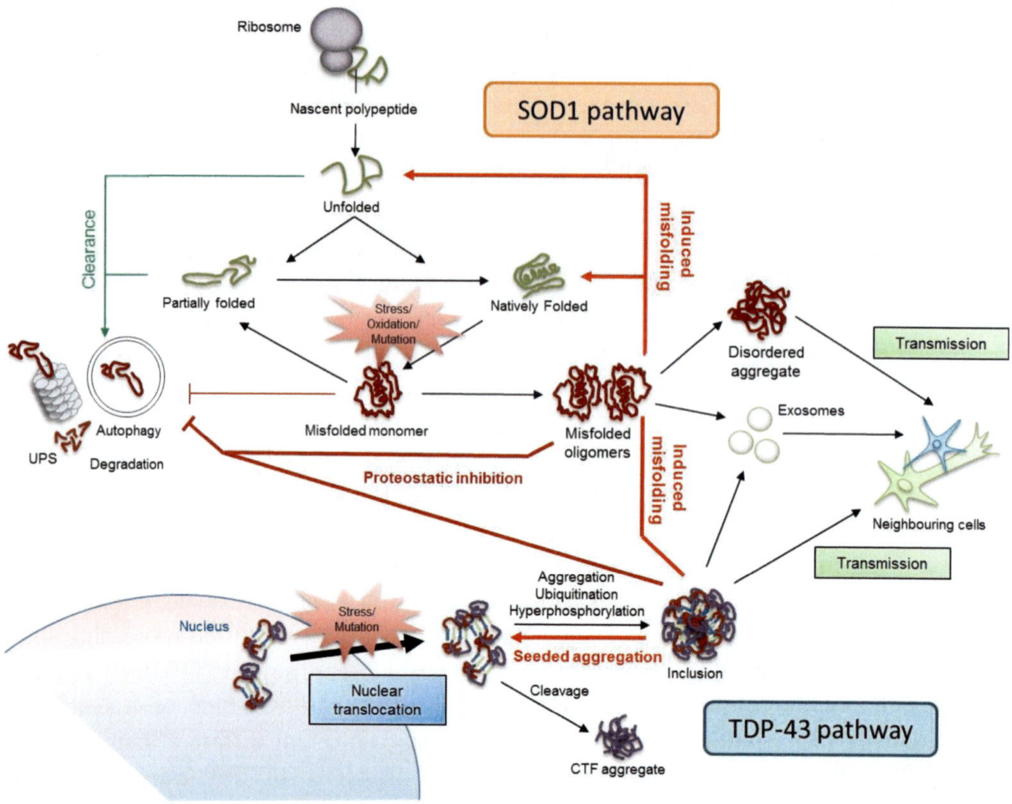

Figure 1. Proposed prion-like mechanisms of misfolded SOD1 and pathological TDP-43 in ALS. Misfolded SOD1, generated through mutation, aberrant oxidation or other cell stressors utilizes post-translational intermediates of WT or mutant SOD1 that remain partially unfolded and susceptible to induced pathological misfolding. Once a misfolded template is present, it can induce subsequent cycles of template-directed misfolding, converting neighbouring native SOD1 molecules into pathological isoforms, which can subsequently form oligomers and aggregates over time. Misfolded SOD1 eventually accumulates in the ER-Golgi system where it can enter the vesicle-mediated secretory pathway, exit the cell *via* exosomes and be taken up by neighbouring cells. Alternatively, large aggregates containing misfolded SOD1 are released and subsequently taken up by neighbouring cells, providing misfolding-competent seed. Misfolded SOD1 itself can act as an inhibitor of both the proteasome and autophagic systems, through as yet identified mechanisms, thereby allowing for aberrantly folded protein to elude proteostasis and build up within the cell. TDP-43 translocation from the nucleus to the cytoplasm can occur *via* mutation or cell stressors. Cytoplasmic TDP-43 has a propensity to aggregate, forming nucleating seeds that recruit other soluble TDP-43 molecules into larger aggregates. Similarly, TDP-43 can be proteolytically cleaved, releasing its CTF, which can form aggregates with other CTFs *via* its prion-like domain. Pathological TDP-43 is known to be released from cells, and has also been detected as a component of exosomes, implicating these vesicles as a mode of transport out of the cell. Evidence also supports a role for pathological TDP-43 in the induction of SOD1 misfolding and dysfunction of the proteostatic machinery.

PRION-LIKE PROPERTIES IN OTHER ALS-ASSOCIATED PROTEINS

Since the initial discovery of TDP-43 involvement in neurodegenerative disease, a host of other RNA-binding proteins, belonging to the heterogeneous ribonucleoprotein family and containing prion-like domains, have been identified and linked to ALS pathobiology. Fused in sarcoma (FUS), a 526 amino-acid RNA-binding transcriptional activator, is structurally and functionally related to TDP-43 [145]. FUS has different binding partners than TDP-43, and the two do not co-localize within pathological inclusions in the cytoplasmic [168, 169] despite their structural, functional and pathological similarities, suggesting the two proteins are involved in pathology *via* distinct, albeit related mechanisms. For example, pathological forms of FUS and TDP-43 have both been observed to induce SOD1 misfolding in cultures cells [23], although the mechanisms for this are currently unknown, in addition to whether or not FUS or TDP-43 acts in a similar fashion in this process.

The C-terminal region of FUS contains a nuclear localization signal (NLS), and glycine-rich domain, while the first 239 amino acids make up a predicted Q/N-rich yeast prion-like domain [147]. Curiously, purified FUS shows a higher propensity to aggregate *in vitro* under native conditions than either SOD1 or TDP-43, requiring only its RNA-binding RRM and glycine-rich RGG domains [169]. The RGG domain of FUS also contains a small prion-like region which opens up the possibility that FUS may self-aggregate using its two prion-like domains [170]. However, FUS mutations that cause ALS are primarily located within the NLS and are believed to primarily contribute to the mislocalization of the protein to the cytoplasm rather than promote misfolding and/or aberrant aggregation [169, 171, 172]. The cytoplasmic accumulation of FUS appears to be enough to induce its aggregation and integration into stress granules (dense foci of RNAs and protein that form in response to certain cell stressors) in cultured neurons [172]. Similar to TDP-43, FUS can be cross-seeded by poly-Q aggregates in cell culture, sequestering the protein into cytoplasmic inclusions in a manner dependent upon its Q/N-rich prion-like domain [156]. Recently, it was shown that the pathogenic FUS mutation, G156E, significantly increases the propensity for both in *vitro* and *in vivo* aggregation of FUS. Spontaneous *in vitro* formation of amyloid-like fibrillar aggregates was observed in mutant but not wild-type FUS, and more importantly, these fibrils served as efficient seeds to trigger the aggregation of wild-type protein [35]. However, at the time of writing this chapter, no experimental evidence has been published demonstrating seeded aggregation of FUS in living cells, although it has been hypothesized that the environment within stress granules, where the concentration of FUS is relatively high may be conducive for the initiation of seeded aggregation, possibly mediated *via* RNAs that could serve as scaffolding molecules [173] and thus not a true prion-like mechanism.

Ewing sarcoma breakpoint region 1 (EWSR1) and TATA-binding protein associated factor 15 (TAF15) are two other proteins that share similar prion-like domain architecture to FUS, are part of the TET family of proteins (reviewed in [174]) and implicated in ALS. TAF15, which serves as a component of the scaffold for assembly of the RNA transcription complex, was identified in a systematic survey used to screen candidates similar to TDP-43 or FUS, which could be involved in ALS [175]. Like other TET family members, TAF15 has a QGSY-rich N-terminal domain which is also predicted to be a prion-like domain [176]. Recent work has demonstrated that TET members bind with each other *via* their N-terminal prion-like domains to form homo- and hetero-complexes, a process which appears to mediate stress granule formation in normal cells, but can be dysregulated in disease resulting in the cytoplasmic inclusions routinely observed in ALS [38]. EWSR1 is an RNA-binding protein also identified in a screen for proteins with prion-like domains, and disease-causing mutations in EWSR1 were discovered in ALS patients [175]. Further work is needed to determine whether TET family members propagate in a prion-like manner in ALS similar to SOD1 or TDP-43, and whether their prion-like domains play a role in this process. The above studies suggest that RNA-binding proteins normally self-associate through their prion-like domains, and that disease-causing mutations in these domains lead to aggregation, perhaps through unregulated polymerization with each other [38]. However, evidence of self-propagation of protein misfolding or intercellular transmission has yet to be published.

Mutations in genes encoding two other RNA-binding proteins with prion-like domains have been identified in an ALS patient. Pathogenic mutations identified in a case of FALS and an inheritable multisystem proteinopathy have been identified in the prion-like domains of heterogeneous nuclear ribonucleoproteins (hnRNPs) A2B1 and A1 [39]. In their wild-type forms, both proteins show a strong tendency to assemble into self-seeding fibrils, although this process is accelerated in the presence of pathological mutations, incorporating wild-type hnRNP into fibrils in a seeded polymerization-type mechanism [39]. Pathological mutations also promote incorporation of hnRNPA1 and hnRNPA2 into stress granules and the formation of cytoplasmic proteinaceous inclusions in a *Drosphila* disease model, recapitulating the human phenotype, demonstrating a direct relationship between dysregulated polymerization of hnRNP proteins and onset of degenerative disease. It has been noted that diseases associated with cytoplasmic inclusions of proteins containing prion-like domains often show the characteristic spatiotemporal spreading of pathology [176] reminiscent of the clinically observed contiguous spread ALS through the neuroaxis [5]. Taken together, RNA binding proteins with prion-like domains may also transmit propagated protein misfolding *via* self-templating polymerization from cell-to-cell in a manner similar to that observed for SOD1, and to a lesser degree TDP-43, although direct evidence of this has yet to be shown in the literature.

Finally, the recent discovery that expansion of a GGGGCC hexanucleotide repeat within the *C9ORF72* gene is the most common mutation in families with ALS or frontotemporal dementia [177] adds another prominent candidate to the list of ALS-associated proteins with peculiar aggregation dynamics. Hexanucleotide expansion in *C9ORF72* is found in nearly 40% of all FALS cases and even up to 7% in SALS [178]. In normal individuals, the hexanucleotide repeat length is typically no longer than 25-30 units, but in ALS patients possessing a *C9ORF72* mutation, repeat length can exceed 700 [179, 180]. C9ORF72-asscoiated ALS cases typically present with TDP-43 aggregation, and p62-positive and TDP-43-negative ubiquitinated inclusions in the cerebellar and hippocampal regions [181, 182]. Mutation within *C9ORF72* results in the subsequent production of aggregating dipeptide-repeat (DPR) proteins [36, 37], which are generated by an alternative type of translation called repeat-associated non-ATG (RAN) translation [183]. DPRs are the primary components of TDP-43-negative inclusions in ALS patients, although the precise role in pathogenesis remains unknown. There is evidence that supports that DPRs can confer toxicity in cultured cells though mechanisms that disrupt RNA biogenesis [184] and protein trafficking [185]. However, it remains to be seen if C9ORF72 DPRs possess any prion-like characteristics prior to their accumulation into inclusions. Considering the prominence of

C9ORF72 mutations among ALS patients, further characterization into the aggregating behaviour of the DRPs and its relevance to ALS pathology is paramount.

USING THE PRION PARADIGM FOR THERAPY DEVELOPMENT

The prion paradigm of ALS offers new opportunities for therapeutic intervention that go beyond simple neuroprotection currently offered by the sole ALS pharmacological therapeutic, riluzole, available on the market. Increased susceptibility to proteolysis of misfolded ALS proteins, such as SOD1 and TDP-43, may expedite their clearance under conditions of enhanced proteasome activation. A similar strategy has been tried in Huntington's disease in which proteasome activators were overexpressed in Huntington patients' skin fibroblasts or mutant huntingtin-expressing striatal neurons [186]. Conversely, interventions may include stabilization of the native conformer of prion-like proteins through the binding of compounds or other biomolecules. In the case of SOD1, monomerization of the native dimer is known to be an early step in misfolding [47], thus molecules that stabilize the native dimer may impede misfolding. Alternatively, small molecules could be utilized to block self-templating of ALS-associated proteins at the site of protein-protein interaction. Although no compounds have yet to be identified that prohibits interactions between the prion-like domains of TDP-43 or FUS, there is crystallographic evidence of specific small molecules binding at or near the Trp32 residue of SOD1 [187], Trp32 being the residue identified as crucial for misfolded SOD1 self-templating and propagated misfolding [28]. Further study will be required to determine whether these compounds effectively inhibit prion-like activity of misfolded SOD1. Other strategies may focus on the transit of misfolded protein through the extracellular environment.

The work by Grad et al., has established that the intercellular transmission of misfolded SOD1 template can be abrogated immunologically through the use of antibodies directed against epitopes that are only exposed when the protein is aberrantly folded [24], demonstrating that misfolded SOD1 is accessible to immunotherapeutic intervention in the extracellular environment. Furthermore, the association of misfolded SOD1 with exosomes appears inconsequential to antibody binding as it was reported that misfolded SOD1 is immunodetectable on the outside of vesicles [24]; this may or may not be analogous to exosome-associated pathological TDP-43 [34]. Immunotherapeutic strategies targeting misfolded isoforms of SOD1 have been investigated *in vivo* with varying results. Passive immunization *via* intracerebroventricular infusion of G93A-SOD1 transgenic mice with monoclonal antibodies that bind epitopes of misfolded SOD1 that are not present in native WTSOD1 successfully reduced levels of misfolded SOD1 by 23% in the spinal cord and modestly prolonged the lifespan of G93A-SOD1 mice [188]. An active immunization strategy targeting monomer/misfolded SOD1 has also been utilized in an attempt to alleviate the burden of pathological SOD1 in neuronal tissue. An antigenic peptide based on the epitope recognized by the SOD1 exposed dimer interface (SEDI) antibody [48] was introduced into G93A-SOD1 or G37R-SOD1 transgenic mice *via* intraperitoneal injection beginning at 6 weeks of age, followed by a series of booster injections, resulting in delayed disease onset, extended disease duration and lifespan, and decreased levels of misfolded conformers of SOD1 in the spinal cord [189]. This study reinforces the key role of misfolded SOD1 in

SOD1-linked ALS pathogenesis and demonstrates the potential of an active immunization approach for the treatment of ALS.

In addition to immunotherapeutic approaches, attempts at targeting misfolded SOD1 through gene therapy have also been experimented with. Adeno-associated virus (AAV)-mediated expression of a DNA construct encoding a secretable single-chain fragment variable antibody, composed of the variable heavy and light chain regions of a monoclonal antibody that specifically recognizes misfolded SOD1, was used to treat G93A-SOD1 transgenic mice, resulting in reduced neuronal stress signals and a decreased load of misfolded SOD1 in spinal cord tissue [190]. Analogous therapeutic strategies have yet to be attempted for other ALS-associated proteins, although other methodologies have been used to target TDP-43 toxicity. For example, suppressor screens in yeast have identified a gene, *DBR1*, which when deleted supresses TDP-43 pathology in yeast and human cells [191], providing a therapeutic target that specifically effects pathological TDP-43, a disease marker in the majority of sporadic ALS cases. Needless to say, exploitation of the prion-like properties of ALS-associated proteins is a *bona fide* area of therapeutic study that will hopefully fill the void of effective treatments that are so desperately needed by the ALS patient community.

Conclusion

Protein misfolding and unfolding is a common occurrence in cells subject to the stresses of a disease state. However, most non-native protein conformations generally do not acquire prion-like properties, thus prions represent a unique type of pathogen. As we learn more about the properties of 'what makes a prion a prion', researchers of neurodegenerative proteinopathies continually demonstrate that the prion paradigm is more common than once thought, extending from the once-mysterious livestock diseases of 'mad cow' and scrapie, and the rare instances of human spongiform encephalopathy (e.g., Creutzfeldt–Jakob disease) to relatively common neurodegenerative diseases of aging such as Alzheimer and Parkinson diseases. Although the uniqueness of prions may be diminished, their biological relevance has never been greater. That being said, to date there is no published experimental evidence demonstrating that any proteinopathy, other than the classical prion diseases, can spread from individual to individual in humans or experimental model systems *via* natural infection pathways such as oral or intravenous inoculation. A recent study examining the use of human growth hormone derived from the cadavers of Alzheimer and Parkinson disease patients reaffirms that person-to-person transmissibility for these diseases is highly unlikely to occur [192]. However, one cannot ignore the more demonstrative observations of facilitated trans-organism disease transmission when intraperitoneal inoculation of misfolded amyloid-beta-enriched brain extract from Alzheimer's patients into transgenic mice induces amyloidosis in the brain, a region considerably non-local to the site of injection [193]. Thus, it is likely that the point of entry of prion-like proteins is crucial for even the slightest chance of interorganismal transmission to occur, if biologically permitted. In the single example of animal-to-animal transmission of motor neuron disease presented in the literature to-date, 'seed' in the form of spinal cord homogenate from pathological G93A-SOD1 mice was introduced *via* spinal and intracerebroventricular injections into G85R-SOD1:YFP transgenic mice within 24 h of birth [32], hardly natural circumstances for infection, but the experiment does show a successful proof-of-concept that, under the right experimental conditions, motor neuron disease can be transmissible. This will no doubt be the first of many subsequent studies investigating *in vivo* transmission of ALS pathology, an important step in understanding the mechanisms of disease progression, which can expectantly lead to therapeutic exploitation. Neurodegenerative diseases of aging, including ALS, represent a dire health concern for developed nations as human lifespans continue to increase due to improving health care and technology. With advancing age comes greater dysfunction of intracellular repair and scavenging mechanisms, contributing to the accumulation of misfolded proteins and the potential seeding of a propagating process [194, 195, 196]. Exploitation of the prion characteristics of ALS may provide the best answer yet to stopping the unrelenting spread of this disease, and other neurodegenerative syndromes.

REFERENCES

[1] Cleveland DW, Rothstein JD (2001) From Charcot to Lou Gehrig: deciphering selective motor neuron death in ALS. *Nat Rev Neurosci* 2: 806-819.

[2] Bradley WG (2009) Updates on amyotrophic lateral sclerosis: improving patient care. *Ann Neurol* 65 Suppl 1: S1-2.

[3] Phukan J, Pender NP, Hardiman O (2007) Cognitive impairment in amyotrophic lateral sclerosis. *Lancet Neurol* 6: 994-1003.

[4] Strong M, Rosenfeld J (2003) Amyotrophic lateral sclerosis: a review of current concepts. *Amyotroph Lateral Scler Other Motor Neuron Disord* 4: 136-143.

[5] Ravits JM, La Spada AR (2009) ALS motor phenotype heterogeneity, focality, and spread: deconstructing motor neuron degeneration. *Neurology* 73: 805-811.

[6] Sekiguchi T, Kanouchi T, Shibuya K, Noto Y, Yagi Y, et al., (2014) Spreading of amyotrophic lateral sclerosis lesions--multifocal hits and local propagation? *J Neurol Neurosurg Psychiatry* 85: 85-91.

[7] Elden AC, Kim HJ, Hart MP, Chen-Plotkin AS, Johnson BS, et al. (2010) Ataxin-2 intermediate-length polyglutamine expansions are associated with increased risk for ALS. *Nature* 466: 1069-1075.

[8] Haverkamp LJ, Appel V, Appel SH (1995) Natural history of amyotrophic lateral sclerosis in a database population. Validation of a scoring system and a model for survival prediction. *Brain* 118 (Pt 3): 707-719.

[9] Renton AE, Chio A, Traynor BJ (2014) State of play in amyotrophic lateral sclerosis genetics. *Nat Neurosci* 17: 17-23.

[10] ALS Mutation Database (2007) http://reseq.biosciencedbc.jp/resequence/SearchDisease.do?targetId=1. The University of Tokyo.

[11] Deng HX, Chen W, Hong ST, Boycott KM, Gorrie GH, et al. (2011) Mutations in UBQLN2 cause dominant X-linked juvenile and adult-onset ALS and ALS/dementia. *Nature* 477: 211-215.

[12] Wu CH, Fallini C, Ticozzi N, Keagle PJ, Sapp PC, et al. (2012) Mutations in the profilin 1 gene cause familial amyotrophic lateral sclerosis. *Nature.*

[13] Stewart H, Rutherford NJ, Briemberg H, Krieger C, Cashman N, et al. (2012) Clinical and pathological features of amyotrophic lateral sclerosis caused by mutation in the C9ORF72 gene on chromosome 9p. Acta Neuropathol 123: 409-417.
[14] Guo W, Chen Y, Zhou X, Kar A, Ray P, et al. (2011) An ALS-associated mutation affecting TDP-43 enhances protein aggregation, fibril formation and neurotoxicity. *Nat Struct Mol Biol* 18: 822-830.
[15] Keller BA, Volkening K, Droppelmann CA, Ang LC, Rademakers R, et al. (2012) Co-aggregation of RNA binding proteins in ALS spinal motor neurons: evidence of a common pathogenic mechanism. *Acta Neuropathol* 124: 733-747.
[16] Maruyama H, Morino H, Ito H, Izumi Y, Kato H, et al. (2010) Mutations of optineurin in amyotrophic lateral sclerosis. *Nature* 465: 223-226.
[17] Kabashi E, Valdmanis PN, Dion P, Rouleau GA (2007) Oxidized/misfolded superoxide dismutase-1: the cause of all amyotrophic lateral sclerosis? *Ann Neurol* 62: 553-559.
[18] Philips T, Robberecht W (2011) Neuroinflammation in amyotrophic lateral sclerosis: role of glial activation in motor neuron disease. *Lancet Neurol* 10: 253-263.
[19] Lagier-Tourenne C, Cleveland DW (2009) Rethinking ALS: the FUS about TDP-43. *Cell* 136: 1001-1004.
[20] Kato S, Takikawa M, Nakashima K, Hirano A, Cleveland DW, et al. (2000) New consensus research on neuropathological aspects of familial amyotrophic lateral sclerosis with superoxide dismutase 1 (SOD1) gene mutations: inclusions containing SOD1 in neurons and astrocytes. *Amyotroph Lateral Scler Other Motor Neuron Disord* 1: 163-184.
[21] Bosco DA, Morfini G, Karabacak NM, Song Y, Gros-Louis F, et al. (2010) Wild-type and mutant SOD1 share an aberrant conformation and a common pathogenic pathway in ALS. *Nat Neurosci* 13: 1396-1403.
[22] Forsberg K, Jonsson PA, Andersen PM, Bergemalm D, Graffmo KS, et al. (2010) Novel antibodies reveal inclusions containing non-native SOD1 in sporadic ALS patients. *PLoS ONE* 5: e11552.
[23] Pokrishevsky E, Grad LI, Yousefi M, Wang J, Mackenzie IR, et al. (2012) Aberrant localization of FUS and TDP43 is associated with misfolding of SOD1 in amyotrophic lateral sclerosis. *PLoS ONE* 7: e35050.
[24] Grad LI, Yerbury JJ, Turner BJ, Guest WC, Pokrishevsky E, et al. (2014) Intercellular propagated misfolding of wild-type Cu/Zn superoxide dismutase occurs via exosome-dependent and -independent mechanisms. *Proc Natl Acad Sci USA* 111: 3620-3625.
[25] Kerman A, Liu HN, Croul S, Bilbao J, Rogaeva E, et al. (2010) Amyotrophic lateral sclerosis is a non-amyloid disease in which extensive misfolding of SOD1 is unique to the familial form. *Acta Neuropathol* 119: 335-344.
[26] Neumann M, Sampathu DM, Kwong LK, Truax AC, Micsenyi MC, et al. (2006) Ubiquitinated TDP-43 in frontotemporal lobar degeneration and amyotrophic lateral sclerosis. *Science* 314: 130-133.
[27] Chia R, Tattum MH, Jones S, Collinge J, Fisher EM, et al. (2010) Superoxide dismutase 1 and tgSOD1 mouse spinal cord seed fibrils, suggesting a propagative cell death mechanism in amyotrophic lateral sclerosis. *PLoS ONE* 5: e10627.
[28] Grad LI, Guest WC, Yanai A, Pokrishevsky E, O'Neill MA, et al. (2011) Intermolecular transmission of superoxide dismutase 1 misfolding in living cells. *Proc Natl Acad Sci USA* 108: 16398-16403.

[29] Munch C, O'Brien J, Bertolotti A (2011) Prion-like propagation of mutant superoxide dismutase-1 misfolding in neuronal cells. *Proc Natl Acad Sci USA* 108: 3548-3553.

[30] Bruijn LI, Houseweart MK, Kato S, Anderson KL, Anderson SD, et al. (1998) Aggregation and motor neuron toxicity of an ALS-linked SOD1 mutant independent from wild-type SOD1. *Science* 281: 1851-1854.

[31] Wang L, Deng HX, Grisotti G, Zhai H, Siddique T, et al. (2009) Wild-type SOD1 overexpression accelerates disease onset of a G85R SOD1 mouse. *Hum Mol Genet* 18: 1642-1651.

[32] Ayers JI, Fromholt S, Koch M, DeBosier A, McMahon B, et al. (2014) Experimental transmissibility of mutant SOD1 motor neuron disease. *Acta Neuropathol* 128: 791-803.

[33] Furukawa Y, Kaneko K, Watanabe S, Yamanaka K, Nukina N (2011) A seeding reaction recapitulates intracellular formation of Sarkosyl-insoluble transactivation response element (TAR) DNA-binding protein-43 inclusions. *J Biol Chem* 286: 18664-18672.

[34] Nonaka T, Masuda-Suzukake M, Arai T, Hasegawa Y, Akatsu H, et al. (2013) Prion-like properties of pathological TDP-43 aggregates from diseased brains. *Cell Rep* 4: 124-134.

[35] Nomura T, Watanabe S, Kaneko K, Yamanaka K, Nukina N, et al. (2014) Intranuclear aggregation of mutant FUS/TLS as a molecular pathomechanism of amyotrophic lateral sclerosis. *J Biol Chem* 289: 1192-1202.

[36] Mori K, Weng SM, Arzberger T, May S, Rentzsch K, et al. (2013) The C9orf72 GGGGCC repeat is translated into aggregating dipeptide-repeat proteins in FTLD/ALS. *Science* 339: 1335-1338.

[37] Ash PE, Bieniek KF, Gendron TF, Caulfield T, Lin WL, et al. (2013) Unconventional translation of C9ORF72 GGGGCC expansion generates insoluble polypeptides specific to c9FTD/ALS. *Neuron* 77: 639-646.

[38] Thomsen C, Grundevik P, Elias P, Stahlberg A, Aman P (2013) A conserved N-terminal motif is required for complex formation between FUS, EWSR1, TAF15 and their oncogenic fusion proteins. *FASEB J* 27: 4965-4974.

[39] Kim HJ, Kim NC, Wang YD, Scarborough EA, Moore J, et al. (2013) Mutations in prion-like domains in hnRNPA2B1 and hnRNPA1 cause multisystem proteinopathy and ALS. *Nature* 495: 467-473.

[40] Beckman JS, Koppenol WH (1996) Nitric oxide, superoxide, and peroxynitrite: the good, the bad, and ugly. *Am J Physiol* 271: C1424-1437.

[41] Rosen DR (1993) Mutations in Cu/Zn superoxide dismutase gene are associated with familial amyotrophic lateral sclerosis. *Nature* 364: 362.

[42] Andersen PM, Sims KB, Xin WW, Kiely R, O'Neill G, et al. (2003) Sixteen novel mutations in the Cu/Zn superoxide dismutase gene in amyotrophic lateral sclerosis: a decade of discoveries, defects and disputes. *Amyotroph Lateral Scler Other Motor Neuron Disord* 4: 62-73.

[43] Das A, Plotkin SS (2013) SOD1 exhibits allosteric frustration to facilitate metal binding affinity. *Proc Natl Acad Sci USA* 110: 3871-3876.

[44] Lindberg MJ, Tibell L, Oliveberg M (2002) Common denominator of Cu/Zn superoxide dismutase mutants associated with amyotrophic lateral sclerosis: decreased stability of the apo state. *Proc Natl Acad Sci USA* 99: 16607-16612.

[45] Ip P, Mulligan VK, Chakrabartty A (2011) ALS-causing SOD1 mutations promote production of copper-deficient misfolded species. *J Mol Biol* 409: 839-852.

[46] Cashman NR CA, Rakhit R, Ostermann JB (2007) Methods and compositions to treat and detect misfolded SOD1 mediated diseases.

[47] Rakhit R, Crow JP, Lepock JR, Kondejewski LH, Cashman NR, et al. (2004) Monomeric Cu,Zn-superoxide dismutase is a common misfolding intermediate in the oxidation models of sporadic and familial amyotrophic lateral sclerosis. *J Biol Chem* 279: 15499-15504.

[48] Rakhit R, Robertson J, Vande Velde C, Horne P, Ruth DM, et al. (2007) An immunological epitope selective for pathological monomer-misfolded SOD1 in ALS. *Nat Med* 13: 754-759.

[49] Rakhit R, Cunningham P, Furtos-Matei A, Dahan S, Qi XF, et al. (2002) Oxidation-induced misfolding and aggregation of superoxide dismutase and its implications for amyotrophic lateral sclerosis. *J Biol Chem* 277: 47551-47556.

[50] Casoni F, Basso M, Massignan T, Gianazza E, Cheroni C, et al. (2005) Protein nitration in a mouse model of familial amyotrophic lateral sclerosis: possible multifunctional role in the pathogenesis. *J Biol Chem* 280: 16295-16304.

[51] Synofzik M, Ronchi D, Keskin I, Basak AN, Wilhelm C, et al. (2012) Mutant superoxide dismutase-1 indistinguishable from wild-type causes ALS. *Hum Mol Genet* 21: 3568-3574.

[52] Shibata N, Hirano A, Kobayashi M, Sasaki S, Kato T, et al. (1994) Cu/Zn superoxide dismutase-like immunoreactivity in Lewy body-like inclusions of sporadic amyotrophic lateral sclerosis. *Neurosci Lett* 179: 149-152.

[53] Chou SM, Wang HS, Komai K (1996) Colocalization of NOS and SOD1 in neurofilament accumulation within motor neurons of amyotrophic lateral sclerosis: an immunohistochemical study. *J Chem Neuroanat* 10: 249-258.

[54] Chou SM, Wang HS, Taniguchi A (1996) Role of SOD-1 and nitric oxide/cyclic GMP cascade on neurofilament aggregation in ALS/MND. *J Neurol Sci* 139 Suppl: 16-26.

[55] Gruzman A, Wood WL, Alpert E, Prasad MD, Miller RG, et al. (2007) Common molecular signature in SOD1 for both sporadic and familial amyotrophic lateral sclerosis. *Proc Natl Acad Sci USA* 104: 12524-12529.

[56] Broom WJ, Greenway M, Sadri-Vakili G, Russ C, Auwarter KE, et al. (2008) 50bp deletion in the promoter for superoxide dismutase 1 (SOD1) reduces SOD1 expression in vitro and may correlate with increased age of onset of sporadic amyotrophic lateral sclerosis. *Amyotroph Lateral Scler* 9: 229-237.

[57] Reaume AG, Elliott JL, Hoffman EK, Kowall NW, Ferrante RJ, et al. (1996) Motor neurons in Cu/Zn superoxide dismutase-deficient mice develop normally but exhibit enhanced cell death after axonal injury. *Nat Genet* 13: 43-47.

[58] Shefner JM, Reaume AG, Flood DG, Scott RW, Kowall NW, et al. (1999) Mice lacking cytosolic copper/zinc superoxide dismutase display a distinctive motor axonopathy. *Neurology* 53: 1239-1246.

[59] Gurney ME, Pu H, Chiu AY, Dal Canto MC, Polchow CY, et al. (1994) Motor neuron degeneration in mice that express a human Cu,Zn superoxide dismutase mutation. *Science* 264: 1772-1775.

[60] Andersen PM, Nilsson P, Ala-Hurula V, Keranen ML, Tarvainen I, et al. (1995) Amyotrophic lateral sclerosis associated with homozygosity for an Asp90Ala mutation in CuZn-superoxide dismutase. *Nat Genet* 10: 61-66.

[61] Bruijn LI, Becher MW, Lee MK, Anderson KL, Jenkins NA, et al. (1997) ALS-linked SOD1 mutant G85R mediates damage to astrocytes and promotes rapidly progressive disease with SOD1-containing inclusions. *Neuron* 18: 327-338.

[62] Cleveland DW (1999) From Charcot to SOD1: mechanisms of selective motor neuron death in ALS. *Neuron* 24: 515-520.

[63] Said Ahmed M, Hung WY, Zu JS, Hockberger P, Siddique T (2000) Increased reactive oxygen species in familial amyotrophic lateral sclerosis with mutations in SOD1. *J Neurol Sci* 176: 88-94.

[64] Beckman JS, Carson M, Smith CD, Koppenol WH (1993) ALS, SOD and peroxynitrite. *Nature* 364: 584.

[65] Beckman JS, Estevez AG, Crow JP, Barbeito L (2001) Superoxide dismutase and the death of motoneurons in ALS. *Trends Neurosci* 24: S15-20.

[66] Cleveland DW, Liu J (2000) Oxidation versus aggregation - how do SOD1 mutants cause ALS? *Nat Med* 6: 1320-1321.

[67] Bendotti C, Marino M, Cheroni C, Fontana E, Crippa V, et al. (2012) Dysfunction of constitutive and inducible ubiquitin-proteasome system in amyotrophic lateral sclerosis: implication for protein aggregation and immune response. *Prog Neurobiol* 97: 101-126.

[68] Bard F, Fox M, Friedrich S, Seubert P, Schenk D, et al. (2012) Sustained levels of antibodies against Abeta in amyloid-rich regions of the CNS following intravenous dosing in human APP transgenic mice. *Exp Neurol* 238: 38-43.

[69] Saxena S, Cabuy E, Caroni P (2009) A role for motoneuron subtype-selective ER stress in disease manifestations of FALS mice. *Nat Neurosci* 12: 627-636.

[70] Urushitani M, Kurisu J, Tsukita K, Takahashi R (2002) Proteasomal inhibition by misfolded mutant superoxide dismutase 1 induces selective motor neuron death in familial amyotrophic lateral sclerosis. *J Neurochem* 83: 1030-1042.

[71] Chen S, Zhang X, Song L, Le W (2012) Autophagy dysregulation in amyotrophic lateral sclerosis. *Brain Pathol* 22: 110-116.

[72] Kabashi E, Agar JN, Strong MJ, Durham HD (2012) Impaired proteasome function in sporadic amyotrophic lateral sclerosis. *Amyotroph Lateral Scler* 13: 367-371.

[73] Prusiner SB (1982) Novel proteinaceous infectious particles cause scrapie. *Science* 216: 136-144.

[74] Pardo CA, Xu Z, Borchelt DR, Price DL, Sisodia SS, et al. (1995) Superoxide dismutase is an abundant component in cell bodies, dendrites, and axons of motor neurons and in a subset of other neurons. *Proc Natl Acad Sci USA* 92: 954-958.

[75] Ratovitski T, Corson LB, Strain J, Wong P, Cleveland DW, et al. (1999) Variation in the biochemical/biophysical properties of mutant superoxide dismutase 1 enzymes and the rate of disease progression in familial amyotrophic lateral sclerosis kindreds. *Hum Mol Genet* 8: 1451-1460.

[76] Saccon RA, Bunton-Stasyshyn RK, Fisher EM, Fratta P (2013) Is SOD1 loss of function involved in amyotrophic lateral sclerosis? *Brain* 136: 2342-2358.

[77] Polling S, Mok YF, Ramdzan YM, Turner BJ, Yerbury JJ, et al. (2014) Misfolded polyglutamine, polyalanine, and superoxide dismutase 1 aggregate via distinct pathways in the cell. *J Biol Chem* 289: 6669-6680.

[78] Prudencio M, Hart PJ, Borchelt DR, Andersen PM (2009) Variation in aggregation propensities among ALS-associated variants of SOD1: correlation to human disease. *Hum Mol Genet* 18: 3217-3226.

[79] Wang J, Xu G, Gonzales V, Coonfield M, Fromholt D, et al. (2002) Fibrillar inclusions and motor neuron degeneration in transgenic mice expressing superoxide dismutase 1 with a disrupted copper-binding site. *Neurobiol Dis* 10: 128-138.

[80] Furukawa Y, Kaneko K, Yamanaka K, O'Halloran TV, Nukina N (2008) Complete loss of post-translational modifications triggers fibrillar aggregation of SOD1 in the familial form of amyotrophic lateral sclerosis. *J Biol Chem* 283: 24167-24176.

[81] Jaarsma D, Haasdijk ED, Grashorn JA, Hawkins R, van Duijn W, et al. (2000) Human Cu/Zn superoxide dismutase (SOD1) overexpression in mice causes mitochondrial vacuolization, axonal degeneration, and premature motoneuron death and accelerates motoneuron disease in mice expressing a familial amyotrophic lateral sclerosis mutant SOD1. *Neurobiol Dis* 7: 623-643.

[82] Fukada K, Nagano S, Satoh M, Tohyama C, Nakanishi T, et al. (2001) Stabilization of mutant Cu/Zn superoxide dismutase (SOD1) protein by coexpressed wild SOD1 protein accelerates the disease progression in familial amyotrophic lateral sclerosis mice. *Eur J Neurosci* 14: 2032-2036.

[83] Deng HX, Shi Y, Furukawa Y, Zhai H, Fu R, et al. (2006) Conversion to the amyotrophic lateral sclerosis phenotype is associated with intermolecular linked insoluble aggregates of SOD1 in mitochondria. *Proc Natl Acad Sci USA* 103: 7142-7147.

[84] Raymond GJ, Bossers A, Raymond LD, O'Rourke KI, McHolland LE, et al. (2000) Evidence of a molecular barrier limiting susceptibility of humans, cattle and sheep to chronic wasting disease. *EMBO J* 19: 4425-4430.

[85] Taylor DM, Gibbs BF, Kabashi E, Minotti S, Durham HD, et al. (2007) Tryptophan 32 potentiates aggregation and cytotoxicity of a copper/zinc superoxide dismutase mutant associated with familial amyotrophic lateral sclerosis. *J Biol Chem* 282: 16329-16335.

[86] Coelho FR, Iqbal A, Linares E, Silva DF, Lima FS, et al. (2014) Oxidation of the tryptophan 32 residue of human superoxide dismutase 1 caused by its bicarbonate-dependent peroxidase activity triggers the non-amyloid aggregation of the enzyme. *J Biol Chem* 289: 30690-30701.

[87] Audet JN, Gowing G, Julien JP (2010) Wild-type human SOD1 overexpression does not accelerate motor neuron disease in mice expressing murine Sod1(G86R). *Neurobiol Dis.*

[88] Prudencio M, Durazo A, Whitelegge JP, Borchelt DR (2009) Modulation of mutant superoxide dismutase 1 aggregation by co-expression of wild-type enzyme. *J Neurochem* 108: 1009-1018.

[89] Horwich AL, Weissman JS (1997) Deadly conformations--protein misfolding in prion disease. *Cell* 89: 499-510.

[90] Wang Q, Johnson JL, Agar NY, Agar JN (2008) Protein aggregation and protein instability govern familial amyotrophic lateral sclerosis patient survival. *PLoS Biol* 6: e170.

[91] Elam JS, Taylor AB, Strange R, Antonyuk S, Doucette PA, et al. (2003) Amyloid-like filaments and water-filled nanotubes formed by SOD1 mutant proteins linked to familial ALS. *Nat Struct Biol* 10: 461-467.

[92] Furukawa Y, Kaneko K, Watanabe S, Yamanaka K, Nukina N (2013) Intracellular seeded aggregation of mutant Cu,Zn-superoxide dismutase associated with amyotrophic lateral sclerosis. *FEBS Lett* 587: 2500-2505.
[93] Witan H, Gorlovoy P, Kaya AM, Koziollek-Drechsler I, Neumann H, et al. (2009) Wild-type Cu/Zn superoxide dismutase (SOD1) does not facilitate, but impedes the formation of protein aggregates of amyotrophic lateral sclerosis causing mutant SOD1. *Neurobiol Dis* 36: 331-342.
[94] Prudencio M, Durazo A, Whitelegge JP, Borchelt DR (2010) An examination of wild-type SOD1 in modulating the toxicity and aggregation of ALS-associated mutant SOD1. *Hum Mol Genet* 19: 4774-4789.
[95] Bruns CK, Kopito RR (2007) Impaired post-translational folding of familial ALS-linked Cu, Zn superoxide dismutase mutants. *EMBO J* 26: 855-866.
[96] Guest WC, Plotkin SS, Cashman NR (2011) Toward a mechanism of prion misfolding and structural models of PrP(Sc): current knowledge and future directions. *J Toxicol Environ Health A* 74: 154-160.
[97] Haass C, Selkoe DJ (2007) Soluble protein oligomers in neurodegeneration: lessons from the Alzheimer's amyloid beta-peptide. *Nat Rev Mol Cell Biol* 8: 101-112.
[98] Kayed R, Head E, Thompson JL, McIntire TM, Milton SC, et al. (2003) Common structure of soluble amyloid oligomers implies common mechanism of pathogenesis. *Science* 300: 486-489.
[99] Lesne S, Koh MT, Kotilinek L, Kayed R, Glabe CG, et al. (2006) A specific amyloid-beta protein assembly in the brain impairs memory. *Nature* 440: 352-357.
[100] Shankar GM, Li S, Mehta TH, Garcia-Munoz A, Shepardson NE, et al. (2008) Amyloid-beta protein dimers isolated directly from Alzheimer's brains impair synaptic plasticity and memory. *Nat Med* 14: 837-842.
[101] El-Agnaf OM, Salem SA, Paleologou KE, Curran MD, Gibson MJ, et al. (2006) Detection of oligomeric forms of alpha-synuclein protein in human plasma as a potential biomarker for Parkinson's disease. *FASEB J* 20: 419-425.
[102] Lashuel HA, Petre BM, Wall J, Simon M, Nowak RJ, et al. (2002) Alpha-synuclein, especially the Parkinson's disease-associated mutants, forms pore-like annular and tubular protofibrils. *J Mol Biol* 322: 1089-1102.
[103] Bellingham SA, Guo BB, Coleman BM, Hill AF (2012) Exosomes: vehicles for the transfer of toxic proteins associated with neurodegenerative diseases? *Front Physiol* 3: 124.
[104] Pant S, Hilton H, Burczynski ME (2012) The multifaceted exosome: biogenesis, role in normal and aberrant cellular function, and frontiers for pharmacological and biomarker opportunities. *Biochem Pharmacol* 83: 1484-1494.
[105] Li CC, Eaton SA, Young PE, Lee M, Shuttleworth R, et al. (2013) Glioma microvesicles carry selectively packaged coding and non-coding RNAs which alter gene expression in recipient cells. *RNA Biol* 10: 1333-1344.
[106] Keller S, Sanderson MP, Stoeck A, Altevogt P (2006) Exosomes: from biogenesis and secretion to biological function. *Immunol Lett* 107: 102-108.
[107] Perez-Gonzalez R, Gauthier SA, Kumar A, Levy E (2012) The exosome secretory pathway transports amyloid precursor protein carboxyl-terminal fragments from the cell into the brain extracellular space. *J Biol Chem* 287: 43108-43115.

[108] Emmanouilidou E, Melachroinou K, Roumeliotis T, Garbis SD, Ntzouni M, et al. (2010) Cell-produced alpha-synuclein is secreted in a calcium-dependent manner by exosomes and impacts neuronal survival. *J Neurosci* 30: 6838-6851.

[109] Danzer KM, Kranich LR, Ruf WP, Cagsal-Getkin O, Winslow AR, et al. (2012) Exosomal cell-to-cell transmission of alpha synuclein oligomers. *Mol Neurodegener* 7: 42.

[110] Fevrier B, Vilette D, Archer F, Loew D, Faigle W, et al. (2004) Cells release prions in association with exosomes. *Proc Natl Acad Sci USA* 101: 9683-9688.

[111] Coleman BM, Hanssen E, Lawson VA, Hill AF (2012) Prion-infected cells regulate the release of exosomes with distinct ultrastructural features. *FASEB J* 26: 4160-4173.

[112] Kim DK, Kang B, Kim OY, Choi DS, Lee J, et al. (2013) EVpedia: an integrated database of high-throughput data for systemic analyses of extracellular vesicles. *J Extracell Vesicles* 2.

[113] Gomes C, Keller S, Altevogt P, Costa J (2007) Evidence for secretion of Cu,Zn superoxide dismutase via exosomes from a cell model of amyotrophic lateral sclerosis. *Neurosci Lett* 428: 43-46.

[114] Urushitani M, Sik A, Sakurai T, Nukina N, Takahashi R, et al. (2006) Chromogranin-mediated secretion of mutant superoxide dismutase proteins linked to amyotrophic lateral sclerosis. *Nat Neurosci* 9: 108-118.

[115] Huttner WB, Gerdes HH, Rosa P (1991) The granin (chromogranin/secretogranin) family. *Trends Biochem Sci* 16: 27-30.

[116] Turner BJ, Atkin JD, Farg MA, Zang DW, Rembach A, et al. (2005) Impaired extracellular secretion of mutant superoxide dismutase 1 associates with neurotoxicity in familial amyotrophic lateral sclerosis. *J Neurosci* 25: 108-117.

[117] Urushitani M, Ezzi SA, Matsuo A, Tooyama I, Julien JP (2008) The endoplasmic reticulum-Golgi pathway is a target for translocation and aggregation of mutant superoxide dismutase linked to ALS. *FASEB J* 22: 2476-2487.

[118] Sundaramoorthy V, Walker AK, Yerbury J, Soo KY, Farg MA, et al. (2013) Extracellular wildtype and mutant SOD1 induces ER-Golgi pathology characteristic of amyotrophic lateral sclerosis in neuronal cells. *Cell Mol Life Sci* 70: 4181-4195.

[119] van Dis V, Kuijpers M, Haasdijk ED, Teuling E, Oakes SA, et al. (2014) Golgi fragmentation precedes neuromuscular denervation and is associated with endosome abnormalities in SOD1-ALS mouse motor neurons. *Acta Neuropathol Commun* 2: 38.

[120] Basso M, Pozzi S, Tortarolo M, Fiordaliso F, Bisighini C, et al. (2013) Mutant copper-zinc superoxide dismutase (SOD1) induces protein secretion pathway alterations and exosome release in astrocytes: implications for disease spreading and motor neuron pathology in amyotrophic lateral sclerosis. *J Biol Chem* 288: 15699-15711.

[121] Roberts K, Zeineddine R, Corcoran L, Li W, Campbell IL, et al. (2013) Extracellular aggregated Cu/Zn superoxide dismutase activates microglia to give a cytotoxic phenotype. *Glia* 61: 409-419.

[122] Horonchik L, Tzaban S, Ben-Zaken O, Yedidia Y, Rouvinski A, et al. (2005) Heparan sulfate is a cellular receptor for purified infectious prions. *J Biol Chem* 280: 17062-17067.

[123] Holmes BB, Devos SL, Kfoury N, Li M, Jacks R, et al. (2013) Heparan sulfate proteoglycans mediate internalization and propagation of specific proteopathic seeds. *Proc Natl Acad Sci USA* 110: E3138-3147.

[124] Legname G, Nguyen HO, Baskakov IV, Cohen FE, Dearmond SJ, et al. (2005) Strain-specified characteristics of mouse synthetic prions. *Proc Natl Acad Sci USA* 102: 2168-2173.

[125] Weichert A, Besemer AS, Liebl M, Hellmann N, Koziollek-Drechsler I, et al. (2013) Wild-type Cu/Zn superoxide dismutase stabilizes mutant variants by heterodimerization. *Neurobiol Dis*.

[126] Lansbury PT, Lashuel HA (2006) A century-old debate on protein aggregation and neurodegeneration enters the clinic. *Nature* 443: 774-779.

[127] Arai T, Hasegawa M, Akiyama H, Ikeda K, Nonaka T, et al. (2006) TDP-43 is a component of ubiquitin-positive tau-negative inclusions in frontotemporal lobar degeneration and amyotrophic lateral sclerosis. *Biochem Biophys Res Commun* 351: 602-611.

[128] Schwab C, Arai T, Hasegawa M, Yu S, McGeer PL (2008) Colocalization of transactivation-responsive DNA-binding protein 43 and huntingtin in inclusions of Huntington disease. *J Neuropathol Exp Neurol* 67: 1159-1165.

[129] Nakashima-Yasuda H, Uryu K, Robinson J, Xie SX, Hurtig H, et al. (2007) Co-morbidity of TDP-43 proteinopathy in Lewy body related diseases. *Acta Neuropathol* 114: 221-229.

[130] Amador-Ortiz C, Lin WL, Ahmed Z, Personett D, Davies P, et al. (2007) TDP-43 immunoreactivity in hippocampal sclerosis and Alzheimer's disease. *Ann Neurol* 61: 435-445.

[131] Kabashi E, Valdmanis PN, Dion P, Spiegelman D, McConkey BJ, et al. (2008) TARDBP mutations in individuals with sporadic and familial amyotrophic lateral sclerosis. *Nat Genet* 40: 572-574.

[132] Sreedharan J, Blair IP, Tripathi VB, Hu X, Vance C, et al. (2008) TDP-43 mutations in familial and sporadic amyotrophic lateral sclerosis. *Science* 319: 1668-1672.

[133] Rutherford NJ, Zhang YJ, Baker M, Gass JM, Finch NA, et al. (2008) Novel mutations in TARDBP (TDP-43) in patients with familial amyotrophic lateral sclerosis. *PLoS Genet* 4: e1000193.

[134] Yokoseki A, Shiga A, Tan CF, Tagawa A, Kaneko H, et al. (2008) TDP-43 mutation in familial amyotrophic lateral sclerosis. *Ann Neurol* 63: 538-542.

[135] Van Deerlin VM, Leverenz JB, Bekris LM, Bird TD, Yuan W, et al. (2008) TARDBP mutations in amyotrophic lateral sclerosis with TDP-43 neuropathology: a genetic and histopathological analysis. *Lancet Neurol* 7: 409-416.

[136] Gitcho MA, Baloh RH, Chakraverty S, Mayo K, Norton JB, et al. (2008) TDP-43 A315T mutation in familial motor neuron disease. *Ann Neurol* 63: 535-538.

[137] Pesiridis GS, Lee VM, Trojanowski JQ (2009) Mutations in TDP-43 link glycine-rich domain functions to amyotrophic lateral sclerosis. *Hum Mol Genet* 18: R156-162.

[138] Sephton CF, Good SK, Atkin S, Dewey CM, Mayer P, 3rd, et al. (2010) TDP-43 is a developmentally regulated protein essential for early embryonic development. *J Biol Chem* 285: 6826-6834.

[139] Wu LS, Cheng WC, Hou SC, Yan YT, Jiang ST, et al. TDP-43, a neuro-pathosignature factor, is essential for early mouse embryogenesis. *Genesis* 48: 56-62.

[140] Johnson BS, Snead D, Lee JJ, McCaffery JM, Shorter J, et al. (2009) TDP-43 is intrinsically aggregation-prone, and amyotrophic lateral sclerosis-linked mutations accelerate aggregation and increase toxicity. *J Biol Chem* 284: 20329-20339.

[141] Polymenidou M, Lagier-Tourenne C, Hutt KR, Huelga SC, Moran J, et al. (2011) Long pre-mRNA depletion and RNA missplicing contribute to neuronal vulnerability from loss of TDP-43. *Nat Neurosci* 14: 459-468.

[142] Vanden Broeck L, Naval-Sanchez M, Adachi Y, Diaper D, Dourlen P, et al. (2013) TDP-43 loss-of-function causes neuronal loss due to defective steroid receptor-mediated gene program switching in Drosophila. *Cell* Rep 3: 160-172.

[143] Barmada S, Finkbeiner S (2010) Bringing SOD1 into the fold. *Nat Neurosci* 13: 1303-1304.

[144] Buratti E, Brindisi A, Giombi M, Tisminetzky S, Ayala YM, et al. (2005) TDP-43 binds heterogeneous nuclear ribonucleoprotein A/B through its C-terminal tail: an important region for the inhibition of cystic fibrosis transmembrane conductance regulator exon 9 splicing. *J Biol Chem* 280: 37572-37584.

[145] Lagier-Tourenne C, Polymenidou M, Cleveland DW (2010) TDP-43 and FUS/TLS: emerging roles in RNA processing and neurodegeneration. *Hum Mol Genet* 19: R46-64.

[146] Alberti S, Halfmann R, King O, Kapila A, Lindquist S (2009) A systematic survey identifies prions and illuminates sequence features of prionogenic proteins. *Cell* 137: 146-158.

[147] Cushman M, Johnson BS, King OD, Gitler AD, Shorter J (2010) Prion-like disorders: blurring the divide between transmissibility and infectivity. *J Cell Sci* 123: 1191-1201.

[148] Kim SH, Shanware NP, Bowler MJ, Tibbetts RS (2010) Amyotrophic lateral sclerosis-associated proteins TDP-43 and FUS/TLS function in a common biochemical complex to co-regulate HDAC6 mRNA. *J Biol Chem* 285: 34097-34105.

[149] Johnson BS, McCaffery JM, Lindquist S, Gitler AD (2008) A yeast TDP-43 proteinopathy model: Exploring the molecular determinants of TDP-43 aggregation and cellular toxicity. Proc Natl Acad Sci U S A 105: 6439-6444.

[150] Liu-Yesucevitz L, Bilgutay A, Zhang YJ, Vanderweyde T, Citro A, et al. (2010) Tar DNA binding protein-43 (TDP-43) associates with stress granules: analysis of cultured cells and pathological brain tissue. *PLoS ONE* 5: e13250.

[151] Udan-Johns M, Bengoechea R, Bell S, Shao J, Diamond MI, et al. (2014) Prion-like nuclear aggregation of TDP-43 during heat shock is regulated by HSP40/70 chaperones. *Hum Mol Genet* 23: 157-170.

[152] Wang IF, Chang HY, Hou SC, Liou GG, Way TD, et al. (2012) The self-interaction of native TDP-43 C terminus inhibits its degradation and contributes to early proteinopathies. *Nat Commun* 3: 766.

[153] Hasegawa M, Arai T, Nonaka T, Kametani F, Yoshida M, et al. (2008) Phosphorylated TDP-43 in frontotemporal lobar degeneration and amyotrophic lateral sclerosis. *Ann Neurol* 64: 60-70.

[154] Robinson JL, Geser F, Stieber A, Umoh M, Kwong LK, et al. (2013) TDP-43 skeins show properties of amyloid in a subset of ALS cases. *Acta Neuropathol* 125: 121-131.

[155] Neumann M, Kwong LK, Sampathu DM, Trojanowski JQ, Lee VM (2007) TDP-43 proteinopathy in frontotemporal lobar degeneration and amyotrophic lateral sclerosis: protein misfolding diseases without amyloidosis. *Arch Neurol* 64: 1388-1394.

[156] Fuentealba RA, Udan M, Bell S, Wegorzewska I, Shao J, et al. (2010) Interaction with polyglutamine aggregates reveals a Q/N-rich domain in TDP-43. *J Biol Chem* 285: 26304-26314.

[157] Aguzzi A, Rajendran L (2009) The transcellular spread of cytosolic amyloids, prions, and prionoids. *Neuron* 64: 783-790.

[158] Hardy J, Selkoe DJ (2002) The amyloid hypothesis of Alzheimer's disease: progress and problems on the road to therapeutics. *Science* 297: 353-356.

[159] Meyer-Luehmann M, Coomaraswamy J, Bolmont T, Kaeser S, Schaefer C, et al. (2006) Exogenous induction of cerebral beta-amyloidogenesis is governed by agent and host. *Science* 313: 1781-1784.

[160] Luk KC, Song C, O'Brien P, Stieber A, Branch JR, et al. (2009) Exogenous alpha-synuclein fibrils seed the formation of Lewy body-like intracellular inclusions in cultured cells. *Proc Natl Acad Sci USA* 106: 20051-20056.

[161] Zhang YJ, Xu YF, Cook C, Gendron TF, Roettges P, et al. (2009) Aberrant cleavage of TDP-43 enhances aggregation and cellular toxicity. *Proc Natl Acad Sci USA* 106: 7607-7612.

[162] van Eersel J, Ke YD, Gladbach A, Bi M, Gotz J, et al. (2011) Cytoplasmic accumulation and aggregation of TDP-43 upon proteasome inhibition in cultured neurons. *PLoS ONE* 6: e22850.

[163] Aguzzi A, Heikenwalder M, Polymenidou M (2007) Insights into prion strains and neurotoxicity. *Nat Rev Mol Cell Biol* 8: 552-561.

[164] Tsuji H, Arai T, Kametani F, Nonaka T, Yamashita M, et al. (2012) Molecular analysis and biochemical classification of TDP-43 proteinopathy. *Brain* 135: 3380-3391.

[165] Hasegawa M, Nonaka T, Tsuji H, Tamaoka A, Yamashita M, et al. (2011) Molecular dissection of TDP-43 proteinopathies. *J Mol Neurosci* 45: 480-485.

[166] Brettschneider J, Del Tredici K, Toledo JB, Robinson JL, Irwin DJ, et al. (2013) Stages of pTDP-43 pathology in amyotrophic lateral sclerosis. *Ann Neurol* 74: 20-38.

[167] Braak H, Brettschneider J, Ludolph AC, Lee VM, Trojanowski JQ, et al. (2013) Amyotrophic lateral sclerosis--a model of corticofugal axonal spread. *Nat Rev Neurol* 9: 708-714.

[168] Huang EJ, Zhang J, Geser F, Trojanowski JQ, Strober JB, et al. (2010) Extensive FUS-immunoreactive pathology in juvenile amyotrophic lateral sclerosis with basophilic inclusions. *Brain Pathol* 20: 1069-1076.

[169] Sun Z, Diaz Z, Fang X, Hart MP, Chesi A, et al. (2011) Molecular determinants and genetic modifiers of aggregation and toxicity for the ALS disease protein FUS/TLS. *PLoS Biol* 9: e1000614.

[170] Gitler AD, Shorter J (2011) RNA-binding proteins with prion-like domains in ALS and FTLD-U. *Prion* 5: 179-187.

[171] Dormann D, Rodde R, Edbauer D, Bentmann E, Fischer I, et al. (2010) ALS-associated fused in sarcoma (FUS) mutations disrupt Transportin-mediated nuclear import. *EMBO J* 29: 2841-2857.

[172] Ito D, Seki M, Tsunoda Y, Uchiyama H, Suzuki N (2011) Nuclear transport impairment of amyotrophic lateral sclerosis-linked mutations in FUS/TLS. *Ann Neurol* 69: 152-162.

[173] Polymenidou M, Cleveland DW (2011) The seeds of neurodegeneration: prion-like spreading in ALS. *Cell* 147: 498-508.

[174] Tan AY, Manley JL (2009) The TET family of proteins: functions and roles in disease. *J Mol Cell Biol* 1: 82-92.

[175] Couthouis J, Hart MP, Shorter J, DeJesus-Hernandez M, Erion R, et al. (2011) A yeast functional screen predicts new candidate ALS disease genes. *Proc Natl Acad Sci USA* 108: 20881-20890.

[176] King OD, Gitler AD, Shorter J (2012) The tip of the iceberg: RNA-binding proteins with prion-like domains in neurodegenerative disease. *Brain Res* 1462: 61-80.

[177] Mackenzie IR, Arzberger T, Kremmer E, Troost D, Lorenzl S, et al. (2013) Dipeptide repeat protein pathology in C9ORF72 mutation cases: clinico-pathological correlations. *Acta Neuropathol.*

[178] Maniecka Z, Polymenidou M (2015) From nucleation to widespread propagation: A prion-like concept for ALS. *Virus Res.*

[179] DeJesus-Hernandez M, Mackenzie IR, Boeve BF, Boxer AL, Baker M, et al. (2011) Expanded GGGGCC hexanucleotide repeat in noncoding region of C9ORF72 causes chromosome 9p-linked FTD and ALS. *Neuron* 72: 245-256.

[180] van Blitterswijk M, Baker MC, DeJesus-Hernandez M, Ghidoni R, Benussi L, et al. (2013) C9ORF72 repeat expansions in cases with previously identified pathogenic mutations. *Neurology* 81: 1332-1341.

[181] Al-Sarraj S, King A, Troakes C, Smith B, Maekawa S, et al. (2011) p62 positive, TDP-43 negative, neuronal cytoplasmic and intranuclear inclusions in the cerebellum and hippocampus define the pathology of C9orf72-linked FTLD and MND/ALS. *Acta Neuropathol* 122: 691-702.

[182] Troakes C, Maekawa S, Wijesekera L, Rogelj B, Siklos L, et al. (2012) An MND/ALS phenotype associated with C9orf72 repeat expansion: abundant p62-positive, TDP-43-negative inclusions in cerebral cortex, hippocampus and cerebellum but without associated cognitive decline. *Neuropathology* 32: 505-514.

[183] Zu T, Liu Y, Banez-Coronel M, Reid T, Pletnikova O, et al. (2013) RAN proteins and RNA foci from antisense transcripts in C9ORF72 ALS and frontotemporal dementia. *Proc Natl Acad Sci USA* 110: E4968-4977.

[184] Kwon I, Xiang S, Kato M, Wu L, Theodoropoulos P, et al. (2014) Poly-dipeptides encoded by the C9orf72 repeats bind nucleoli, impede RNA biogenesis, and kill cells. *Science* 345: 1139-1145.

[185] May S, Hornburg D, Schludi MH, Arzberger T, Rentzsch K, et al. (2014) C9orf72 FTLD/ALS-associated Gly-Ala dipeptide repeat proteins cause neuronal toxicity and Unc119 sequestration. *Acta Neuropathol* 128: 485-503.

[186] Seo H, Sonntag KC, Kim W, Cattaneo E, Isacson O (2007) Proteasome activator enhances survival of Huntington's disease neuronal model cells. *PLoS ONE* 2: e238.

[187] Wright GS, Antonyuk SV, Kershaw NM, Strange RW, Samar Hasnain S (2013) Ligand binding and aggregation of pathogenic SOD1. *Nat Commun* 4: 1758.

[188] Gros-Louis F, Soucy G, Lariviere R, Julien JP (2010) Intracerebroventricular infusion of monoclonal antibody or its derived Fab fragment against misfolded forms of SOD1 mutant delays mortality in a mouse model of ALS. *J Neurochem* 113: 1188-1199.

[189] Liu HN, Tjostheim S, Dasilva K, Taylor D, Zhao B, et al. (2012) Targeting of monomer/misfolded SOD1 as a therapeutic strategy for amyotrophic lateral sclerosis. *J Neurosci* 32: 8791-8799.

[190] Patel P, Kriz J, Gravel M, Soucy G, Bareil C, et al. (2014) Adeno-associated virus-mediated delivery of a recombinant single-chain antibody against misfolded superoxide dismutase for treatment of amyotrophic lateral sclerosis. *Mol Ther* 22: 498-510.

[191] Armakola M, Higgins MJ, Figley MD, Barmada SJ, Scarborough EA, et al. (2012) Inhibition of RNA lariat debranching enzyme suppresses TDP-43 toxicity in ALS disease models. *Nat Genet* 44: 1302-1309.
[192] Irwin DJ, Abrams JY, Schonberger LB, Leschek EW, Mills JL, et al. (2013) Evaluation of potential infectivity of Alzheimer and Parkinson disease proteins in recipients of cadaver-derived human growth hormone. *JAMA Neurol* 70: 462-468.
[193] Eisele YS, Obermuller U, Heilbronner G, Baumann F, Kaeser SA, et al. (2010) Peripherally applied Abeta-containing inoculates induce cerebral beta-amyloidosis. *Science* 330: 980-982.
[194] Soti C, Csermely P (2003) Aging and molecular chaperones. *Exp Gerontol* 38: 1037-1040.
[195] Hipkiss AR (2006) Accumulation of altered proteins and ageing: causes and effects. *Exp Gerontol* 41: 464-473.
[196] Basaiawmoit RV, Rattan SI (2010) Cellular stress and protein misfolding during aging. *Methods Mol Biol* 648: 107-117.

In: The Prion Phenomena in Neurodegenerative Diseases ISBN: 978-1-63483-399-8
Editors: Giuseppe Legname and Gabriele Giachin

Chapter 10

PRIONS IN YEAST: THINKING OUTSIDE OF THE BRAIN

***Polina Drozdova*[1,3,*] *and Andrew Matveenko*[1,2,3]**
[1]Dept. of Genetics and Biotechnology,
Saint Petersburg State University, St. Petersburg, Russia
[2]St. Petersburg Branch, Vavilov Institute of General Genetics of the Russian Academy of Sciences, St. Petersburg, Russia
[3]Laboratory of Amyloid Biology, St. Petersburg State University,
St. Petersburg, Russia

ABSTRACT

During the last decade prion-related phenomena were shown to be more widespread than it was initially thought. Prions and prion-like factors were discovered not only in mammals but in other Metazoa and several fungal species. Studies on the budding yeast *Saccharomyces cerevisiae*, a well-known model organism, were crucial for this understanding.

Unicellularity of yeast permits self-templating protein conformations to behave as heritable traits. This is why the first yeast prions had been discovered as non-Mendelian cytoplasmic elements long before the prion hypothesis was proved and acknowledged. After the seminal article published in 1994 by Reed Wickner and suggesting the prion nature of two such elements the prion biology skyrocketed. The rapid progress in the field benefited from this species being easy to cultivate and manipulate, as well as from immense knowledge in yeast genetics and molecular biology accumulated to date. Yeast prions were also implied to be molecular diseases similar to the mammalian amyloids but further studies questioned this concept.

Since the beginning of yeast prionology about a dozen of yeast proteins were proved to be prions, with more than a hundred proteins suggested as prion candidates. Interestingly, many of these proteins contribute to the regulation of gene expression, often on a global scale. This suggests a functional role of prion conversion in cellular homeostasis. There is another line of evidence supporting this thesis: some natural factors like ethanol or oxygen concentration induce or inhibit formation of particular yeast

* E-mail address: drozdovapb@gmail.com

prions. These data propose a role for prions in adaptation. At least three prions found in wild populations of *S. cerevisiae* also support this idea. Moreover, under certain conditions prion-containing cells gain advantage in growth or survival. This implies that different prions may sharply increase phenotypic variation within the clonal population, which in turn may raise the survival rate of this particular clone under varying conditions. Thus, prion conversion may contribute to the so-called "bet-hedging" strategy. Heat shock proteins also play a major role in prion propagation, and that might be one of the mechanisms by which environmental factors control prion conversion.

In this chapter we first discuss the complexity and ambiguity of the prion problem. Then we highlight the common features of yeast prions and characterize known mechanisms controlling prion life cycle. Finally, we describe the diversity of fungal prions and prion-like elements and disclose the usefulness of yeast as a model to study amyloids *in vivo*.

1. INTRODUCTION

Prions and related phenomena were first described and studied in the context of mammalian diseases. However, phenomena based on the principle of "conformational infectivity" turned out to be more widespread. Infectivity of prions, which is basically the ability of one protein conformation to force its own structure on other molecules of the same protein species, leads to conformational disorders in multicellular organisms (see [1]). In animals, prions and prion-like amyloids are primarily found and studied in non-dividing tissues and are observed as terminal phenotypes. But what kind of a trait would it manifest in a unicellular organism? When prions appear in microbial cells they are transmitted during cell divisions thus enabling prion-related phenotype to persist in generations, i.e., leading to establishment of heritable traits (see [2]). These exact phenomena were discovered for several fungal species and are most extensively studied in baker's yeast *Saccharomyces cerevisiae*.

This species has been exploited by humans and co-evolved with us for thousands of years [3]. It has a short life cycle, is easily cultivated, stable in both haploid and diploid states which simplifies the genetic analysis [4], and *S. cerevisiae* genome was the first completely sequenced eukaryotic genome [5]. All these qualities make yeast an excellent model organism for studying diverse biological problems including prions. Yeast studies further benefit from the existence of *Saccharomyces* Genome Database integrating genomic data, annotation, functional information and helpful tools for analysis [6, 7].

The prion problem is complex and ambiguous. Even the terminology issue is still unsolved. The necessary and sufficient features for a protein to be called a prion are still under debate. The word "prion" had been originally introduced to describe an infectious agent of mammalian transmissible spongiform encephalopathies (TSEs), i.e., what we now call PrP^{Sc}. When many other proteins were found to behave like PrP^{Sc}, the term was expanded.

The known basis of prion phenomena in mammals resides on the properties of amyloid aggregates. Amyloids are fibrillar aggregates enriched in β-sheets. Amyloids are able to "grow" by addition of soluble monomers at the termini of fibril. Specific fluorescent dyes like thioflavin T (ThT) selectively bind amyloid aggregates and thus are commonly used to study the dynamics of fibril formation. It occurred that most, but not all, yeast prions are also amyloid-based (see [8]), and the new data raised new issues.

First, does amyloid mean prion? Not necessarily. The term "amyloid" refers to physicochemical properties of a protein, while "prion" is a purely biological term that implies the *in vivo* infectivity of a protein conformation. *I.e.*, only infectious amyloids are prions. Then what about non-amyloid prions? Despite their similarity to amyloid prions, the mechanisms of their propagation are physiologically different. These are usually referred to as prion-like determinants but can occasionally be called prions, depending on our definition of "prion."

Second, it is still unclear whether an infectious agent, i.e., amyloid or other self-templating conformation, or the protein itself which can have multiple conformations with at least one being infectious, should be called prion. But what does an "infectious protein" mean? The main characteristics that define prions are their abilities, first, to convert other molecules of the same protein species into prion state and, second, to transmit self-templating conformations to other cells. Combined, these processes ensure stable presence of the prion in successive generations of cells, and that is called prion propagation.

Third, PrP^{Sc} causes neurodegenerative diseases while yeast prions are extrachromosomal heritable elements. Still, yeast prions are often described as diseases, and some generally accepted terms in yeast prion biology reflect this "negative" attitude. E.g., elimination of a prion from culture is called "curing" [9]. There are two polar opposite points of view on whether yeast prions are good or bad (see Section 7).

Fourth, yeast is a well-studied and convenient model system for studying recombinant proteins. Coupled with developed methods of studying yeast prions, it allows investigation of prions and amyloids from other species. There are examples of heterologous and chimeric proteins from *Podospora anserina* [10, 11], *Aplysia californica* [12], *Drosophila melanogaster* [13], human and other mammals [14, 15], that behave as prions in *S. cerevisiae*. Should we consider them prions? Moreover, one of yeast prions was shown to propagate in *Caenorhabditis elegans* [16] and mouse cell cultures [17] raising even more questions about the limitations of the term.

2. WICKNER'S GENETIC CRITERIA OF YEAST PRIONS

As the knowledge about the *S. cerevisiae* genome grew, evidence about mitochondrial DNA and viruses, i.e., cytoplasmic genetic elements not linked to the chromosomal DNA, was also accumulating. However, some cytoplasmic "mutations" could not be mapped in these structures (see [18, 19]). This led to the discovery of first yeast prions many years before the prion concept was proved and acknowledged. Almost half a century ago two unusual genetic determinants were independently described, [*PSI*$^+$] [20] and [*URE3*] [21].

The [*PSI*$^+$] (or Ψ factor) was discovered as a nonsense suppressor by Brian Cox in 1965 [20]. [*URE3*] was discovered by Francois Lacroute in 1971 [21] during studies of uracil biosynthesis in yeast. Both were described as cytoplasmically encoded dominant mutations [21, 22]. A chromosomal *ure2* mutant was unable to maintain [*URE3*] even though it displayed the same phenotype [23]. This was the crucial finding that allowed determination of the true nature of [*URE3*] and all the other prions afterwards (see [2, 19]).

In early 1990s, the data concerning [PSI^+] was accumulating. In 1993, Yury O. Chernoff and coworkers found that overexpression of *SUP35* dramatically increased the frequency of [PSI^+] induction [24].

Table 1. Prions and prion-like genetic elements in fungi discovered so far

Fungal prions (in alphabetic order)	Protein	Protein function	Q/N enrichment	Amyloid formation/ Hsp104 requirement	References
[β]	Prb1	vacuolar protease B	no	no/no	[29]
[*C*]*	PaASK1	MAPKKK	yes**	no/n.d.	[30, 31]
[GAR^+]	n.d.	n.a.	n.a.	no/no	[32]
[*Het-s*]*	Het-s	vegetative incompatibility	no	yes/yes***	[33]
[ISP^+]	Sfp1	transcriptional regulation (ribosome biogenesis)	yes	n.d./no	[34, 35]
[MCA^+] †	Mca1	Metacaspase	yes	yes#/n.d.	[36–38]
[MOD^+]	Mod5	tRNA modification (tRNA isopenteny ltransferase)	no	yes/yes	[39]
[$MOT3^+$]	Mot3	transcriptional regulation	yes	yes/yes	[40]
[NSI^+]	n.d.	n.a.	n.a.	n.a./yes	[41]
[$NUP100^+$]	Nup100	nuclear pore formation	yes	yes/yes	[42]
[OCT^+]	Cyc8	transcriptional regulation	yes	yes#/yes	[43]
[PIN^+]/ [RNQ^+]	Rnq1	unknown	yes	yes/yes	[44, 45]
[PSI^+]	Sup35	translation termination (release factor eRF3)	yes	yes/yes	[9, 20]
[SWI^+]	Swi1	chromatin remodeling	yes	yes/yes	[46]
[*URE3*]	Ure2	transcriptional regulation (nitrogen metabolism)	yes	yes/yes	[9, 21]

*, A *Podospora anserina* trait.
**, Q-rich sequence of PaASK1 does not contribute to [*C*] propagation.
***, PaHsp104 inactivation does not cause immediate loss of [*Het-s*] due to the coenocytic structure of the organism but makes impossible its transmission during meiosis [47].
†, original paper retracted.
#, Only ThT fluorescence of the purified protein and detergent resistance are confirmed [40].
n.d., not determined.
n.a., non-applicable.

Parallel group led by Michael D. Ter-Avanesyan showed that manifestation of [PSI^+] strongly required the N-terminal domain of Sup35 [25]. Independently, after carrying out analogous experiments on [*URE3*], Reed B. Wickner suggested prion properties for [*URE3*] and [PSI^+] in his seminal article [9]. He also proposed the genetic criteria for identifying prions in fungi.

These criteria are as follows [18]:

- Reversible curing. Curing usually refers to loss of prion after mild guanidinium chloride (GuHCl) treatment which was first shown for [*PSI*$^+$] [26]. As proved later, GuHCl-driven elimination is due to inactivation of Hsp104 (see Section 3.2). What distinguishes prions from other cytoplasmic elements is their ability to reappear *de novo* after elimination at constant rates which are higher than those of the spontaneous mutations.
- Overproduction of the corresponding protein ("prion determinant" hereafter) increases the rate of prion appearance which is also called prion induction. The more protein there is in the cell, the higher the chance of acquiring infectious conformation and thus developing the corresponding prion phenotype.
- The gene encoding the structural protein is necessary for prion appearance and propagation while mutations in this gene can mimic the prion phenotype. The latter means that the protein may be inactivated either by prion conversion or mutation both leading to similar phenotypes.

Since proposing prion nature of [*PSI*$^+$] and [*URE3*] about a dozen new fungal prions or prion-like genetic elements have been discovered (Table 1; see [27, 28]). There are also many prion candidates that require additional studies.

3. Common Characteristics of Yeast Prions

As the set of known yeast prions grew, it became possible to distinguish other unifying (as well as varying) features.

3.1. Yeast Prion Domains and Amino Acid Composition

A distinctive feature of most prion proteins is a minimal region that is called prion domain (PrD) and is sufficient for prion maintenance but does not influence canonical functions of the corresponding protein. For amyloid prions, this domain includes the amyloid core. PrDs are often N- or C-terminal. Thus, PrDs are stacked into an amyloid fibril with the functional domain hanging over around it. Amyloid nature provides an explanation for existence of different prion strains, or variants. Since the core of amyloid fibrils can vary in length or in folding pattern, it occurred that assembly into different structures may result in diverse phenotypes of prion-bearing cells [48–51]. The aggregation of yeast prion proteins was shown not only *in vitro* [44, 52-54] but also *in vivo*. If fused with fluorescent proteins, prion proteins in aggregated state form fluorescent foci. It was first shown for [*PSI*$^+$] [55] and subsequently became a routine method for proving aggregation and for studying characteristics of known and putative prions. Amyloid aggregates of [*URE3*] and [*PSI*$^+$] have also been visualized in cells with electron microscopy [56-58]. As a rule, PrDs are enriched in glutamine (Q) and asparagine (N) residues (Q/N-rich) (Figure 1A,B).

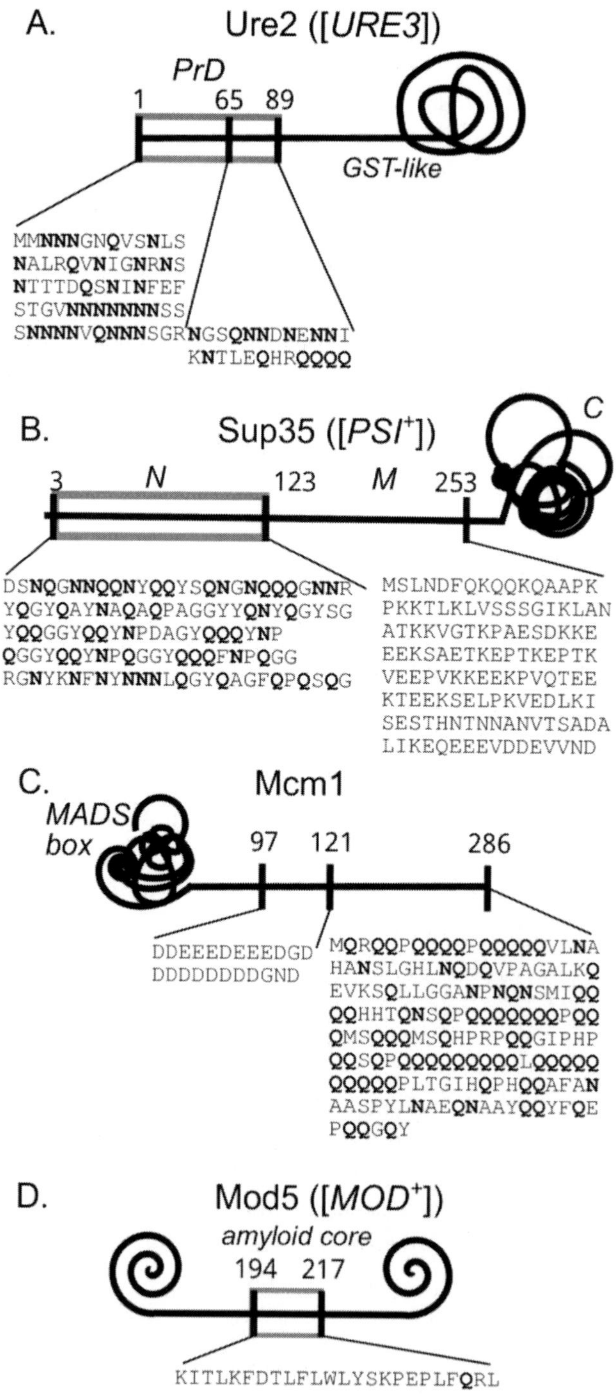

Figure 1. Domain architecture and amino acid sequence of the PrDs and linker domains of Ure2 (A), Sup35 (B), Mcm1 (C) and Mod5 (D). Q (glutamine) and N (asparagine) residues in PrDs are in bold. Scribbled lines indicate structured non-prion domains of the proteins (schematics are generated with Inkscape). See Section 3.1 for details.

Interestingly, the prion domains of Ure2 or Sup35 with randomly shuffled residues still enable the respective proteins to form amyloid fibrils *in vitro* and prions *in vivo* [59, 60]. Thus, not the sequence but the amino acid composition determines prion properties. Functional domains and PrDs are typically separated with a linker domain, a region that is thought to act as a flexible "leash" that holds the PrD to the amyloid core. Still, meeting all the aforementioned requirements does not guarantee prion properties (see [61]). E.g., Mcm1 is similar to Sup35 in its domain architecture: it consists of C-terminal Q/N-rich domain, middle D/E-rich region (K/E-rich in Sup35) and N-terminal domain, the latter being sufficient for DNA binding and regulation of transcription [62, 63] (Figure 1C). However, no prion properties for Mcm1 have been found [40]. In contrast, Mod5 does not possess any Q/N-rich region but forms amyloid aggregates *in vitro* and a *bona fide* prion [*MOD*$^+$] *in vivo* [39] (Figure 1D).

Even though PrDs are thought to be dispensable for canonical function of the protein there are data contradicting this notion. E.g., N-domain of Ure2 may be important for stability of the whole protein [64], and N-domain of Sup35 is shown to interact both physically and functionally with Pab1 (Poly(A)-Binding protein) during translation [65] and with Pub1 in a tubulin-associated complex [15]. Both may be evolutionarily conserved, since analogous interactions are shown for mammalian homologs of Sup35 and Pab1 or Pub1 [15, 67].

3.2. Yeast Prion Propagation by Cytosolic Chaperones

Having the ability to form amyloids is not enough for a protein to propagate as a prion. In order to be infectious, prion aggregates must not only grow but also divide and be transmitted into daughter cells. Responsible for dismantling of large aggregates into transmissible particles (also known as propagons) are cellular chaperone machinery components. In yeast and bacteria three major classes of chaperones, Hsp100, Hsp70 and Hsp40, are responsible for dissolving aggregates.

Hsp104 is the main disaggregase, or "crowbar." It is an AAA+ class ATPase that performs its functions as a ring-like hexamer [68]. Hsp104 plays a key role in heat stress response in yeast [69, 70]. At the same time, Hsp104 is required for propagation of all known amyloid yeast prions (see [27, 42, 39]) which explains prion curing by GuHCl at mM concentrations since it is shown to inactivate Hsp104 [71, 72]. *Escherichia coli* has an Hsp100 homolog called ClpB which executes the same function [73]. However, ClpB cannot substitute for Hsp104 in yeast and, reversely, Hsp104 cannot substitute for ClpB in bacteria [74]. The reason is inability of ClpB to interact with yeast Hsp70, which is crucial for disaggregation machinery to operate [75, 76]. Hsp104 homolog found in plants also contributes to thermotolerance [77] and even substitutes for Hsp104 in yeast [78, 79], but no homolog is known in Metazoa [68].

Six nuclear/cytosolic Hsp70 chaperones are known in mammals, and the same number is found in two groups of cytosolic Hsp70s in yeast, Ssa and Ssb (see [80]). Out of the four genes in *S. cerevisiae* that encode Hsp70-Ssa proteins at least one is required for viability [81]. All the Ssa proteins are highly similar, with Ssa1 and Ssa2 being 99% identical [82]. However, they differently affect prion propagation. E.g., additional copies of *SSA1* but not *SSA2* cure [*URE3*] [83] while deletion of *SSA2* but not *SSA1* destabilizes [*URE3*] [84]. In strains constitutively expressing only one of the four *SSA* genes, prion propagation depends not only on the particular *SSA* gene but also on the prion studied ([*PSI*$^+$] or [*URE3*]) [85]. Nearly identical Ssb1 and Ssb2 are normally ribosome-associated and thought to aid in the cotranslational folding [86]. Interestingly, depletion of Ssb promotes [*PSI*$^+$] appearance *de novo* [87] while its abundance has an anti-prion effect [88, 89]. The former can be explained by increasing rate of misfolding of the prion protein while the latter leads to increase in cytoplasmic fraction of Ssb proteins that interfere with Ssa's binding prion aggregates [90].

Hsp40s, or J-proteins, are essential partners of Hsp70s that define the functional specificity and stimulate the ATPase activity of Hsp70. There are 22 known J-proteins in *S. cerevisiae* that are known or predicted to work in almost every compartment of the cell (see [91]). Major cytosolic J-proteins are Sis1 and Ydj1. Sis1 is the only Hsp40 that is absolutely necessary for propagation of at least four prions. *SIS1* is an essential gene, so its deletion is impossible. Its depletion causes rapid loss of [*PIN*$^+$], [*URE3*], and [*SWI*$^+$] but very slow loss of [*PSI*$^+$] [92, 93]. Recent data confirm that [*PSI*$^+$] is less dependent on defects in Sis1 than other prions [94–96]. Sis1 activity is regulated not only by heat stress since at least two sorting factors, Btn2 and Cur1, are known to regulate Sis1 abundance in cytoplasm [97]. Btn2 and Cur1 overproduction is also shown to cure [*URE3*] [98], and the curing is alleviated by additional Sis1 coexpression [99]. The role of Ydj1 in prion propagation differs from that of Sis1 though they partially share functions in thermotolerance [100, 101]. Overexpression of *YDJ1* cures [*URE3*] [102] and some variants of [*PIN*$^+$] [103] or chimeric [*PSI*$^+_{PS}$] [104].

Most of the data contribute to the idea that propagation of amyloid prions is driven by the same machinery that dissolves heat-denatured aggregates. In summary: Hsp40 (Sis1 or Ydj1) recognizes an amyloid (Figure 2, 3A) and recruits Hsp70. Formation of an aggregate-associated Hsp70/Hsp40 complex (Figure 2, 3B) allows Hsp104 to bind and to perform its disaggregation activity (Figure 2, 3C). The whole process leads to fragmentation of prion fibrils which enables infectious particles, or propagons, to persist after numerous cell divisions [75, 76].

This underlies the unifying model of prion propagation as it progresses through successive stages of amyloid prion life cycle [105] (Figure 2).

1. *De novo* appearance of prion seed.
2. Growth of amyloid fibril, conversion of native proteins into amyloid conformation.
3. Fibril fragmentation by disaggregation machinery and formation of propagons.
4. Repeat 2 and 3.
5. Dispersion of propagons into daughter cells.
6. Repeat 2-5 in each daughter cell.

Thus, growth and division of prion aggregates coupled with growth and division of yeast cells can be summarized in the prion life cycle model [105], and the same principle may be applied to prion propagation in mammalian cells [106]. While mechanisms of stages 2 and 3 are being successfully investigated in yeast, little is known about 1 and 5. There are multiple pieces of evidence about conditions that elevate frequency of appearance of particular prions (see Section 4).

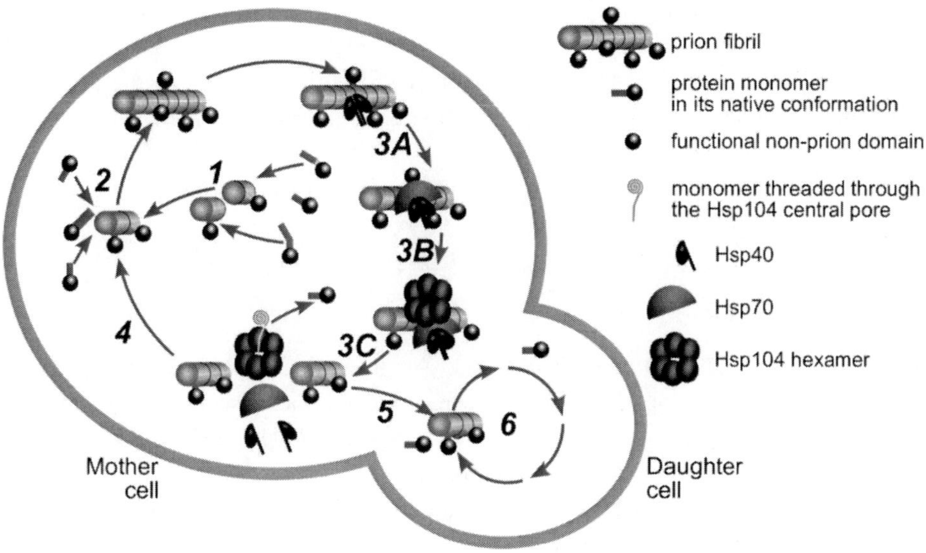

Figure 2. The life cycle of amyloid prions. Schematic view of amyloid formation (1), growth (2), fragmentation (3A-C) and transmission (5). See Section 3.2 for details about each step.

Known mechanisms of transmission of propagons to daughter cells are controversial. First of all, several pathways of asymmetric segregation of amyloids between mother and daughter cells are proposed [107–109] and they basically counteract propagon transmission. The nature of propagons is also a matter of debates, although the data so far suggest they might correspond to small oligomeric amyloid fibrils [58, 107].

4. The Diversity of Yeast Prions

S. cerevisiae is not the only fungal species examined for prions. Extensive research led to discovery of at least two prion-like traits in filamentous fungus *Podospora anserina*.

The first one, [*Het-s*], is the prion form of the Het-s protein [33] which plays an important role in vegetative incompatibility, a programmed cell death reaction that takes place upon fusion of hyphae with different genotypes (see [110]). The C-terminal 71 amino acids of the Het-s protein comprise the prion domain [111], which is able to propagate the [*Het-s*]$_y$ prion when expressed as a GFP-fusion in *S. cerevisiae* [10]. An interesting feature of [*Het-s*] is the existence of a single prion variant (see [112]). It is consistent with the results of NMR studies that returned a 3D model suggesting only one stable amyloid structure [113]. [*Het-s*] is considered to be advantageous. More than 90% of wild *Podospora anserina het-s* populations were screened as [*Het-s*] [114].

Another prion-like determinant found in *Podospora* is called [*C*] [30]. It cannot propagate without the MAPKKK gene *PaASK1* and arises at higher frequencies after its overexpression. The [*C*] phenotype differs from that of *PaASK1* mutants suggesting that the protein is not inactivated. [*C*] may confer active state of the enzyme that propagates via self-phosphorylation although it requires confirmation [31].

Another trait implied to propagate by the similar principle was discovered in yeast. It was named [*β*] and it is self-activating form of the vacuolar protease B, encoded by *PRB1*. Like [*C*] phenotype is the opposite of *PaASK1* mutants, [*β*] is the opposite of the *PRB1* deletion phenotype [29] that suggests it might be a common characteristic intrinsic to all traits based on self-activating enzymes.

Further, we will focus on the conventional and well-studied determinants.

4.1. [*PSI*$^+$]

[*PSI*$^+$] is a dominant omnipotent nonsense suppressor [20]. It is usually monitored in mutants defective in adenine biosynthesis, which are red because of accumulation of the adenine precursor which transforms into a red pigment [115]. *ade1-14* and *ade2-1* are suppressed when translation termination (release) factors malfunction (see [116]). If accumulated in [*PSI*$^+$] aggregates, Sup35 is unable to provide adequate translation termination leading to stop codon read-through [9, 117]. Thus, *ade1-14* or *ade2-1* [*PSI*$^+$] cells acquire a fraction of full length Ade1 or Ade2 protein, and thus accumulate less red pigment and form pink or white colonies (see [116]). Early studies of [*PSI*$^+$] with genetic methods identified dominant mutations termed *PNM* ([*PSI*$^+$]-No-More) that abolished [*PSI*$^+$] propagation. The *PNM2-1* allele was later shown to be a missense mutation in *SUP35* N-domain [118] while *PNM1* corresponded to a mutation in *HSP104* (see [116]).

Sup35 comprises three domains: N, M and C (Figure 1B). The C-domain is translation termination factor eRF3, which is essential and does not require other two domains to function [118]. Functions of the M-domain are poorly understood while the N-domain is the PrD of Sup35 [119, 120].

[*PSI*$^+$] is the only prion known to disappear after *HSP104* overexpression. The dynamics of the loss of [*PSI*$^+$] drastically differs from the one during Hsp104 inactivation by GuHCl [121, 122]. Independent works elucidated the mechanism. The N-domain of Hsp104, as well as a motif in the Sup35 M-domain, are necessary for curing by Hsp104 overexpression [76, 123, 124]. Thus, it is safe to conclude that, when the N-domain of Hsp104 directly binds the M-domain of Sup35, Hsp104 becomes unable to perform its functions, as for disaggregation to occur Hsp104 must be sequestered by Hsp70/Hsp40. Thus, direct binding of Hsp104 is thought to be non-productive for the disaggregation activity of Hsp104 [76]. There is more to the mechanism as the requirement for cofactors was shown [125]. [*PSI*$^+$] is destabilized by mild heat shock, which is explained by more rapid elevation of Hsp104 levels than of those of Hsp70 and Hsp40. This mechanism is unique for [*PSI*$^+$] since elevation of Hsp104 levels does not cure other yeast prions [126].

[*PSI*$^+$] was the first yeast prion with diverse variants described [127]. They differ in strength, which correlates with the efficiency of nonsense suppression and is inversely related to the level of Sup35 that remains soluble. Strains bearing weak [*PSI*$^+$] are pink while those with strong [*PSI*$^+$] are white [127]. To explain how prion variants acquire different strength, an analytical model was proposed. According to it, the strength of a prion variant is a function of the rates of protein synthesis, fibril growth and fibril division [49]. The actual mechanism seems to be more complex since there are data that variants of [*PSI*$^+$] differ in their sensitivity to the Hsp40 chaperones [94, 95]. Although some [*PSI*$^+$] variants (so-called "suicidal [*PSI*$^+$]") were found to be deleterious [128], read-through of natural stop codons may confer selective advantage to yeast cells in population. Indeed, it was found that translational read-throughs of natural stop codons may occur in [*PSI*$^+$] strains [129], so [*PSI*$^+$] might serve as a mechanism to increase survival under unstable conditions [130].

[*PSI*$^+$] is unstable in presence of high concentrations of KCl, ethylene glycol [131], dimethyl sulfoxide, ethanol or methanol [26]. Various stressful conditions increase the frequency of [*PSI*$^+$] formation [130]; especially, influence of oxidative stress has been a subject of particular interest [132]. With all that in mind, it is no surprise that the [*PSI*$^+$] prion was found in wild yeast strains though quite rarely [133]. *S. cerevisiae* is not the only species known to propagate [*PSI*$^+$] since the Sup35 homolog from *Kluyveromyces lactis* can form a prion in both *K. lactis* and *S. cerevisiae* [134]. [*PSI*$^+$] was also discovered in a natural isolate of *Saccharomyces bayanus* [133].

4.2. [*URE3*]

[*URE3*], formed by Ure2, was the first trait to be proposed as prion [9]. Ure2 normally inhibits transcription of nitrogen catabolism genes by preventing several transcriptional activators from entering the nucleus [135] and was also shown to exhibit glutathione peroxidase activity *in vitro* [136].

Ure2 can be subdivided into two domains. The N-terminal part of the protein corresponds to the prion domain: the region 1-89 is Q/N-rich, and the subregion 1-65 is sufficient for induction and maintenance of the prion (Figure 1A) while the C-terminal part of the protein can fully compensate for the *URE2* deletion [137, 138].

Whether Ure2 is fully inactivated upon prionization is unclear. The changes in global transcriptome in [*URE3*] cells compared to the *ure2* mutants can be attributed to residual activity of Ure2 in the [*URE3*] strains [139]. At the same time, *in vitro* experiments showed that fibrils of Ure2 formed *in vitro* preserved the enzymatic activity of monomeric Ure2, though on reduced levels. A possible reconciliation for these data is that aggregation of Ure2 inhibits its interaction with transcription factors by steric means but does not inhibit its enzymatic activity [136, 140].

Like [*PSI*$^+$], [*URE3*] may exist in other fungal species. E.g., [*URE3*] can definitely arise spontaneously in *Saccharomyces uvarum* (*S. bayanus*) [141] and can be induced in *Candida albicans* [142].

4.3. [*PIN*$^+$] ([*RNQ*$^+$])

SUP35 overexpression does not always lead to [*PSI*$^+$] induction but the ability to induce [*PSI*$^+$] (namely, Pin$^+$ phenotype) requires another prion, hence the name [*PIN*$^+$] (PSI INduction) [143]. Independent studies revealed a prion-like behaviour of Rnq1 [44], and Rnq1 was proved to be [*PIN*$^+$] determinant [45].

[*PIN*$^+$] is mysterious. First, the Rnq1 function is still unclear: it is shown to affect sporulation through an unknown mechanism [144] but it is possible that facilitating aggregation of other amyloids is the main function of Rnq1, which makes [*PIN*$^+$] a functional prion. Second, elevated Rnq1 causes very inefficient induction of [*PIN*$^+$] [45] while the rate of *de novo* appearance of [*PIN*$^+$] is much higher than that for other prions [138, 145, 146] which may explain why [*PIN*$^+$] is more often found in natural *S. cerevisiae* populations [133, 147]. Well-known for its first sequenced genome *S. cerevisiae* strain S288C and its derivatives also happened to be [*PIN*$^+$] [44, 148] which allowed to reveal genes necessary for [*PIN*$^+$] propagation [148].

Rnq1 is commonly divided into two domains: N-terminal non-prion domain and Q/N-rich C-terminal PrD. However, deletion of the first 100 amino acids or various mutations in the N-terminal domain are shown to interfere with [*PSI*$^+$] propagation on [*PIN*$^+$] background [149, 150] or destabilize [*PIN*$^+$] itself [149, 151].

4.4. [*SWI*$^+$]

Swi1, the protein determinant of [*SWI*$^+$], is a component of the chromatin remodeling SWI/SNF complex that regulates the transcription of carbon source utilization genes [152]. Similar to *swi1* mutations, [*SWI*$^+$] affects metabolism of raffinose, galactose and glycerol by making yeast unable to metabolize these non-fermentable sugars. The Swi1 protein comprises three domains: N (N-rich N-terminal domain), Q (Q-rich middle domain) and C. The last one is sufficient to ensure the function of the protein in carbon source utilization [46], while the very N-terminal part of the protein is sufficient for [*SWI*$^+$] propagation. The function of the middle region of the protein is still unclear [153].

There is no data about presence of [*SWI*$^+$] in wild populations, but it seems unlikely because of narrow range of growth temperatures suited for stable [*SWI*$^+$] propagation and its high sensitivity to changes in balance of cellular chaperones [93].

4.5. [*OCT*$^+$]

The [*OCT*$^+$] prion is formed by Cyc8 [43], a component of transcriptional repression Cyc8-Tup1 complex. Similar to [*SWI*$^+$], [*OCT*$^+$] affects carbon source utilization. In order to assimilate lactate, working electron transport chain is required with cytochrome C as its essential component. Cyc8 inhibits many genes including *CYC7* that encodes the minor isoform of cytochrome C [154]. If Cyc8 is inactivated by mutation or by conversion into prion form ([*OCT*$^+$]), such cells are capable of growing on lactate even in the absence of Cyc1, the major cytochrome C isoform [155]. There is evidence that Cyc8 is not fully inactivated in the [*OCT*$^+$] state as derepression of at least five Cyc8-controlled genes is significantly lower in [*OCT*$^+$] than in *cyc8Δ* cells [43].

4.6. [*MOT3*$^+$]

This prion was identified in a massive targeted search for prionogenic proteins in yeast [40]. Mot3, the protein determinant of [*MOT3*$^+$], is a zinc finger protein mainly regulating transcription of anaerobic genes [156]. Mot3 might be the main regulator in the cellular response to oxygen availability. [*MOT3*$^+$] was shown to be regulated by conditions similar to what happens during wine production. Excess of ethanol increases [*MOT3*$^+$] appearance rates, which may contribute to stress conditions affecting protein homeostasis. This prion is eliminated in response to hypoxia due to Mot3 downregulation. [*MOT3*$^+$] also plays an important role in control of multicellularity in yeast populations by promoting biofilm formation and may be advantageous under certain conditions [157]. This idea is further supported by the fact that this prion was found in 6 out of 96 strains from the natural populations [133].

4.7. [*MOD*$^+$]

Mod5, the determinant of [*MOD*$^+$], was identified as a factor that templates prionization of Q62-Sup35 and as a Pin$^+$ factor. Mod5 regulates ergosterol biosynthesis and also functions as a tRNA isopentenyltransferase [39]. [*MOD*$^+$] is yet another prion involved in control of translation. Though there is no direct evidence of its involvement in regulation of translational fidelity, the *MOD5* gene was originally identified by a mutation suppressing a dominant (tRNA) suppressor [158]. Moreover, *MOD5* was identified as a chromosomal [*PSI*$^+$] antagonist [19] despite being a [*PSI*$^+$]-inducing factor [39]. Also, similar to [*PSI*$^+$], [*MOD*$^+$] is sensitive to *HSP104* overexpression even though it is not completely cured by it [39].

[*MOD*$^+$] exemplifies an advantageous prion. Propagation of [*MOD*$^+$] not only elevates the level of ergosterol but also increases the resistance to a spectrum of antifungal agents, such as microtubule inhibitor nocodazole and a number of ergosterol biosynthesis inhibitors, two of which, fluconazole and ketoconazole, increase the rate of spontaneous appearance of [*MOD*$^+$] [39].

In contrast to most known yeast prion proteins but similar to mammalian PrP^{Sc} and *Podospora* Het-s, the Mod5 amyloid core region lacks Q/N-rich sequences (Figure 1D). Thus, [*MOD*$^+$] may serve as a good model for studying PrP^{Sc} [159].

4.8. [*ISP*$^+$]

[*ISP*$^+$] was identified serendipitously during studies of translation termination in yeast [34]. Like [*PSI*$^+$], some *sup35* mutations lead to nonsense suppression. Investigating suppressor qualities of the *sup35-10* and *sup35-25* mutants revealed that they conform to two alternative states: either suppressor or non-suppressor. Intense passaging on GuHCl-containing media lets the suppressor phenotype turn into non-suppressor with relatively high frequency of reversion. The determinant was designated [*ISP*$^+$], that technically stands for "Inversion of Suppressor Phenotype" and also reflects that the observed phenotype is [*PSI*$^+$]-reversed [34].

[*ISP*$^+$] is shown to be the prion form of transcriptional regulator Sfp1, and its unique property is nuclear localization of prion aggregates [35]. Besides, [*ISP*$^+$] propagation does not depend on Hsp104 [34]. Sfp1 is known regulator of ribosome biogenesis genes and ribosomal protein genes [160] and might also function in elongation of transcription [161]. Intriguingly, the consequences of the *SFP1* deletion and presence of [*ISP*$^+$] are utterly different both in terms of phenotypic changes [35] and in terms of their effect on the cell transcriptome [162]. So, the role of Sfp1 in [*ISP*$^+$] formation is still oblique. The [*ISP*$^+$] phenotype is supposedly mediated by changes in *SUP35* expression [163]. Compared to both [*isp*$^-$] and *sfp1Δ* strains,

[ISP^+] strains grow faster under optimal conditions and are less sensitive to some translation inhibitors which underlies the advantageousness of the trait [34, 35].

4.9. [GAR^+]

The [GAR^+] prion could be an excellent example of a functional prion if its prion nature were firmly established. This heritable trait also influences carbon source utilization. Like [ISP^+], [GAR^+] is cured by GuHCl but does not depend on Hsp104. Maintenance of [GAR^+] is linked to *PMA1* and *STD1* but the exact determinant is unknown. Authors also provide evidence that [GAR^+] propagation does not involve amyloid aggregation [32], which classifies [GAR^+] as a prion-like element. Interestingly, the [GAR^+] phenotype cannot only arise *de novo* in yeast cells but it can also stem from interaction of yeast and bacteria. The bacterial component responsible for the induction of [GAR^+] was filtered from cells but has not been reliably identified [164]. Intriguingly, a trait indistinguishable from [GAR^+] exists in many yeast species, even in those lacking homologs of Std1 [165].

4.10. [$NUP100^+$]

Some yeast proteins, e.g., GLFG-rich nucleoporins, contain domains that are naturally enriched in Q/N residues. One such nucleoporin, Nup116, has been previously identified as a Pin^+ factor [45], and four more proteins were identified as potentially prionogenic [40, 166]. The study of prion properties of yeast GLFG-rich nucleoporins started with an observation that they can form two distinct types of cytosolic aggregates one of which was amyloid-like [167]. Further investigation showed that at least one of these proteins, Nup100, formed a genuine prion but no associated phenotype was found [42]. Possible prion properties of other nucleoporins give a fascinating perspective of discovering a novel prion network involved in nuclear transport regulation.

4.11. [NSI^+]

The [NSI^+] phenotype resembles that of [PSI^+], hence the name (Nonsense Suppression Inducer), but it was found in a strain lacking Sup35 PrD. [NSI^+] is cured by Hsp104 inactivation, but, unlike [PSI^+], not by *HSP104* overexpression [41]. Interestingly, while mimicking [PSI^+] phenotype in nonsense suppression, [NSI^+] also mimics [SWI^+] phenotype in carbon source utilization conferring decrease in growth on galactose and glycerol. The exact prion determinant for [NSI^+] is still unknown but a screen identified the *VTS1* gene that, although proved not to be the [NSI^+] determinant, almost perfectly recapitulates the [NSI^+] phenotype [168]. Furthermore, *VTS1* expression is higher in [NSI^+] strains, which suggests some link between *VTS1* and the putative [NSI^+] determinant [169].

4.12. [*MCA*$^+$]

The prion of yeast metacaspase Mca1 (or Yca1), [*MCA*$^+$], had been reported, but then the paper was retracted [36, 37]. But even saying nothing about the original paper, there are at least three independent lines of evidence that can be interpreted as describing the prion properties of Mca1. First, the protein was identified as a potential prion in a global screen for prion candidates, and it was shown to form amyloid fibrils *in vitro* and aggregates *in vivo*, but did not confer to [*PSI*$^+$]-like phenotype and did not form detergent-resistant aggregates *in vivo* when its putative PrD was fused to Sup35C [40]. The second work partially explained the inconsistencies as it showed that the occurrence of [*PSI*$^+$]-like phenotype depends on the length of N-terminal extension of the protein which may vary because of the presence of alternative translation starts upstream the conventional coding sequence. Also MC- instead of C-fusion was used, but no evidence that the observed phenotype was GuHCl-curable was presented [38]. And finally, after short-term heat shock Mca1 was shown to form foci that colocalized with Hsp104. Moreover, Mca1 interacts with Hsp70-Ssa, Ydj1 and some other proteins that participate in disaggregation. Also Mca1 was predominantly found in insoluble protein fraction but truncations or mutations in the putative PrD led to its redistribution into soluble fraction [170]. The data are interpreted as Mca1 taking part in the aggregate control machinery but the prion properties might also explain the observed effects.

It should be noted that no strains or plasmids from the original study were used in the three works mentioned, which implies that the results were obtained independently. Thus, even though there is no consecutive evidence that Mca1 forms a prion in yeast, yet it is still a prion candidate and a novel [*MCA*$^+$] prion might be rediscovered.

5. HETEROLOGOUS PRION INTERACTION

Prions can coexist, cooperate and interact with each other. There are two models, the cross-seeding and the titration models, that describe positive and negative prion-prion interactions, or how prions enhance or inhibit each other. The cross-seeding model proposes a physical interaction of heterologous prion proteins during prion induction or, more specifically, that a pre-existing amyloid facilitates formation of another amyloid. The titration model proposes that the aggregated proteins interact indirectly via cellular cofactors, e.g., chaperone machinery components, which may have opposing effects on different proteins ([171], see [172]).

The cross-seeding model is supported by the study of Pin$^+$ factors that concluded that either overproduction of several Q/N-rich proteins or the presence of other prions facilitates heterologous prion formation. The [*PIN*$^+$] prion was identified as a factor essential for effective [*PSI*$^+$] and [*URE3*] induction. Moreover, both [*PSI*$^+$] and [*URE3*] facilitated induction of [*PIN*$^+$]. A systematic screen for Pin$^+$ factors identified 11 genes that facilitate [*PSI*$^+$] induction when overexpressed [45]. Products of two of these genes, Swi1 and Cyc8, were later shown to form prions (See Sections 4.4 and 4.5). Not only *SWI1* overexpression but the [*SWI*$^+$] prion itself promotes [*PSI*$^+$] formation, albeit less efficiently than [*PIN*$^+$]. While [*SWI*$^+$] also facilitates induction of [*PIN*$^+$] *de novo*, and even better than [*PSI*$^+$] does, Swi1 overproduction fails to do so, leading to formation of non-prion Rnq1 aggregates [66].

The role of [*PIN*$^+$] seems to be one of a universal "seeder." Rnq1 aggregates are suggested to occupy the IPOD compartment [173], and [*PIN*$^+$]-dependent aggregation might start in there [57, 174]. Rnq1 thus promotes aggregation of many Q/N-rich proteins including yeast prions. There are only two notable exceptions, namely Sfp1 and Mot3. While [*PIN*$^+$]-independent prionization of Sfp1 is expected since [*ISP*$^+$] aggregates are predominantly localized in the nucleus, which spatially isolates them from [*PIN*$^+$] [35], *de novo* formation of [*MOT3*$^+$], not requiring any known Pin$^+$ factors, is unique among conventional yeast prions. That may also be the reason why [*MOT3*$^+$] appears in wild populations [40, 133].

However, several lines of evidence suggest that cross-seeding does not explain even all positive prion-prion interactions while cases of negative prion-prion interactions have also been described. First, various mutations in non-prion domain of Rnq1 inhibit [*PSI*$^+$] formation [150, 151]. Second, the formation of [*PSI*$^+$] is not facilitated by non-Q/N-rich aggregates, which was shown for transthyretin, α-synuclein and synphilin-1 [175], but there are exceptions. E.g., overexpression of Mod5 induces formation of [*PSI*$^+$] without physical interaction with Sup35. A possible explanation may be sequestering of chaperones from the newly formed Sup35 aggregates that allows them to turn into prion seeds [174] and that is the essence of titration model. Third, induction of [*Het-s*]$_y$ may occur in [*pin*$^-$] strains but [*PIN*$^+$] presence increases its rate approximately twofold [10]. The mechanism is still unveiled and, while cross-seeding cannot be ruled out, [*PIN*$^+$] may titrate Sis1 which is shown to cure [*Het-s*]$_y$ when overabundant [176].

The most surprising case of negative prion-prion interactions is the observation that several [*PIN*$^+$] variants can destabilize and even eliminate weak [*PSI*$^+$] variants, even those variants that they originally templated. The reverse also occurs and soon after induction [*PSI*$^+$] persists but [*PIN*$^+$] is lost [177]. [*PSI*$^+$] and [*URE3*] were also shown to be antagonists. Not only they destabilize each other but they inhibit *de novo* formation of each other. Antagonism between [*PSI*$^+$] and [*URE3*] is explained by cellular response model, particularly, presence of [*PSI*$^+$] increases expression of Ssa1 which is known to selectively destabilize the [*URE3*] prion [83,103]. The co-existence of the two prions also results in increased *HSP104* expression, which is, *vice versa*, known to selectively cure [*PSI*$^+$] [178]. The model can be considered a variation of the titration model but with more complex cofactor-prion interdependence.

An interesting phenomenon was found out during investigation of a mammalian stress granule component Tia1 in yeast. Apart from constituting transmissible amyloid aggregates by itself, Tia1 overexpression inhibits induction of [*PSI*$^+$] by forming Tia1/Sup35 amyloid oligomers, that are arranged into lines colocalized with tubulin. Q/N-rich domains of Sup35 and Tia1 or its yeast homolog Pub1 are shown to interact with each other in a tubulin-associated complex that might play an important role in translation machinery interactions with cytoskeleton. Pub/Tia forming co-prion with Sup35 basically contributes to cross-seeding model, but at the same time it antagonizes [*PSI*$^+$] formation which constitutes negative interactions. This is the first evidence of *in vivo* amyloid comprising two heterologous proteins [15].

Negative interactions may also occur via cross-seeding-like mechanism, which underlies the capping model. According to it, protein monomers may bind pre-existing heterologous aggregates without subsequent nucleation of the heterologous amyloid. Instead, this blocks ends of pre-existing fibrils preventing them from growing. This model explains how the

PNM2 mutation can cause the loss of [*PSI*$^+$], and it also explains some cases of interspecies prion transmission barriers (see [179]).

While even unrelated proteins can form co-prions, even homologs from related species often fail to do so. The phenomenon is called interspecies prion transmission barrier and it confers a good model for studying mechanisms of prion transmission between different species that is an important problem for mammalian prion biology. So far, only the [*PSI*$^+$] and [*URE3*] prions were extensively investigated in this aspect.

Sup35 homologs from many species can form prions in *S. cerevisiae* but not all of them can transmit the prion state to native *S. cerevisiae* Sup35. Most data obtained from using N or NM-domains from different species fused to MC or C-domains from *S. cerevisiae*, respectively, conclude that Sup35 homologs from almost any species might potentially form a [*PSI*$^+$] prion if the prion domain is Q/N-rich. Still, *S. cerevisiae* [*PSI*$^+$] variants are unable to retain the prion when the N-domain comes from the majority of other species [e.g., 104, 134, 180-184]. Notable exceptions are homologs from closely related to *S. cerevisiae* species *S. bayanus* and *S. paradoxus* which can both maintain pre-existing [*PSI*$^+$] in *S. cerevisiae* cells and infect *S. cerevisiae* with the prion formed by chimeric proteins themselves [184]. Sup35 from *C. albicans* showed the ability to propagate *S. cerevisiae*-derived [*PSI*$^+$] but not the other way around. This is the manifestation of the asymmetry of interspecies barriers, which is quite common [186]. During coexpression aggregates from *K. lactis* are shown to colocalize with *S. cerevisiae* Sup35 although that does not result in prion transmission which suggests that capping mechanism may provide explanation for at least some cases of the interspecies barriers [134].

Similar experiments for [*URE3*] showed that Ure2 homologs from various species differ both in the ability to form prion in *S. cerevisiae* and to transmit the prion state to the native Ure2, and these abilities do not strictly correlate with the identity of the amino acid sequence [141, 142, 185–188].

6. How to Discover New Prions?

6.1. Phenotypic Approach

Discovery of [*PSI*$^+$] and [*URE3*] was a happy coincidence that allowed to establish the universality of prion concept. This led to targeted search for new proteins with presumed characteristics. Phenotypic approach, employing search for phenocopies of mutations, enabled the discovery of [*ISP*$^+$] [34] and [*GAR*$^+$] [32]. Later, application of a high-throughput version of such approach revealed a bunch of GuHCl-reversible phenotypes suggesting that different yeast strains contain a number of unveiled prions [133]. A disadvantage of this approach is the compulsory subsequent identification of the genetic element responsible for this trait which can be cumbersome.

An extension of the phenotypic approach, fusions of potentially prionogenic proteins or their regions with C or MC-domain of Sup35, employs the [*PSI*$^+$] phenotype to monitor prionization of other proteins [44, 171]. This approach may lead to controversial results.

First, either too weak or too strong aggregation of the putative prion protein is likely to be overlooked because the former cannot be distinguished from no-aggregation phenotype while the latter may simply be lethal.

Second, different constructs may give conflicting results, e.g., the New1 Q/N-rich domain fused to MC-Sup35 forms a prion [*NU*$^+$] that resembles [*PSI*$^+$] [171] but expression of an analogous fusion of truncated New1 with C-Sup35 led to unstable but GuHCl non-curable suppressor phenotype [40] while New1 itself seems not to form a prion (see [189]).

6.2. *In Silico* Approaches

Extended phenotypic approaches require candidate proteins. So, an analysis of the whole yeast proteome predicting prionogenic proteins was needed. Most yeast prion proteins are Q/N-rich, so the first attempt to screen for prion proteins and to classify them was performed by Melissa D. Michelitsch and Jonathan S. Weissman with an algorithm searching for the longest Q/N-only stretch. It resulted in finding 107 proteins with Q/N-rich regions in the *Saccharomyces cerevisiae* proteome [166]. The second attempt was performed by Paul M. Harrison and Mark Gerstein with a more complex algorithm and defined 167 proteins with such potential prion domains [190]. The third was Simon Alberti and coworkers who used a hidden Markov model to identify candidate prions (a list of 178 proteins) and experimentally validated one of them, Mot3 [40]. Interestingly, these three lists demonstrate a significant overlap sharing a total of 73 proteins (Figure 3). Moreover, all known Q/N-rich prion proteins — Sup35, Rnq1, Ure2, Swi1, Mot3, Cyc8, Sfp1, and Nup100 — fell into each of these lists.

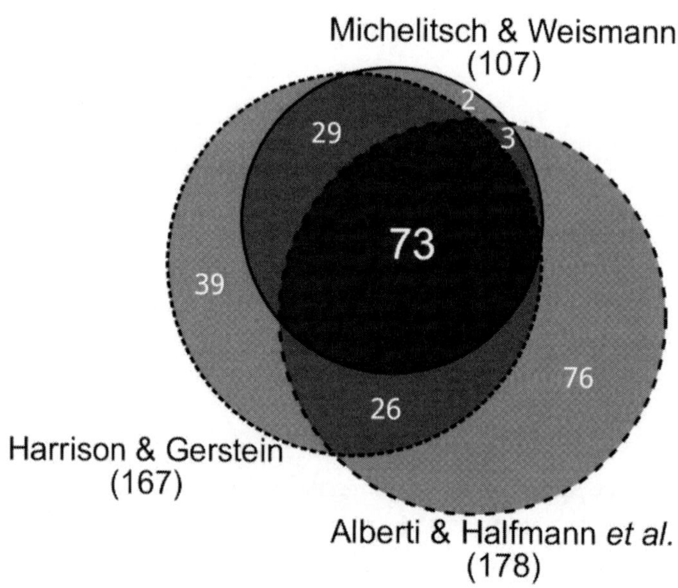

Figure 3. Overlapping lists of potentially prionogenic proteins derived from three independent analyses of the yeast proteome. See Section 6.2 for details. The analysis was performed with R [191].

6.3. Screening for Aggregation-Prone Proteins

Since almost all known prions show amyloid properties, a number of methods was developed to determine whether the protein in question can form aggregates *in vitro* or *in vivo*. Visualizing fluorescent foci in cell is the easiest way to detect an aggregated protein *in vivo*. This is routinely done by producing the protein or its PrD fused with a fluorescent protein. However, a protein may occupy a particular compartment indistinguishable from an aggregate or be titrated into heterologous aggregates, so the method does not guarantee aggregation properties of a candidate even if tested positive.

Other methods employ physical properties of aggregates. Sup35 was shown to be enriched in high molecular weight fraction in [PSI^+], but not in [psi^-] cells with ultracentrifugation followed by polyacrylamide gel electrophoresis [135]. Then, a method to directly visualize weight distribution of prion aggregates was invented. It was called SDD-AGE standing for semi-denaturing detergent agarose gel electrophoresis. Amyloids cannot enter standard polyacrylamide gels and slowly enter agarose gels. This allows total protein fraction to be separated into oligomers and monomers [192]. SDD-AGE is now widely used and has been applied to explore known prions in wild yeast strains. And indeed, [PSI^+], [PIN^+] and [$MOT3^+$] were found [133].

Together with test for *in vitro* amyloid fibril assembly of recombinant proteins, all methods listed were successfully implemented in the fundamental research by Alberti et al., which gave extensive characteristics of potentially prionogenic proteins and suggested the most promising candidates [40]. The vast body of data generated in this study as well as data obtained in other studies is accumulated in PrionHome database [193].

Recently, a novel method for identification of cellular amyloids was introduced [194]. It is based on resistance of amyloids to detergents. Purification of detergent-resistant aggregate fractions is followed by labeling proteins and separation in 2D-DIGE. Different labels allow comparison of aggregated proteins followed by their identification with mass spectrometry. The method is called PSIA (Proteomic Screening for Identification of Amyloid proteins) and it is universal as it may be adapted to screening for amyloids in any organism including human [194].

7. Are Yeast Prions Functional?

The diseases that derive from existence of human amyloids and seemingly regulatory functions of known yeast prions lead to controversy in an attempt to evaluate the pros and cons of the prionization phenomena. So, are prions functional? Two opposing points of view prevail:

- Prions are diseases (see [195]).
- Prions are advantageous (see [196]).

Here we briefly review commonly used arguments.

1. There are many prions involved in the regulation of gene expression. At least three known prions are involved in regulation of translational fidelity; [MOD^+] may be the fourth.

Changing the accuracy of translation on the one hand increases variability of protein molecules, and that can lead to both gain of new functions or restoration of functions lost due to mutations or pseudogene formation. On the other hand, it can decrease the activities of conservative proteins. Such controversy allows us to call it neither an advantage nor a disadvantage. Six known prions contribute to regulation of transcription. Their targets include carbon source utilization genes in the case of [*GAR*$^+$], [*SWI*$^+$], [*OCT*$^+$], and [*MOT3*$^+$] as well as catabolite repression genes for [*URE3*] and [*GAR*$^+$]. Transcription factors appearing to be prions is not an accidental phenomenon since yeast Q/N-rich proteins are enriched in regulators of transcription [190]. Heterologous prion interactions support the existence of additional level of transcriptional regulation as aggregation-prone transcription factors may activate or inactivate each other. However, the cascades of aggregation are stochastic on every step, and so the outcome could hardly be predicted: in extreme cases, protein may fail to aggregate or fail to promote aggregation of its functional partner or, even worse, its total inactivation may fail to support viability as proposed for suicidal [*PSI*$^+$] variants [128]. To our current knowledge, regulation of gene expression by prion state of transcription factors is too uncertain, and thus, its advantageousness is questionable.

2. Several prions ([*PSI*$^+$], [*PIN*$^+$] and [*MOT3*$^+$]) were found in wild yeast strains [133]. Only one of three targeted screens revealed [*PSI*$^+$] and [*MOT3*$^+$] that appear in about 1.5 and 9% of strains analyzed, respectively. [*URE3*] was searched for in 70 strains but was not found. [*PIN*$^+$] seems to be one of the most frequently found prion in non-laboratory strains [133, 147, 197], which might be explained by high rates of its *de novo* appearance (see [198]). Moreover, search for GuHCl-curable phenotypic traits unveiled many putative prions in wild strains. Notably, several of those strains showed difference in growth on non-fermentable carbon sources [133]. The fact can be also interpreted in both ways. One viewpoint is that natural yeast prions are a very rare occasion and thus contribute to diseases, unlike *Podospora* [*Het-s*] that is advantageous and ubiquitous (see [199]). Another viewpoint is that the presence of "wild" prions itself argues for their usefulness. The rare appearance does not pose a problem since prions might become advantageous under stressful conditions, and thus there is no need to maintain them all the time [196].

3. However, prions as a phenomenon may be advantageous *per se*, as existence of traits that enforce reversible phenotypic change may increase phenotypic variability and help yeast cells thrive under unpredictable conditions [200]. This evolutionary strategy is called "bet-hedging" — increasing phenotypic variability at the cost of sacrificing mean fitness [201, 202]. No obvious arguments against prions as bet-hedging agents have been presented, but no proof as well. Mathematical prediction draws the conclusion that [*PSI*$^+$] may be fixed due to its effect on evolvability only if environmental change makes nonsense suppression adaptive at a frequency of at least once every million years [203].

4. This raises the question whether prion properties are evolutionarily conserved or appear by chance. As discussed above, not all fungal species, even closely related to *S. cerevisiae*, can propagate prions analogous to those in *S. cerevisiae*. Still, [*PSI*$^+$] and [*URE3*] found in *K. lactis* and *C. albicans*, respectively [134, 142], that are evolutionarily more distant than members of *Saccharomyces sensu stricto* unable to propagate the traits, suggest conservation of prion forming ability. But conservation of prion properties may represent a side effect of conservation of the PrD non-prion function [188]. Indeed, Sup35 and Ure2 PrDs correspond to several processes [64, 65]. The controversy remains about Rnq1 as its prion form may be functional. The *RNQ1* gene is conserved only in eight species

closely related to *S. cerevisiae* [204], so [*PIN*$^+$] may be a relatively novel trait. Further investigations on evolutionary conservation of [*PIN*$^+$]-forming might elucidate the uncertainties.

5. In terms of functional state of the protein, prion conversion often contributes to the "loss of function" and thus is assumed to be deleterious [195]. But there are several counter arguments. First, the inactivation is usually partial (e.g., [*PSI*$^+$], [*OCT*$^+$]) [128, 43]. Second, for some prions, consequences of prionization are not equivalent to deletion ([β], [*ISP*$^+$], [*PIN*$^+$]) [29, 35, 45].

6. Several prions are proved to be advantageous under certain conditions. Examples are prions linked to carbon source utilization, since it is possible for them to affect survival rates in the wild. E.g., [*MOT3*$^+$] is advantageous, and it is induced and inhibited by conditions that might allow optimal usage of its phenotype [157]. Yet, the conditions that are usually tested are restricted to laboratory use only. The same applies to prions that can be detected by phenotype only on the mutant backgrounds (e.g., [*PSI*$^+$], [*ISP*$^+$], [*URE3*], [*OCT*$^+$]). Then, being advantageous or not becomes irrelevant if the required genotype correlates with decreased fitness.

The dispute whether prions are good or bad seems inconsistent. From ecological perspective, traits like prions make yeast more of a generalist and less a specialist. So, the "goodness" of a trait depends upon the certain ecological niche and the degree of variability of environmental factors. Thus, any prion may prove to be advantageous or disadvantageous depending on circumstances.

CONCLUSION

To conclude, no argument presented is sufficient to prove or disprove advantageousness of the yeast prion phenomena. The facts concerning at least two determinants being adaptive cannot be ignored. Those are [*Het-s*] and [*MOT3*$^+$] from *P. anserina* and *S. cerevisiae*, respectively. Indeed, one cannot assume all other prions to be advantageous based solely on two proven cases, but their existence envisions that other prions that will be discovered in a not too distant future may also contribute to adaptive functions. Recent discovery of [*MOD*$^+$] as non-Q/N rich amyloid prion [39] and the fact that dozens of unknown prions were found in wild strains [133] gives much ground for optimism. Functional amyloids found in yeast (Whi3) [205] and Metazoa (CPEB, Orb2) [12, 13] add to the spectrum of phenomena that are subjects of investigations in the prion field. Novel discoveries also suggest that there is still much we do not know about the diversity and complexity of prion phenomena in nature.

ACKNOWLEDGMENTS

The authors would like to acknowledge all the authors whose papers we could not cite because of space limitations. We are grateful to our colleagues from the Department of Genetics and Biotechnology (Saint Petersburg State University), especially to Ludmila Mironova for the opportunity to write this review and valuable comments. We also thank Stanislav Bondarev for productive discussions, Stanislav Bondarev, Anton Gurkov, Polina

Lipaeva, Yury Barbitoff and Mikhail Belousov for critical reading of the manuscript and useful comments. The authors acknowledge RFBR for research grants 13-04-00645, 14-04-31265 and Saint Petersburg State University for research grants 0.37.696.2013, 1.50.2218.2013, 1.37.291.2015.

REFERENCES

[1] S.B. Prusiner, *Proc. Natl. Acad. Sci.*, 95, 13363 (1998).
[2] R.B. Wickner, *J. Biol. Chem.*, 287, 14432 (2012).
[3] J.-L. Legras, D. Merdinoglu, J.-M. Cornuet, and F. Karst, *Mol. Ecol.*, 16, 2091 (2007).
[4] F. Sherman and C. Lawrence, Saccharomyces, in: Ed. R.C. King, Bact. Bacteriophages, Fungi, Springer US, Boston, MA (1974), pp. 359–393.
[5] A. Goffeau, B.G. Barrell, H. Bussey, R.W. Davis, B. Dujon, H. Feldmann, F. Galibert, J.D. Hoheisel, C. Jacq, M. Johnston, E.J. Louis, H.W. Mewes, Y. Murakami, P. Philippsen, H. Tettelin, and S.G. Oliver, *Science*, 274, 546 (1996).
[6] R. Balakrishnan, M.A. Harris, R. Huntley, K. Van Auken, and J.M. Cherry, *Database (Oxford)*, 2013, bat054 (2013).
[7] J.M. Cherry, E.L. Hong, C. Amundsen, R. Balakrishnan, G. Binkley, E.T. Chan, K.R. Christie, M.C. Costanzo, S.S. Dwight, S.R. Engel, D.G. Fisk, J.E. Hirschman, B.C. Hitz, K. Karra, C.J. Krieger, S.R. Miyasato, R.S. Nash, J. Park, M.S. Skrzypek, et al., *Nucleic Acids Res.*, 40, D700 (2012).
[8] U. Baxa, *Curr. Alzheimer Res.*, 5, 308 (2008).
[9] R.B. Wickner, *Science*, 264, 566 (1994).
[10] V. Taneja, M.-L. Maddelein, N. Talarek, S.J. Saupe, and S.W. Liebman, *Mol. Cell*, 27, 67 (2007).
[11] V. Mathur, V. Taneja, Y. Sun, and S.W. Liebman, *Mol. Biol. Cell.*, 21, 1449 (2010).
[12] K. Si, S. Lindquist, and E.R. Kandel, *Cell*, 115, 879 (2003).
[13] A. Majumdar, W.C. Cesario, E. White-Grindley, H. Jiang, F. Ren, M.R. Khan, L. Li, E.M.-L. Choi, K. Kannan, F. Guo, J. Unruh, B. Slaughter, and K. Si, *Cell*, 148, 515 (2012).
[14] A.A. Rubel, T.A. Ryzhova, K.S. Antonets, Y.O. Chernoff, and A.P. Galkin, *Prion*, 7, 469 (2013).
[15] X. Li, J.B. Rayman, E.R. Kandel, and I.L. Derkatch, *Mol. Cell*, 1 (2014).
[16] C.I. Nussbaum-Krammer, K.-W. Park, L. Li, R. Melki, and R.I. Morimoto, *PLoS Genet.*, 9, e1003351 (2013).
[17] J.P. Hofmann, P. Denner, C. Nussbaum-Krammer, P.-H. Kuhn, M.H. Suhre, T. Scheibel, S.F. Lichtenthaler, H.M. Schätzl, D. Bano, and I.M. Vorberg, *Proc. Natl. Acad. Sci. U. S. A.*, 110, 5951 (2013).
[18] R.B. Wickner, *Annu. Rev. Genet.*, 30, 109 (1996).
[19] M.F. Tuite and B.S. Cox, *Prion*, 1, 101 (2007).
[20] B.S. Cox, *Genetics*, 20, 505 (1965).
[21] F. Lacroute, *J. Bacteriol.*, 106, 519 (1971).
[22] B.S. Cox, M.F. Tuite, and C.S. McLaughlin, *Yeast*, 4, 159 (1988).
[23] M. Aigle and F. Lacroute, *Mol. Gen. Genet.*, 136, 327 (1975).

[24] Y.O. Chernoff, I.L. Derkach, and S.G. Inge-Vechtomov, *Curr. Genet.*, 24, 268 (1993).

[25] M.D. Ter-Avanesyan, V.V. Kushnirov, A.R. Dagkesamanskaya, S.A. Didichenko, Y.O. Chernoff, S.G. Inge-Vechtomov, and V.N. Smirnov, *Mol. Microbiol.*, 7, 683 (1993).

[26] M.F. Tuite, C.R. Mundy, and B.S. Cox, *Genetics*, 98, 691 (1981).

[27] E.T. Crow and L. Li, *Semin. Cell Dev. Biol.*, 22, 452 (2011).

[28] G.L. Staniforth and M.F. Tuite, Fungal prions, in: Prog. Mol. Biol. Transl. Sci., 1st ed., Elsevier Inc., (2012), pp. 417–56.

[29] B.T. Roberts and R.B. Wickner, *Genes Dev.*, 17, 2083 (2003).

[30] P. Silar, V. Haedens, M. Rossignol, and H. Lalucque, *Genetics*, 151, 87 (1999).

[31] S. Kicka and P. Silar, *Genetics*, 166, 1241 (2004).

[32] J.C.S. Brown and S. Lindquist, *Genes Dev.*, 23, 2320 (2009).

[33] V. Coustou, C. Deleu, S. Saupe, and J. Begueret, *Proc. Natl. Acad. Sci. U. S. A.*, 94, 9773 (1997).

[34] K.V. Volkov, A.Y. Aksenova, M.J. Soom, K.V. Osipov, A.V. Svitin, C. Kurischko, I.S. Shkundina, M.D. Ter-Avanesyan, S.G. Inge-Vechtomov, and L.N. Mironova, *Genetics*, 160, 25 (2002).

[35] T. Rogoza, A. Goginashvili, S. Rodionova, M. Ivanov, O. Viktorovskaya, A. Rubel, K. Volkov, and L. Mironova, *Proc. Natl. Acad. Sci. U. S. A.*, 107, 10573 (2010).

[36] J. Nemecek, T. Nakayashiki, and R.B. Wickner, *Proc. Natl. Acad. Sci. U. S. A.*, 106, 1892 (2009).

[37] J. Nemecek, T. Nakayashiki, and R.B. Wickner, *Proc. Natl. Acad. Sci. U. S. A.*, 108, 10022 (2011).

[38] M. Erhardt, R.D. Wegrzyn, and E. Deuerling, *PLoS One*, 5, e9929 (2010).

[39] G. Suzuki, N. Shimazu, and M. Tanaka, *Science*, 336, 355 (2012).

[40] S. Alberti, R. Halfmann, O. King, A. Kapila, and S. Lindquist, *Cell*, 137, 146 (2009).

[41] A.F. Saifitdinova, A.A. Nizhnikov, A.G. Lada, A. a Rubel, Z.M. Magomedova, V. V Ignatova, S.G. Inge-Vechtomov, and A.P. Galkin, *Curr. Genet.*, 56, 467 (2010).

[42] R. Halfmann, J.J.R. Wright, S. Alberti, S. Lindquist, and M. Rexach, *Prion*, 6, 391 (2012).

[43] B.K. Patel, J. Gavin-Smyth, and S.W. Liebman, *Nat. Cell Biol.*, 11, 344 (2009).

[44] N. Sondheimer and S. Lindquist, *Mol. Cell*, 5, 163 (2000).

[45] I.L. Derkatch, M.E. Bradley, J.Y. Hong, and S.W. Liebman, *Cell*, 106, 171 (2001).

[46] Z. Du, K.-W. Park, H. Yu, Q. Fan, and L. Li, *Nat. Genet.*, 40, 460 (2008).

[47] L. Malato, S. Dos Reis, L. Benkemoun, R. Sabaté, S.J. Saupe, *Mol Biol Cell*, 18, 4803 (2007)

[48] C. King, *J. Mol. Biol.*, 307, 1247 (2001).

[49] M. Tanaka, S.R. Collins, B.H. Toyama, and J.S. Weissman, *Nature*, 442, 585 (2006).

[50] F. Shewmaker, D. Kryndushkin, B. Chen, R. Tycko, and R.B. Wickner, *Biochemistry*, 48, 5074 (2009).

[51] S.A. Bondarev, V.V. Shchepachev, A.V. Kajava, and G.A. Zhouravleva, *J. Biol. Chem.*, 288, 28503 (2013).

[52] J.R. Glover, a S. Kowal, E.C. Schirmer, M.M. Patino, J.J. Liu, and S. Lindquist, *Cell*, 89, 811 (1997).

[53] C.-Y. King, P. Tittmann, H. Gross, R. Gebert, M. Aebi, and K. Wuthrich, *Proc. Natl. Acad. Sci.*, 94, 6618 (1997).

[54] M. Schlumpberger, H. Wille, M.A. Baldwin, D.A. Butler, I. Herskowitz, and S.B. Prusiner, *Protein Sci.*, 9, 440 (2000).
[55] M.M. Patino, J.J. Liu, J.R. Glover, and S. Lindquist, *Science*, 273, 622 (1996).
[56] V.V. Speransky, K.L. Taylor, H.K. Edskes, R.B. Wickner, and A.C. Steven, *J. Cell Biol.*, 153, 1327 (2001).
[57] J. Tyedmers, S. Treusch, J. Dong, J.M. McCaffery, B. Bevis, and S. Lindquist, *Proc. Natl. Acad. Sci. U. S. A.*, 107, 8633 (2010).
[58] S. Kawai-Noma, C.-G. Pack, T. Kojidani, H. Asakawa, Y. Hiraoka, M. Kinjo, T. Haraguchi, H. Taguchi, and A. Hirata, *J. Cell Biol.*, 190, 199 (2010).
[59] E. Ross, U. Baxa, and R. Wickner, *Mol. Cell. Biol.*, 24, 7206 (2004).
[60] E.D. Ross, H.K. Edskes, M.J. Terry, and R.B. Wickner, *Proc. Natl. Acad. Sci. U. S. A.*, 102, 12825 (2005).
[61] Z. Du, *Prion*, 5, 311–6 (2011).
[62] C. Christ and B.K. Tye, *Genes Dev.*, 5, 751 (1991).
[63] M. Primig, H. Winkler, and G. Ammerer, *EMBO J.*, 10, 4209 (1991).
[64] F. Shewmaker, L. Mull, T. Nakayashiki, D.C. Masison, and R.B. Wickner, *Genetics*, 176, 1557 (2007).
[65] B. Cosson, A. Couturier, S. Chabelskaya, D. Kiktev, S. Inge-Vechtomov, M. Philippe, and G. Zhouravleva, *Mol. Cell. Biol.,* 22, 3301 (2002).
[66] Z. Du and L. Li, *Genetics*, 197, 685 (2014).
[67] B. Cosson, N. Berkova, A. Couturier, S. Chabelskaya, M. Philippe, and G. Zhouravleva, *Biol. Cell*, 94, 205 (2002).
[68] B. Bösl, V. Grimminger, and S. Walter, *J. Struct. Biol.*, 156, 139 (2006).
[69] Y. Sanchez and S. Lindquist, *Science*, 248, 1112 (1990).
[70] S. Lindquist and G. Kim, *Proc. Natl. Acad. Sci. U. S. A.*, 93, 5301 (1996).
[71] V. Grimminger, K. Richter, A. Imhof, J. Buchner, and S. Walter, *J. Biol. Chem.*, 279, 7378 (2004).
[72] L. Nowicki, P. Leźnicki, E. Morawiec, N. Litwińczuk, and K. Liberek, *Cell Stress Chaperones*, 17, 361 (2012).
[73] C.L. Squires, S. Pedersen, B.M. Ross, and C. Squires, *J. Bacteriol.*, 173, 4254 (1991).
[74] K.A. Tipton, K.J. Verges, and J.S. Weissman, *Mol. Cell*, 32, 584 (2008).
[75] M. Miot, M. Reidy, S.M. Doyle, J.R. Hoskins, D.M. Johnston, O. Genest, M.-C. Vitery, D.C. Masison, and S. Wickner, *Proc. Natl. Acad. Sci. U. S. A.*, 108, 6915 (2011).
[76] J. Winkler, J. Tyedmers, B. Bukau, and A. Mogk, *J. Cell Biol.*, 198, 387 (2012).
[77] C. Queitsch, S.W. Hong, E. Vierling, and S. Lindquist, *Plant Cell*, 12, 479 (2000).
[78] E.C. Schirmer, S. Lindquist, and E. Vierling, *Plant Cell*, 6, 1899 (1994).
[79] Y.R. Lee, R.T. Nagao, and J.L. Key, *Plant Cell*, 6, 1889 (1994).
[80] D. Sharma and D.C. Masison, *Protein Pept. Lett.*, 16, 571 (2009).
[81] M. Werner-Washburne, D.E. Stone, and E.A. Craig, *Mol. Cell. Biol.*, 7, 2568 (1987).
[82] W.R. Boorstein, T. Ziegelhoffer, and E.A. Craig, *J. Mol. Evol.*, 38, 1 (1994).
[83] C. Schwimmer and D. Masison, *Mol. Cell. Biol.*, 22, 3590 (2002).
[84] B.T. Roberts, H. Moriyama, and R.B. Wickner, *Yeast*, 21, 107 (2004).
[85] D. Sharma and D.C. Masison, *Genetics*, 179, 1301 (2008).
[86] C. Pfund, P. Huang, N. Lopez-Hoyo, and E.A. Craig, *Mol. Biol. Cell*, 12, 3773 (2001).
[87] Y.O. Chernoff, G.P. Newnam, J. Kumar, K. Allen, and a D. Zink, *Mol. Cell. Biol.*, 19, 8103 (1999).

[88] V.V. Kushnirov, D.S. Kryndushkin, M. Boguta, V.N. Smirnov, and M.D. Ter-Avanesyan, *Curr. Biol.*, 10, 1443 (2000).
[89] K.D. Allen, R.D. Wegrzyn, T.A. Chernova, S. Müller, G.P. Newnam, P.A. Winslett, K.B. Wittich, K.D. Wilkinson, and Y.O. Chernoff, *Genetics*, 169, 1227 (2005).
[90] D.A. Kiktev, M.M. Melomed, C.D. Lu, G.P. Newnam, and Y.O. Chernoff, *Mol. Microbiol.*, (2015).
[91] P. Walsh, D. Bursać, Y.C. Law, D. Cyr, and T. Lithgow, *EMBO Rep.*, 5, 567 (2004).
[92] T. Higurashi, J.K. Hines, C. Sahi, R. Aron, and E.A. Craig, *Proc. Natl. Acad. Sci. U. S. A.*, 105, 16596 (2008).
[93] J.K. Hines, X. Li, Z. Du, T. Higurashi, L. Li, and E.A. Craig, *PLoS Genet.*, 7, e1001309 (2011).
[94] K.C. Stein and H.L. True, *Mol. Microbiol.*, 93, 1156 (2014).
[95] J.M. Harris, P.P. Nguyen, M.J. Patel, Z.A. Sporn, and J.K. Hines, *PLoS Genet.*, 10, e1004510 (2014).
[96] M. Reidy, R. Sharma, S. Shastry, B.-L. Roberts, I. Albino-Flores, S. Wickner, and D.C. Masison, *PLoS Genet.*, 10, e1004720 (2014).
[97] L. Malinovska, S. Kroschwald, M.C. Munder, D. Richter, and S. Alberti, *Mol. Biol. Cell*, 23, 3041 (2012).
[98] D.S. Kryndushkin, F. Shewmaker, and R.B. Wickner, *EMBO J.*, 27, 2725 (2008).
[99] R.B. Wickner, E. Bezsonov, and D. a Bateman, *Proc. Natl. Acad. Sci. U. S. A.*, 111, E2711 (2014).
[100] M.M. Luke, A. Sutton, and K.T. Arndt, *J. Cell Biol.*, 114, 623 (1991).
[101] A.J. Caplan and M.G. Douglas, *J. Cell Biol.*, 114, 609 (1991).
[102] H. Moriyama, H.K. Edskes, and R.B. Wickner, *Mol. Cell. Biol.*, 20, 8916 (2000).
[103] M.E. Bradley, H.K. Edskes, J.Y. Hong, R.B. Wickner, and S.W. Liebman, *Proc. Natl. Acad. Sci. U. S. A.*, 99, 16392 (2002).
[104] V.V. Kushnirov, N.V. Kochneva-Pervukhova, M.B. Chechenova, N.S. Frolova, and M.D. Ter-Avanesyan, *EMBO J.*, 19, 324 (2000).
[105] Y. Inoue, *Protein Pept. Lett.*, 16, 271 (2009).
[106] J. Hofmann and I. Vorberg, *Prion*, 7, 369 (2013).
[107] S. Kawai-Noma, C.-G. Pack, T. Tsuji, M. Kinjo, and H. Taguchi, *Genes Cells*, 14, 1045 (2009).
[108] B. Liu, L. Larsson, A. Caballero, X. Hao, D. Oling, J. Grantham, and T. Nyström, *Cell*, 140, 257 (2010).
[109] Y. Wang, A.B. Meriin, N. Zaarur, N. V Romanova, Y.O. Chernoff, C.E. Costello, and M.Y. Sherman, *FASEB J.*, 23, 451 (2009).
[110] S.J. Saupe, *Semin. Cell Dev. Biol.*, 22, 460 (2011).
[111] A. Balguerie, S. Dos Reis, C. Ritter, S. Chaignepain, B. Coulary-Salin, V. Forge, K. Bathany, I. Lascu, J.-M. Schmitter, R. Riek, and S.J. Saupe, *EMBO J.*, 22, 2071 (2003).
[112] S.J. Saupe and A. Daskalov, *PLoS Pathog.*, 8, e1002687 (2012).
[113] C. Wasmer, A. Lange, H. Van Melckebeke, A.B. Siemer, R. Riek, and B.H. Meier, *Science*, 319, 1523 (2008).
[114] A.J.M. Debets, H.J.P. Dalstra, M. Slakhorst, B. Koopmanschap, R.F. Hoekstra, and S.J. Saupe, *Proc. Natl. Acad. Sci. U. S. A.*, 109, 10432 (2012).
[115] C.C. Lindegren and G. Lindegren, *Proc. Natl. Acad. Sci. U. S. A.*, 33, 314 (1947).
[116] M.F. Tuite and B.S. Cox, *Methods*, 39, 9 (2006).

[117] M. Firoozan, C.M. Grant, J.A. Duarte, and M.F. Tuite, *Yeast*, 7, 173 (1991).
[118] S.M. Doel, S.J. McCready, C.R. Nierras, and B.S. Cox, *Genetics*, 137, 659 (1994).
[119] M.D. Ter-Avanesyan, A.R. Dagkesamanskaya, V.V. Kushnirov, and V.N. Smirnov, *Genetics*, 137, 671 (1994).
[120] S.V. Paushkin, V.V. Kushnirov, V.N. Smirnov, and M.D. Ter-Avanesyan, *EMBO J.*, 15, 3127 (1996).
[121] S.S. Eaglestone, L.W. Ruddock, B.S. Cox, and M.F. Tuite, *Proc. Natl. Acad. Sci. U. S. A.*, 97, 240 (2000).
[122] R.D. Wegrzyn, K. Bapat, G.P. Newnam, A.D. Zink, and Y.O. Chernoff, *Mol. Cell. Biol.*, 21, 4656 (2001).
[123] G.-C. Hung and D.C. Masison, *Genetics*, 173, 611 (2006).
[124] C.W. Helsen and J.R. Glover, *J. Biol. Chem.*, 287, 542 (2012).
[125] B. Moosavi, J. Wongwigkarn, and M.F. Tuite, *Yeast*, 27, 167 (2010).
[126] G.P. Newnam, J.L. Birchmore, and Y.O. Chernoff, *J. Mol. Biol.*, 408, 432 (2011).
[127] I.L. Derkatch, Y.O. Chernoff, V.V. Kushnirov, S.G. Inge-Vechtomov, and S.W. Liebman, *Genetics*, 144, 1375 (1996).
[128] R.P. McGlinchey, D. Kryndushkin, and R.B. Wickner, *Proc. Natl. Acad. Sci. U. S. A.*, 108, 5337 (2011).
[129] O. Namy, G. Duchateau-Nguyen, and J.-P. Rousset, *Mol. Microbiol.*, 43, 641 (2002).
[130] J. Tyedmers, M.L. Madariaga, and S. Lindquist, *PLoS Biol.*, 6, e294 (2008).
[131] A. Singh, C. Helms, and F. Sherman, *Proc. Natl. Acad. Sci. U. S. A.*, 76, 1932 (1979).
[132] T.C. Sideri, K. Stojanovski, M.F. Tuite, and C.M. Grant, *Proc. Natl. Acad. Sci. U. S. A.*, 107, 6394 (2010).
[133] R. Halfmann, D.F. Jarosz, S.K. Jones, A. Chang, A.K. Lancaster, and S. Lindquist, *Nature*, 482, 363 (2012).
[134] T. Nakayashiki, K. Ebihara, H. Bannai, and Y. Nakamura, *Mol. Cell*, 7, 1121 (2001).
[135] T.S. Cunningham, *J. Biol. Chem.*, 275, 14408 (2000).
[136] M. Bai, J.-M. Zhou, and S. Perrett, *J. Biol. Chem.*, 279, 50025 (2004).
[137] D.C. Masison, M.-L. Maddelein, and R.B. Wickner, *Proc. Natl. Acad. Sci.*, 94, 12503 (1997).
[138] M.-L. Maddelein and R.B. Wickner, *Mol. Cell. Biol.*, 19, 4516 (1999).
[139] E.D. Ross and R.B. Wickner, *Yeast*, 21, 963 (2004).
[140] U. Baxa, V. Speransky, A.C. Steven, and R.B. Wickner, *Proc. Natl. Acad. Sci. U. S. A.*, 99, 5253 (2002).
[141] N. Talarek, L. Maillet, C. Cullin, and M. Aigle, *Genetics*, 171, 23 (2005).
[142] H.K. Edskes and R.B. Wickner, *Eukaryot. Cell*, 12, 551 (2013).
[143] I. Derkatch, M. Bradley, P. Zhou, Y.O. Chernoff, and S.W. Liebman, *Genetics*, 147, 507 (1997).
[144] G. Orlowska-Matuszewska and D. Wawrzycka, *Biochem. Biophys. Res. Commun.*, 340, 190 (2006).
[145] T.C. Sideri, N. Koloteva-Levine, M.F. Tuite, and C.M. Grant, *J. Biol. Chem.*, 286, 38924 (2011).
[146] A.K. Lancaster, J.P. Bardill, H.L. True, and J. Masel, *Genetics*, 184, 393 (2010).
[147] T. Nakayashiki, C.P. Kurtzman, H.K. Edskes, and R.B. Wickner, *Proc. Natl. Acad. Sci. U. S. A.*, 102, 10575 (2005).

[148] A.L. Manogaran, V.M. Fajardo, R.J.D. Reid, R. Rothstein, and S.W. Liebman, *Yeast*, 27, 159 (2010).
[149] H. Kurahashi, S. Shibata, M. Ishiwata, and Y. Nakamura, *Genes Cells*, 14, 659 (2009).
[150] H. Kurahashi, K. Oishi, and Y. Nakamura, *Prion*, 5, 305 (2011).
[151] K.C. Stein and H.L. True, *PLoS Genet.*, 10, e1004337 (2014).
[152] W. Wang, *Curr. Top. Microbiol. Immunol.*, 274, 143 (2003).
[153] E.T. Crow, Z. Du, and L. Li, *Mol. Cell. Biol.*, 31, 3436 (2011).
[154] J.A. Downie, J.W. Stewart, N. Brockman, A.M. Schweingruber, and F. Sherman, *J. Mol. Biol.*, 113, 369 (1977).
[155] F. Sherman, H. Taber, and W. Campbell, *J. Mol. Biol.*, 13, 21 (1965).
[156] O. Sertil, R. Kapoor, B. Cohen, N. Abramova, and D. Lowry, *Nucleic Acids Res.*, 31, 5831 (2003).
[157] D.L. Holmes, A.K. Lancaster, S. Lindquist, and R. Halfmann, *Cell*, 153, 153 (2013).
[158] H. Laten, J. Gorman, and R.M. Bock, *Nucleic Acids Res.*, 5, 4329 (1978).
[159] G. Suzuki and M. Tanaka, *Prion*, 7, 109 (2013).
[160] P. Jorgensen, I. Rupes, J.R. Sharom, L. Schneper, J.R. Broach, M. Tyers, *Genes Dev.*, 18(20), 2491 (2004).
[161] F. Gómez-Herreros, L. de Miguel-Jiménez, M. Morillo-Huesca, L. Delgado-Ramos, M.C. Muñoz-Centeno, and S. Chávez, *Nucleic Acids Res.*, 40, 6508 (2012).
[162] P. Drozdova, T. Rogoza, E. Radchenko, P. Lipaeva, and L. Mironova, *FEMS Yeast Res.*, 14, 1160 (2014).
[163] E. Radchenko, T. Rogoza, M. Khokhrina, P. Drozdova, and L. Mironova, *Prion*, 5, 317 (2011).
[164] D.F. Jarosz, J.C.S. Brown, G.A. Walker, M.S. Datta, W.L. Ung, A.K. Lancaster, A. Rotem, A. Chang, G.A. Newby, D.A. Weitz, L.F. Bisson, and S. Lindquist, *Cell*, 158, 1083 (2014).
[165] D.F. Jarosz, A.K. Lancaster, J.C.S. Brown, and S. Lindquist, *Cell*, 158, 1072 (2014).
[166] M.D. Michelitsch and J.S. Weissman, *Proc. Natl. Acad. Sci. U. S. A.*, 97, 11910 (2000).
[167] J. Yamada, J.L. Phillips, S. Patel, G. Goldfien, A. Calestagne-Morelli, H. Huang, R. Reza, J. Acheson, V. V Krishnan, S. Newsam, A. Gopinathan, E.Y. Lau, M.E. Colvin, V.N. Uversky, and M.F. Rexach, *Mol. Cell. Proteomics*, 9, 220 (2010).
[168] A.A. Nizhnikov, Z.M. Magomedova, A.A. Rubel, A.M. Kondrashkina, S.G. Inge-Vechtomov, and A.P. Galkin, *Curr. Genet.*, 58, 35 (2012).
[169] A.A. Nizhnikov, A.M. Kondrashkina, and A.P. Galkin, *Genetika*, 49, 1155 (2013).
[170] R.E.C. Lee, S. Brunette, L.G. Puente, and L.A. Megeney, *Proc. Natl. Acad. Sci. U. S. A.*, 107, 13348 (2010).
[171] L.Z. Osherovich and J.S. Weissman, *Cell*, 106, 183 (2001).
[172] L.Z. Osherovich and J.S. Weissman, *Dev. Cell*, 2, 143 (2002).
[173] D. Kaganovich, R. Kopito, and J. Frydman, *Nature*, 454, 1088 (2008).
[174] F. Arslan, J.Y. Hong, V. Kanneganti, S.-K. Park, and S.W. Liebman, *PLoS Genet.*, 11, e1004814 (2015).
[175] I.L. Derkatch, S.M. Uptain, T.F. Outeiro, R. Krishnan, S.L. Lindquist, and S.W. Liebman, *Proc. Natl. Acad. Sci. U. S. A.*, 101, 12934 (2004).
[176] V. Mathur, C. Seuring, R. Riek, S.J. Saupe, and S.W. Liebman, *Mol. Cell. Biol.*, 32, 139 (2012).
[177] M.E. Bradley and S.W. Liebman, 51, 1629 (2004).

[178] Y.O. Chernoff, S.L. Lindquist, B. Ono, S.G. Inge-Vechtomov, and S.W. Liebman, *Science*, 268, 880 (1995).
[179] I.L. Derkatch and S.W. Liebman, *Prion*, 1, 161 (2007).
[180] Y.O. Chernoff, A.P. Galkin, E. Lewitin, T.A. Chernova, G.P. Newnam, and S.M. Belenkiy, *Mol. Microbiol.*, 35, 865 (2000).
[181] P. Chien and J.S. Weissman, 410, 223 (2001).
[182] B. Chen, G.P. Newnam, and Y.O. Chernoff, 104, 2791 *Proc. Natl. Acad. Sci. U. S. A.* (2007).
[183] E.G. Afanasieva, V.V. Kushnirov, M.F. Tuite, and M.D. Ter-Avanesyan, 286, 15773 (2011).
[184] H.K. Edskes, H.J. Khamar, C.-L. Winchester, A.J. Greenler, A. Zhou, R.P. McGlinchey, A. Gorkovskiy, and R.B. Wickner, *Genetics*, 198, 605 (2014).
[185] A. Baudin-Baillieu, E. Fernandez-Bellot, F. Reine, E. Coissac, and C. Cullin, *Mol. Biol. Cell*, 14, 3449 (2003).
[186] H.K. Edskes, L.M. McCann, A.M. Hebert, and R.B. Wickner, *Genetics*, 181, 1159 (2009).
[187] H.K. Edskes, A. Engel, L.M. McCann, A. Brachmann, H.-F. Tsai, and R.B. Wickner, *Genetics*, 188, 81 (2011).
[188] R. Al Safadi, N. Talarek, N. Jacques, and M. Aigle, *FEMS Yeast Res.*, 11, 151 (2011).
[189] S.M. Uptain and S. Lindquist, *Annu. Rev. Microbiol.*, 56, 703 (2002).
[190] P.M. Harrison and M. Gerstein, *Genome Biol.*, 4, R40 (2003).
[191] R Core Team, (2013).
[192] D.S. Kryndushkin, I.M. Alexandrov, M.D. Ter-Avanesyan, and V.V. Kushnirov, *J. Biol. Chem.*, 278, 49636 (2003).
[193] D. Harbi, M. Parthiban, D.M.A. Gendoo, S. Ehsani, M. Kumar, G. Schmitt-Ulms, R. Sowdhamini, and P.M. Harrison, *PLoS One*, 7, e31785 (2012).
[194] A.A. Nizhnikov, A.I. Alexandrov, T.A. Ryzhova, O.V. Mitkevich, A.A. Dergalev, M.D. Ter-Avanesyan, and A.P. Galkin, *PLoS One*, 9, e116003 (2014).
[195] R.B. Wickner, H.K. Edskes, D. Kryndushkin, R. McGlinchey, D. Bateman, and A. Kelly, *Semin. Cell Dev. Biol.*, 22, 469 (2011).
[196] G.A. Newby and S. Lindquist, *Trends Cell Biol.*, 23, 251 (2013).
[197] A.C. Kelly, B. Busby, and R.B. Wickner, *Genetics*, 197, 1007 (2014).
[198] S.W. Liebman and Y.O. Chernoff, *Genetics*, 191, 1041 (2012).
[199] R.B. Wickner, H.K. Edskes, D.A. Bateman, A.C. Kelly, A. Gorkovskiy, Y. Dayani, and A. Zhou, *Biochemistry*, 52, 1514 (2013).
[200] H.L. True and S.L. Lindquist, *Nature*, 407, 477 (2000).
[201] D. Cohen, *J. Ecol.*, 56, 219 (1968).
[202] J. Seger and H. Brockmann, *Oxford Surv. Evol. Biol.*, 4, 182 (1987).
[203] J. Masel and A. Bergman, *Evolution*, 57, 1498 (2003).
[204] L.B. Harrison, Z. Yu, J.E. Stajich, F.S. Dietrich, and P.M. Harrison, *J. Mol. Biol.*, 368, 273 (2007).
[205] F. Caudron and Y. Barral, *Cell*, 155, 1244 (2013).

In: The Prion Phenomena in Neurodegenerative Diseases ISBN: 978-1-63483-399-8
Editors: Giuseppe Legname and Gabriele Giachin

Chapter 11

FUNCTIONAL PRIONS: THE CASE STUDY OF *APLYSIA*

Eric R. Kandel[1,2,3,4,*]
[1]Kavli Institute for Brain Science
[2]Zuckerman Mind Brain Behavior Institute
[3]Department of Neuroscience
[4]Howard Hughes Medical Institute
College of Physicians and Surgeons of Columbia University,
New York State Psychiatric Institute, New York, New York, US

ABSTRACT

Studies on the factors that lead to the maintenance of long-term memory and the underlying synaptic plasticity have revealed a novel regulator of local protein synthesis at the synapse, the cytoplasmic polyadenylation element-binding protein (CPEB). This protein turns out to have the properties of a prion protein. It exists in two states: a soluble state and an aggregated state. The aggregated state is self-sustaining both in yeast cells and in neurons. But CPEB differs from pathogenic prions that underlie degenerative disease of the nervous system in two ways: 1) The convergence from the soluble to an aggregated form is triggered by a physiological signal – in this case serotonin, a modulatory transmitter released during learning; and 2) The aggregated form does not kill the cells but has a beneficial function. In the case of long-term memory for sensitization in *Aplysia* it serves to regulate local protein synthesis and to maintain the growth of new synaptic connections.

INTRODUCTION: THE MAINTENANCE OF LONG-TERM MEMORY

My colleagues and I have been studying the marine snail *Aplysia,* which has a simple nervous system that makes it highly suitable for studying the neuronal mechanisms of

* Correspondence: erk5@columbia.edu

reflexes at the cellular and the molecular level. Specifically, *Aplysia* has simple withdrawal reflexes that can be modified by different forms of learning. We have focused on the gill-withdrawal reflex.

The gill is an external respiratory organ, which is covered by a sheet of skin called the mantle shelf, which ends in a fleshy spout called the siphon. If one applies a weak tactile stimulus to the siphon it elicits a brisk withdrawal of the gill underneath the mantle shelf (Figure 1).

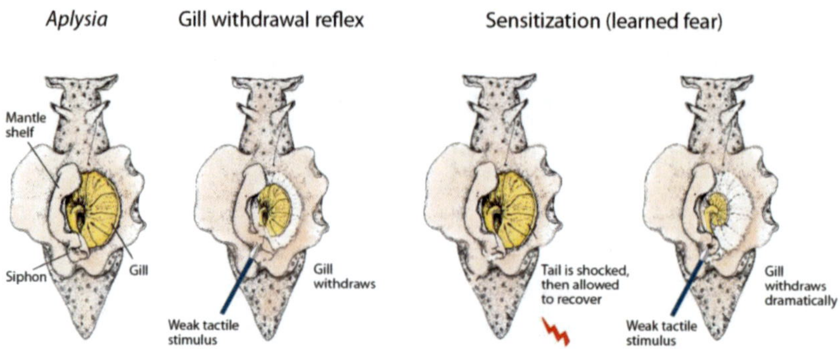

Figure 1. The gill withdrawal reflex of the marine snail *Aplysia* can undergo sensitization, a form of learned fear.

This gill withdrawal reflex can be modified by various forms of learning. We have focused in particular on sensitization - a form of learned fear. A shock applied to the tail scares the animal. As a result, the same weak tactile stimulus that had produced a modest withdrawal reflex of the gill now produces a much more powerful withdrawal. The memory for this noxious event varies as a function of a number of training trials. If one applies a single tail shock it produces a short-term form of sensitization that lasts for minutes. But if one repeats the tail shock training five times it produces a long-term form of sensitization that lasts for days or weeks.

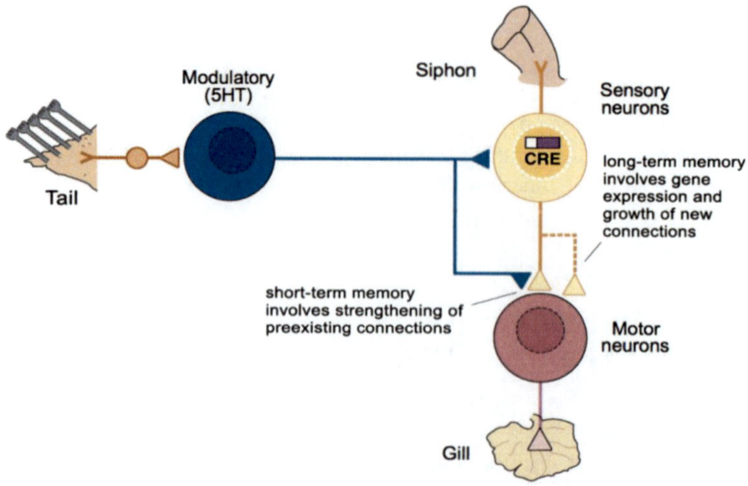

Figure 2. The gill withdrawal reflex reveals short- and long-term memory.

Synaptic plasticity, the ability of neurons to modulate the strength and structure of their synapses, is a key mechanism contributing to learning and memory storage. The neural circuit of the gill withdrawal reflex has an important monosynaptic component (Figure 2). The sensory neurons that innervate the siphon make direct connections to the motor neuron that move the gill. Like behavioral memory, synaptic plasticity between the sensory and motor neurons has at least two temporally distinct forms: a short-term form lasting minutes and a long-term form lasting days or weeks (Figure 2). These temporally distinct forms of learning-related synaptic plasticity have distinct molecular requirements; the short-term form depends on the covalent modifications of pre-existing proteins and the strengthening of pre-existing connections, whereas the long-term forms require gene expression, the synthesis of new proteins and the remodeling of pre-existing synapses as well as the formation of new synaptic connections. Since long-term synaptic plasticity requires transcription and therefore the nucleus, a compartment of the nerve cell that is in principle, in contact with every synapse of the neuron (Figure 3), it raises the question of whether all long-term changes must necessarily be cell-wide or can long-term changes be transcriptionally dependent, yet restricted to some synapses and not others?

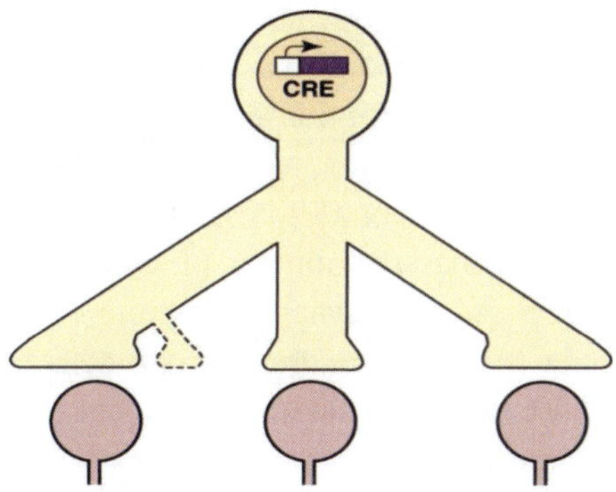

Figure 3. Activation of the nucleus during the formation of long-term memory poses the question of whether long-term changes can be synapse specific.

To address this question, Kelsey Martin and her colleagues [1] developed a culture system in *Aplysia*, where a single bifurcated sensory neuron of the gill-withdrawal reflex was plated in contact with two spatially separated gill motor neurons (Figure 4).

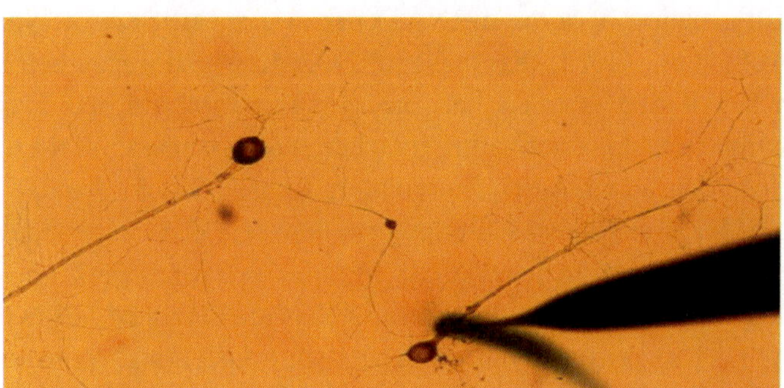

Figure 4. Microcultures of individual neurons of the gill-withdrawal reflex for studying synapse-specific plasticity [1].

In this culture system, application of a single pulse of serotonin (5-HT), the modulatory neurotransmitter released *in vivo* by interneurons activated during learning, to one of the two sets of synapses results in a synapse-specific short-term facilitation of pre-existing connections that lasts for minutes. Application of five pulses of 5-HT, designed to simulate the spaced behavioral training that leads to long-term memory, to one of the two synapses, also elicited synapse-specific long-term facilitation (LTF) that lasts for three or more days. Whereas the short-term form does not require new protein synthesis, the long-term form requires both cAMP Response Element-Binding protein (CREB)-dependent transcription in the nucleus and local protein synthesis at activated synapses. Moreover, the synapse-specific long-term facilitation initiated in one branch can be captured at the other by application of only a single pulse of 5-HT (which by itself is capable of producing only synapse-specific short-term facilitation) (Figure 5A).

These experiments, as well as parallel experiments by Frey and Morris in the hippocampus [2], demonstrate that individual synapses can undergo long-term synaptic changes independently and that these changes persist for more than 24 hours. Thus, long-term facilitation and its associated structural changes are synapse-specific. Moreover, this synapse specificity requires CREB-1 expression in the presynaptic sensory neurons. These findings imply that signals are sent not only from the synapse back to the nucleus [3, 4], but also from the nucleus to specific synapses, i.e., the molecular dialog required for synapse-specific long-term memory is bidirectional. Once transcription has been initiated, newly synthesized gene products, both mRNA molecules and proteins, have to be delivered to the specific synapses whose activation originally triggered the gene expression. To explain how this specificity can be achieved efficiently, despite the massive number of synapses in a single neuron, several research groups [2, 4, 5] proposed the synaptic capture, or tagging, hypothesis. This hypothesis states that the products of gene expression are delivered to synapses throughout the cell, but are only used at those synapses that have been tagged or marked by their previous learning-related activity [1, 2, 4, 6, 7, 8].

What is the molecular nature of the synaptic *mark*? Casadio et al., [7] examined this question and found that the *mark* has at least two components: (1) a PKA-dependent component needed for the initial capture of synapse-specific facilitation and for the growth of new synaptic connections, and (2) a rapamycin-sensitive, local protein synthesis dependent component needed for the maintenance of long-term facilitation and for the stabilization of synaptic growth beyond 24 hrs (Figure 5B and Figure 5C).

Since mRNAs are made in the cell body and then presumably shipped to all terminals, the need for the local translation of some mRNAs only at a specific set of synapses and not at others suggested to Si et al., (2003) that these mRNAs may be dormant before they reach the site of translation [9]. If that is true, then the synaptic *mark* for stabilization might be a regulator of translation capable of activating translationally dormant mRNAs.

In searching for such a translational regulator, Kausik Si and Kandel [10] focused on cytoplasmic polyadenylation element binding protein (CPEB), a molecule that activates dormant mRNAs in other biological contexts (Figure 6). Earlier work on *Xenopus* oocytes had revealed that some translationally dormant mRNAs are activated following elongation of their poly(A) tail [11]. This polyadenylation-dependent translational control requires two cis-acting elements at the 3'UTR of the mRNAs, a polyadenylation sequence AAUAAA, and a cytoplasmic polyadenylation element (CPE) with a general structure of UUUUUAU [12] that is regulated by a CPE binding protein, CPEB [13, 14].

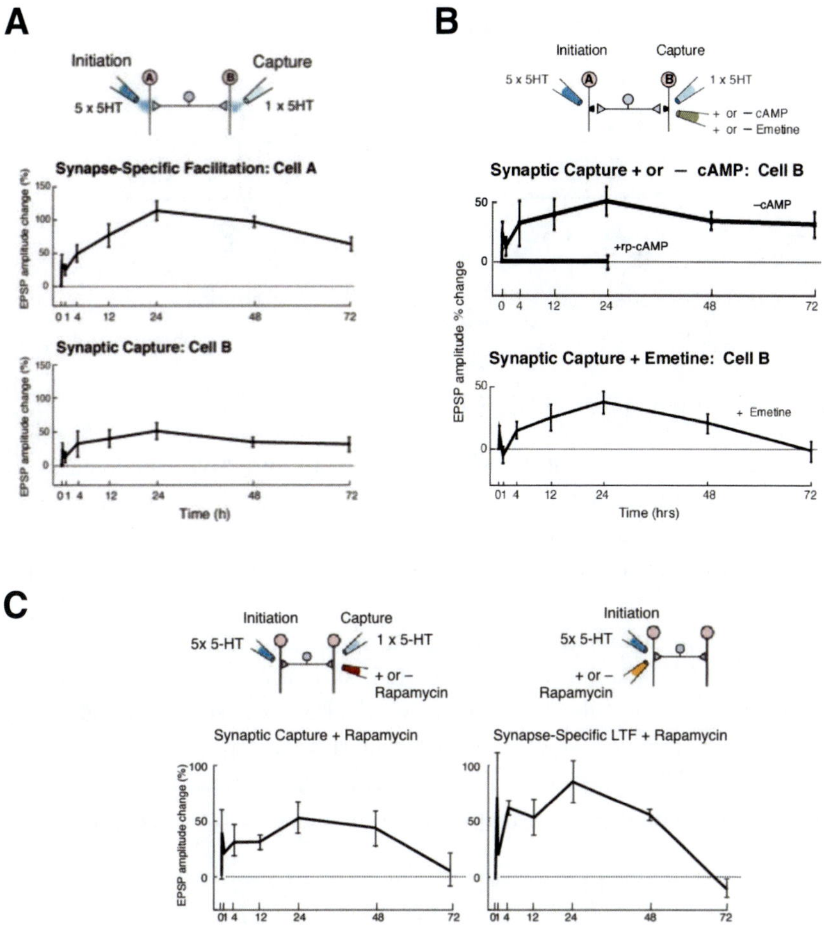

Figure 5. Synapse-specific facilitation (A); there are two molecular components to the “synaptic” mark (B); rapamycin, a selective inhibitor of protein synthesis, also blocks the growth-dependent late phase of LTF (C) both at the site of capture (left) and at the site of initiation (right) [1, 7].

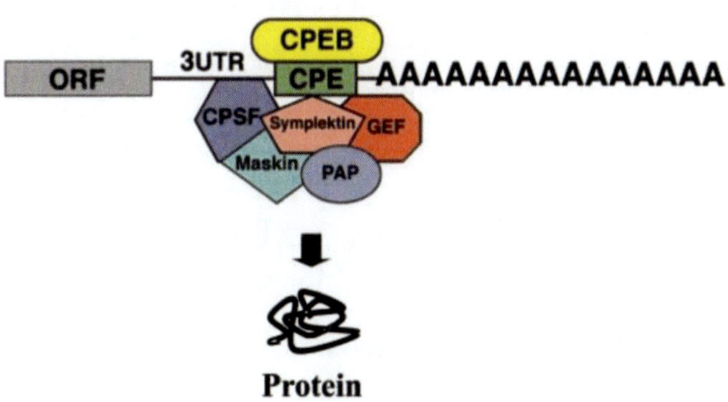

Figure 6. The cytoplasmic polyadenylation element binding protein can activate dormant mRNA.

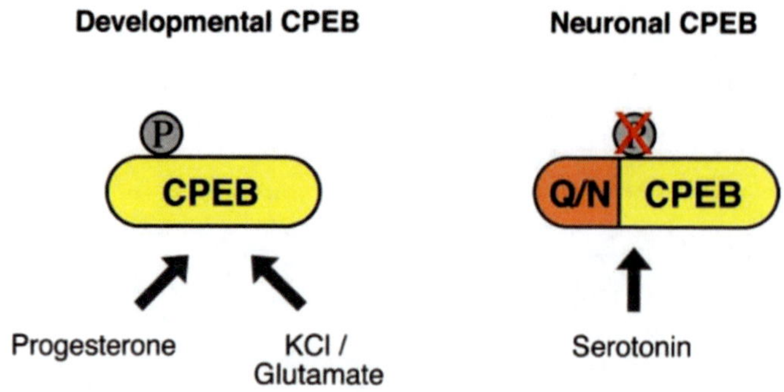

Figure 7. There are two isoforms of CPEB in *Aplysia*.

CPEB has four important features which made it an attractive candidate as a synapse-specific mark for stabilization: (1) it is activated through an extracellular signal; (2) it activates mRNAs that are translationally dormant [15, 16]; (3) its localization can be spatially restricted [15, 17, 18]; and (4) a number of mRNAs targeted by CPEB are involved in cellular growth [19, 20].

Kausik Si therefore searched for a homolog in *Aplysia* and found, in addition to the developmental form of CPEB that Richter had studied, a new form that had novel properties [9, 10] (Figure 7). It was not phosphorylated by an aurora kinase and it had an unusual N-terminus. ApCPEB is induced at the sensory neuron synapse by one pulse of 5-HT and blocking this form of CPEB by means of an antisense oligonucleotide at a marked (active) synapse prevents the maintenance, but not the initiation, of long-term synaptic facilitation (Figure 8).

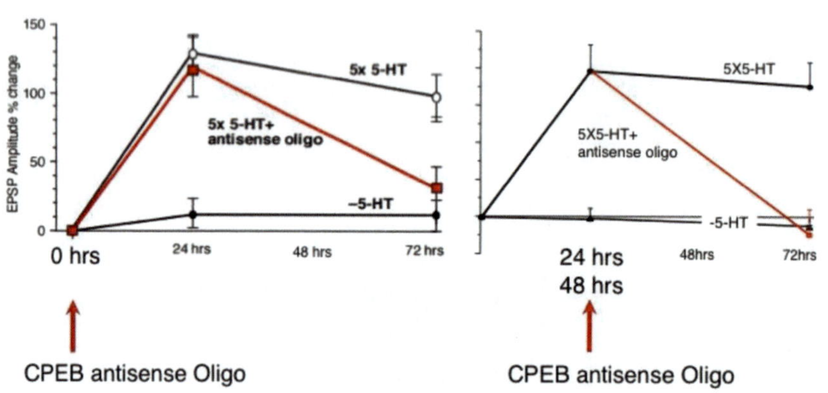

Figure 8. Persistent activity of CPEB is needed for the maintenance of LTF.

ApCPEB has a remarkable N-terminus

How does ApCPEB remain active for the long-term in the absence of further synaptic stimulation? A remarkable feature of the *Aplysia* form of CPEB is that its N-terminus is enriched in polar residues – glutamine and asparagine – characteristic of the prion domain of yeast prion proteins (Figure 9).

As Stanley Prusiner first showed, prion-like proteins are self-replicating structures. Indeed, Si et al., have found in yeast and in *Aplysia* that this prion domain endows the *Aplysia* CPEB with similar self-sustaining properties (Figure 10).

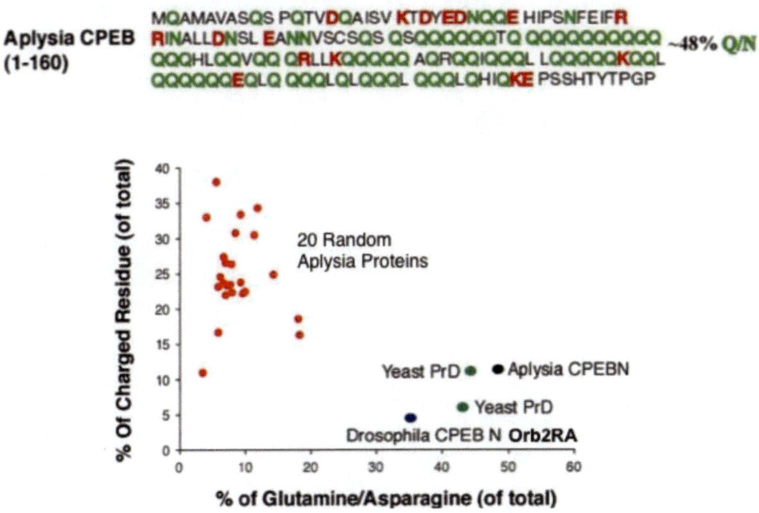

Figure 9. The N-terminal end of *Aplysia* CPEB has a prion-like domain [10].

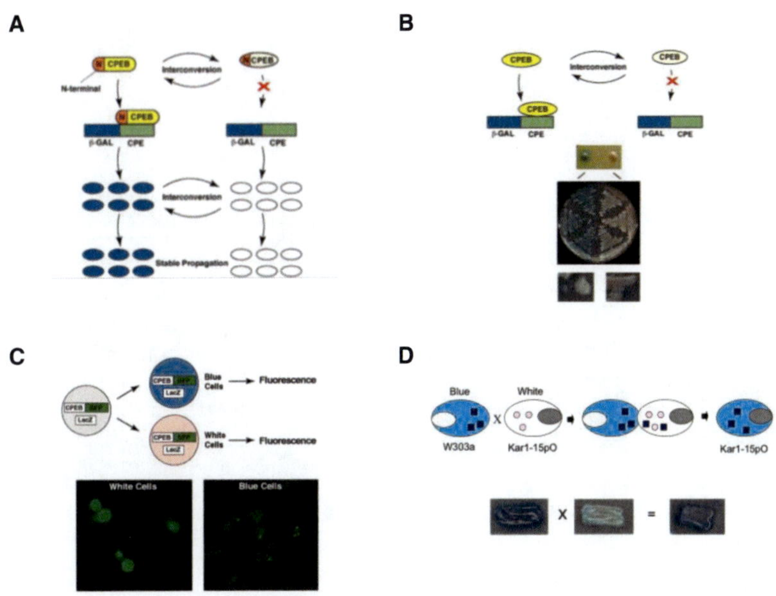

Figure 10. ApCPEB has properties of a prion in yeast. The full-length CPEB protein can exist in two functional conformational states (A); the two states are interconvertible (B); *Aplysia* CPEB forms aggregates: Multimeric structures in blue cells (C); the aggregates are heritable: Dominant cytoplasmic inheritance of the blue state. Protein from blue cells recruit and convert the protein from the white cells in a self-perpetuating manner (D).

The full-length protein can exist in two functional conformational states: monomeric and aggregated. The aggregated form is heritable. The protein from the aggregated cells can recruit and convert the monomeric protein in a self-perpetuating manner. But unlike other prions found to date, which are pathogenic, the *Aplysia* CPEB is functional: the active, self-perpetuating form of the protein does not kill cells, but rather controls synapse-specific translation. Notably, the persistence of long-term memory in *Drosophila* and in mice were subsequently also found to involve CPEB [21, 22, 23] (Figure 11A and Figure 11B).

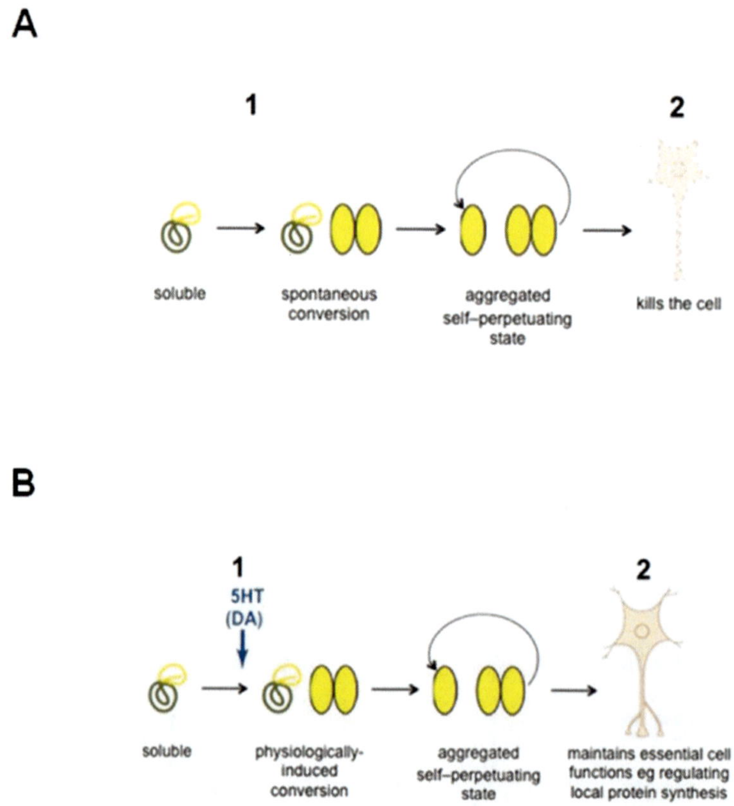

Figure 11. Conventional prions are characterized by two features: they spontaneously convert to a self-perpetuating state, and they kill the cell (A). Functional prions differ from conventional prions in that the conversion to the self-perpetuating state is physiologically induced, and the prions act to help maintain the essential functions of the cell (B).

Conventional and Functional Prions

Although first identified as disease – causing agents in people, proteins with prion properties were found subsequently in yeast and fungi suggesting that prion-like proteins might be more prevalent than initially anticipated [24, 25, 26, 27, 28, 29, 30].

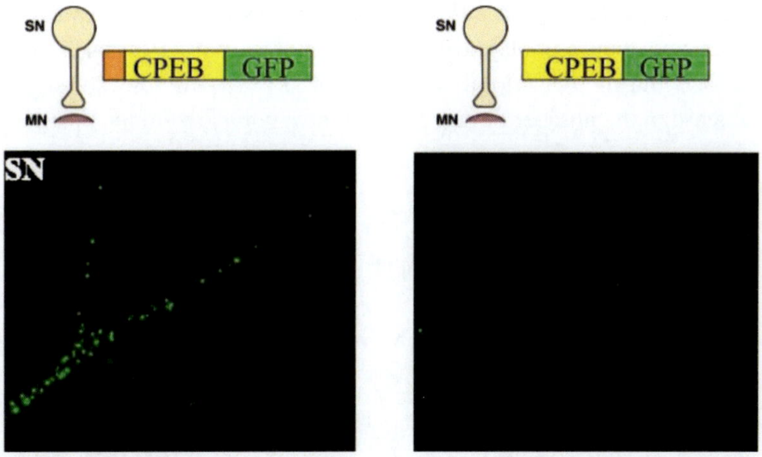

Figure 12. ApCPEB exists in two forms in sensory neurons. Overexpression of ApCPEB causes aggregation. This is lost when the prion domain is deleted [31].

Based on the prion-like properties of ApCPEB in yeast, Si et al., [9, 10, 31] outlined a model for the perpetuation of synapse-specific long-term functional and structural changes and the consequent persistence of memory storage. They proposed that at the synapse ApCPEB can assume at least two conformational states: monomeric and multimeric. In a naïve synapse, ApCPEB is monomeric and either less active or acts as a repressor. Synaptic activation leads to the conversion of ApCPEB to a dominant, self-perpetuating, multimeric state. However, unlike conventional prions, the dominant state of ApCPEB is either more active or devoid of the repressive function of the basal state. This dominant state is locally restricted and creates a self-sustaining synaptic mark limited to the specific set of synapses that have been activated. This leads to sustained period of translation over time at the activated synapse that allows for the long-term maintenance of the functional and structural synaptic changes. A test of this hypothesis requires an experimental analysis in neurons that addresses four questions: First, does ApCPEB have the properties of a self-perpetuating prion-like protein in neurons? Second, is the prion-like conversion from a soluble to an aggregated form modulated by synaptic stimulation? Third, is ApCPEB active in the aggregated, prion-like state? Finally, is the prion-like state of ApCPEB required for the maintenance of long-term facilitation? Si and Kandel et al., found that in the presynaptic sensory neurons of *Aplysia* both the exogenously expressed and the endogenous *Aplysia* CPEB exist in two states, one of which is multimeric. The exogenous multimers in the sensory neuron result from a homotypic interaction of ApCPEB. The exogenous multimers are amyloidogenic and self-sustaining. These features are consistent with ApCPEB having prion-like properties in the sensory neuron. This aggregation is lost by deletion of the N-terminal prion domain (Figure 12).

Multimerization of *Aplysia* CPEB Is Regulated by 5-HT

All known examples of prion-like conversions are stochastic in nature. However, our model postulates that the conversion of ApCPEB to the multimeric state should be regulated by synaptic activity. To address this question (Si. et al., 2003; 2010) expressed ApCPEB-

EGFP in the sensory-motor neuron co-culture, waited 48 hr for the expression to reach a steady-state level, and then stimulated the cells with five pulses of 5-HT, the modulatory transmitter released during behavioral learning (Figure 13). In the stimulated cells they observed an increase in the number of detectable puncta compared to the unstimulated cells.

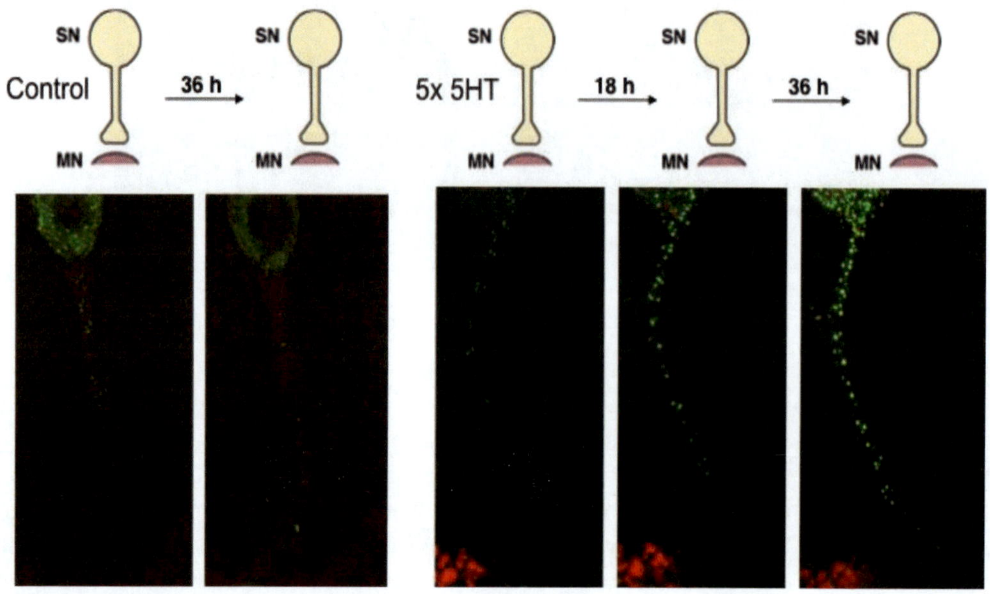

Figure 13. The conversion of CPEB is regulated by 5HT. Stimulation with 5HT, which increases the level of the CPEB, changes the amount and distribution of the aggregated CPEB [31].

An Antibody That Preferentially Recognizes the Multimeric ApCPEB Blocks Persistence of Synaptic Facilitation

If ApCPEB indeed acts as an active multimer, then one would predict that inhibition of the endogenous multimeric form of ApCPEB should destabilize the maintenance of long-term facilitation. To test this prediction Si. et al., (2010) took advantage of the antibody 464 (Ab464) that preferentially binds the multimeric form of *Aplysia* CPEB and injected this antibody into the sensory cell of sensory-motor neuron co-cultures (Figure 14). They assumed that binding of antibody to the protein would either inhibit or diminish its activity. Injection of the Ab464 interferes neither with basal synaptic transmission nor with long-term facilitation measured at 24 hr post-bath application of five pulses of 5-HT. However, unlike the control cells, synaptic facilitation failed to persist beyond 24 hrs in Ab464-injected cells. These results indicate that the multimeric form of *Aplysia* CPEB is involved in long-term stabilization of activity-dependent change in synaptic efficacy.

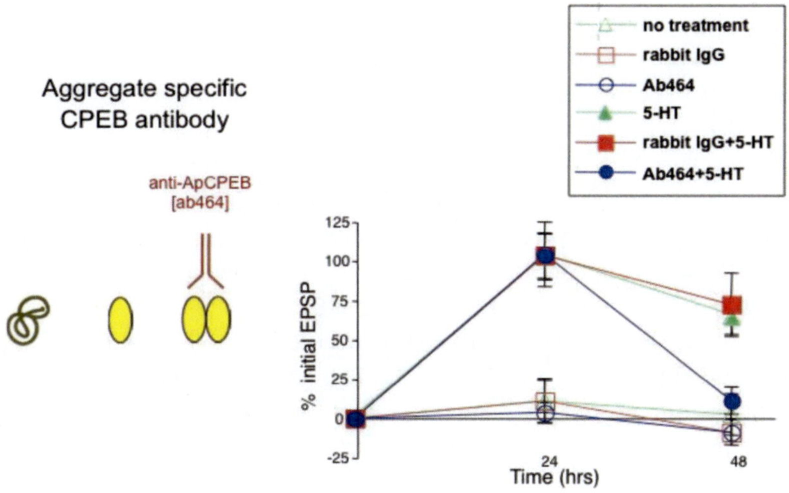

Figure 14. Injection into sensory neurons of ApCPEB antibody (Ab464), that recognizes only the aggregated and not the soluble form of CPEB, selectively blocks the maintenance of LTF.

Destabilization and Restabilization of Long-Term Memory

Ample data now indicate that in many types of memory, the reactivation of the long-term trace upon its retrieval can result in transient destabilization of the trace that may lead to its change. This is commonly construed in terms of a process of "reconsolidation" [32, 33], which shares mechanisms with consolidation, and will be discussed later in this chapter. Reconsolidation also has been demonstrated in *Aplysia* [34, 35]. This allows dissection of its mechanisms in identified neurons and synapses. Particularly, the question can be investigated whether the same synapses that are involved in encoding and storing the memory trace also are those that are destabilized and restabilized after synaptic reactivation that accompanies memory retrieval? Or are new and different synapses recruited?

Lee and his colleagues [34] have addressed this issue in the gill-withdrawal reflex in *Aplysia* and found that indeed, many of the same sensory-motor synapses that store long-term facilitation are destabilized by protein degradation during reactivation and restabilized by protein synthesis afterwards. This cellular change parallels the behavioral performance on memory retrieval. This finding indicates that the long-term memory trace, once formed, remains potentially dynamic even in simple reflexes at the level of the individual neurons and synapses that have encoded the memory in the first place.

The Maintenance of Long-Term Facilitation Is Gated Presynaptically by microRNA 22 Acting Directly on CPEB and Indirectly on Atypical PKC (aPKC)

The identification of CPEB as a functional prion-like molecule with a role in synaptic plasticity first in *Aplysia* and subsequently in *Drosophila* and mice [9, 10, 21, 31, 36, 37, 50, 51, 53] raises a number of biological questions regarding the regulation of its structural and functional dynamics in response to physiological stimuli. Structural, genetic and cell biological studies have highlighted regulatory mechanisms intrinsic to the structure of this protein, as well as extrinsic regulatory mechanisms based on post-translational modifications [37, 38, 39, 40]. Since the conformational transitions of CPEB, like those of other Q/N-rich prions, are dependent on the expression level of the protein, it is of interest to understand how the expression level of CPEB is dynamically regulated in neurons in response to synaptic signals. Si et al., [9] have described a mechanism controlling the post-transcriptional up-regulation of CPEB triggered by the neurotransmitter serotonin at the onset of long-term facilitation. Interference with this up-regulation is sufficient to block the long-term maintenance of long-term facilitation after induction [10].

Fuimara et al., [52] have identified a neuron-specific microRNA, miRNA-22 (miR-22), that inhibits CPEB mRNA through multiple 3'UTR binding sites and is down-regulated by serotonin. Inhibition of miR-22 simulates serotonin's effect, increasing CPEB levels and enhancing long-term facilitation. Conversely, miR-22 overexpression down-regulates CPEB and impairs long-term facilitation.

miR-22 also indirectly down-regulates presynaptic expression of aPKC, which has a role in long-term facilitation. A novel, extended 3'-UTR of aPKC mRNA contains one low-affinity miR-22 binding site but is not directly regulated by miR-22. However, the UTR contains several CPE elements and undergoes polyadenylation *in vivo*.

This would also be consistent with previous studies in *Drosophila* that had identified the *Drosophila* aPKC mRNA as a target for Orb2, the orthologue of *Aplysia* CPEB [41]. miR-22 is expressed in presynaptic sensory neurons but not in motor neurons. However, pharmacological experiments have studied the activity of aPKC/M in synaptic plasticity in the postsynaptic compartment, both in vertebrates and in *Aplysia* [42, 43]. Using genetic approaches based on the selective presynaptic overexpression of wild type and dominant negative forms of the kinase, Fuimara et al., have now further studied the role of this kinase in the presynaptic compartment. They find that aPKC also acts presynaptically in the maintenance of long-term facilitation. Thus the 5-HT/miR-22 pathway controls the maintenance phase of long-term facilitation through CPEB and through a downstream target with synergistic functions.

Taken together, the results of these experiments support a model in which the presynaptic 5-HT-dependent down-regulation of miR-22 promotes the upregulation and activation of CPEB and downstream targets, including an atypical PKC, which function synergistically in the maintenance of learning-related long-term synaptic plasticity.

Structure Insights into Functional Prions

The functional prion ApCPEB has an alpha-helix rich structure in its soluble form and a beta-sheet structure in its aggregated form very much as does the pathogenic form.

But importantly, functional NMR studies by Raveendra et al., also reveal that the functional prion domain is not solely composed of beta sheets but also has a novel mixed structure containing helical and random coil stretches [44].

This mixed structure view is consistent with the independent bioinformatics and mutagenesis studies by Fiumara et al., that predict that the glutamine rich prion domain of ApCPEB has a propensity to form alpha-helical coiled-coil structures [38].

This mixed structure model has the advantage of beta sheet rigidity necessary for a translational machine model and the flexibility of the coiled- coil needed for regulation.

The coiled-coils of the prion domains are stacked together, exposed, and free to bind mRNAs on the surface of the beta sheet fiber axis – scaffold. This can allow the coordinated translation of the population of interrelated mRNAs required for stabilization of synaptic growth. Thus, this structure gives us some preliminary insights into how CPEB aggregates can coordinate the polyadenylation of multiple RNAs required for stabilization.

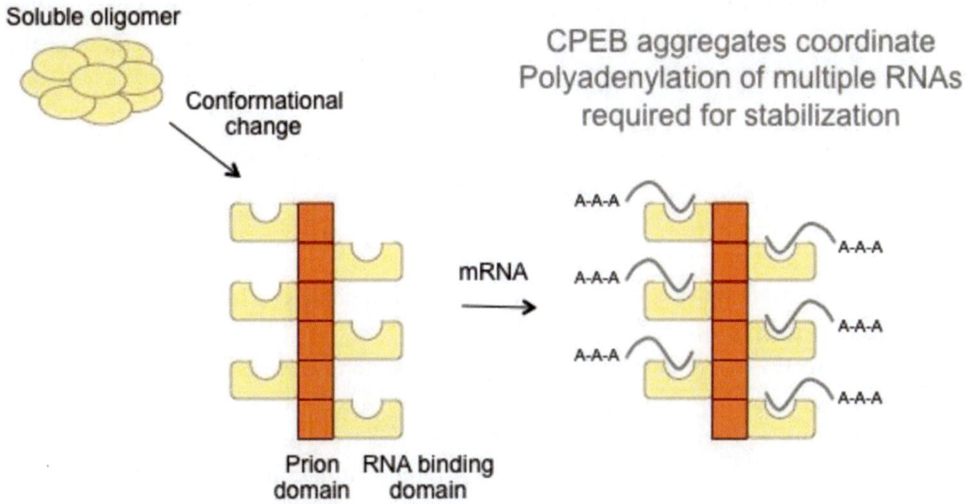

Figure 15. Functional prions are likely to have a distinctive regulatable structure. The coiled coils of the prion domains are stacked together, exposed, and free to bind mRNAs on the surface of the beta sheet fiber axis – scaffold. This can allow the coordinated translation of the population of interrelated mRNAs required for stabilization of synaptic growth [38, 39].

An Overall View

Are Neuronal CPEBs a New Class of Functional Prion-Like Proteins?

All proteins that multimerize in the cell are clearly not prions. There also are many instances when multimerization of a protein can be changed in response to external signals such as polymerization of actin [45]. ApCPEB forms self-sustaining multimers with the properties of an amyloid. But are these features sufficient to categorize ApCPEB as a prion-like protein?

The term prion has taken on two meanings. The first derives from the unique disease causing properties of the PrP protein PrP^{Sc}. One of the most remarkable aspects of the prion disease is the ability of the PrP^{Sc} protein to be absorbed in the digestive system to enter the circulation, cross the blood brain barrier, and enter the central nervous system where the protein propagates the disease. By this definition of infectivity, only PrP^{Sc} and no other protein, including yeast or fungal prions, can be categorized as prions [46]. The second definition of prion is mechanistic and is based on the ability of the disease-causing state of the protein to induce its own conformational state onto the non-disease-causing form of the protein, resulting in self-propagation. This second feature of the prion disease is more general [47] and is manifested by a number of yeast proteins and at least one fungal protein [25, 26, 28, 29, 48]. We now have found that the self-propagation is manifested by *Aplysia* neuronal CPEB. It is possible that the ability of a prion-like protein to assume a self-propagating conformational state is part of an evolutionarily conserved molecular mechanism that can create two distinct activity states from a single polypeptide [48, 49]. In the case of the prion disease, the PrP protein has acquired additional features that result in its remarkable infectivity. We would suggest that the *Aplysia* CPEB might be representative of a new class of proteins that utilize a self-perpetuating multimeric state to create self-sustaining altered activity states in the cell in response to specific stimuli.

References

[1] Martin KC, Casadio A, Zhu H, Yaping E, Rose JC, et al., (1997) Synapse-specific, long-term facilitation of aplysia sensory to motor synapses: a function for local protein synthesis in memory storage. *Cell* 91: 927-938.

[2] Frey U, Morris RG (1997) Synaptic tagging and long-term potentiation. *Nature* 385: 533-536.

[3] Lee SH, Lim CS, Park H, Lee JA, Han JH, et al. (2007) Nuclear translocation of CAM-associated protein activates transcription for long-term facilitation in Aplysia. *Cell* 129: 801-812.

[4] Martin KC, Michael D, Rose JC, Barad M, Casadio A, et al. (1997) MAP kinase translocates into the nucleus of the presynaptic cell and is required for long-term facilitation in Aplysia. *Neuron* 18: 899-912.

[5] Michael D, Martin KC, Seger R, Ning MM, Baston R, et al. (1998) Repeated pulses of serotonin required for long-term facilitation activate mitogen-activated protein kinase in sensory neurons of Aplysia. *Proceedings of the National Academy of Sciences of the United States of America* 95: 1864-1869.

[6] Barco A, Alarcon JM, Kandel ER (2002) Expression of constitutively active CREB protein facilitates the late phase of long-term potentiation by enhancing synaptic capture. *Cell* 108: 689-703.

[7] Casadio A, Martin KC, Giustetto M, Zhu H, Chen M, et al. (1999) A transient, neuron-wide form of CREB-mediated long-term facilitation can be stabilized at specific synapses by local protein synthesis. *Cell* 99: 221-237.

[8] Dudek SM, Fields RD (2002) Somatic action potentials are sufficient for late-phase LTP-related cell signaling. *Proc Natl Acad Sci USA* 99: 3962-3967.

[9] Si K, Giustetto M, Etkin A, Hsu R, Janisiewicz AM, et al. (2003) A neuronal isoform of CPEB regulates local protein synthesis and stabilizes synapse-specific long-term facilitation in Aplysia. *Cell* 115: 893-904.

[10] Si K, Lindquist S, Kandel ER (2003) A neuronal isoform of the aplysia CPEB has prion-like properties. *Cell* 115: 879-891.

[11] McGrew LL, Dworkin-Rastl E, Dworkin MB, Richter JD (1989) Poly(A) elongation during Xenopus oocyte maturation is required for translational recruitment and is mediated by a short sequence element. *Genes Dev* 3: 803-815.

[12] Fox CA, Sheets MD, Wickens MP (1989) Poly(A) addition during maturation of frog oocytes: distinct nuclear and cytoplasmic activities and regulation by the sequence UUUUUAU. *Genes Dev* 3: 2151-2162.

[13] Gebauer F, Richter JD (1996) Mouse cytoplasmic polyadenylylation element binding protein: an evolutionarily conserved protein that interacts with the cytoplasmic polyadenylylation elements of c-mos mRNA. *Proc Natl Acad Sci USA* 93: 14602-14607.

[14] Hake LE, Richter JD (1994) CPEB is a specificity factor that mediates cytoplasmic polyadenylation during Xenopus oocyte maturation. *Cell* 79: 617-627.

[15] Schroeder KE, Condic ML, Eisenberg LM, Yost HJ (1999) Spatially regulated translation in embryos: asymmetric expression of maternal Wnt-11 along the dorsal-ventral axis in Xenopus. *Dev Biol* 214: 288-297.

[16] Stebbins-Boaz B, Hake LE, Richter JD (1996) CPEB controls the cytoplasmic polyadenylation of cyclin, Cdk2 and c-mos mRNAs and is necessary for oocyte maturation in Xenopus. *EMBO J* 15: 2582-2592.

[17] Bally-Cuif L, Schatz WJ, Ho RK (1998) Characterization of the zebrafish Orb/CPEB-related RNA binding protein and localization of maternal components in the zebrafish oocyte. *Mech Dev* 77: 31-47.

[18] Tan L, Chang JS, Costa A, Schedl P (2001) An autoregulatory feedback loop directs the localized expression of the Drosophila CPEB protein Orb in the developing oocyte. *Development* 128: 1159-1169.

[19] Chang JS, Tan L, Wolf MR, Schedl P (2001) Functioning of the Drosophila orb gene in gurken mRNA localization and translation. *Development* 128: 3169-3177.

[20] Groisman I, Jung MY, Sarkissian M, Cao Q, Richter JD (2002) Translational control of the embryonic cell cycle. *Cell* 109: 473-483.

[21] Keleman K, Kruttner S, Alenius M, Dickson BJ (2007) Function of the Drosophila CPEB protein Orb2 in long-term courtship memory. *Nat Neurosci* 10: 1587-1593.

[22] Majumdar A, Cesario WC, White-Grindley E, Jiang H, Ren F, et al. (2012) Critical role of amyloid-like oligomers of Drosophila Orb2 in the persistence of memory. *Cell* 148: 515-529.

[23] Rajasethupathy P, Antonov I, Sheridan R, Frey S, Sander C, et al. (2012) A role for neuronal piRNAs in the epigenetic control of memory-related synaptic plasticity. *Cell* 149: 693-707.

[24] Wickner RB (1994) [URE3] as an altered URE2 protein: evidence for a prion analog in Saccharomyces cerevisiae. *Science* 264: 566-569.

[25] Wickner RB, Masison DC, Edskes HK (1995) [PSI] and [URE3] as yeast prions. *Yeast* 11: 1671-1685.

[26] Coustou V, Deleu C, Saupe S, Begueret J (1997) The protein product of the het-s heterokaryon incompatibility gene of the fungus Podospora anserina behaves as a prion analog. *Proc Natl Acad Sci USA* 94: 9773-9778.

[27] Prusiner SB (1998) Prions. *Proc Natl Acad Sci USA* 95: 13363-13383.

[28] Sondheimer N, Lindquist S (2000) Rnq1: an epigenetic modifier of protein function in yeast. *Mol Cell* 5: 163-172.

[29] Derkatch IL, Bradley ME, Hong JY, Liebman SW (2001) Prions affect the appearance of other prions: the story of [PIN(+)]. *Cell* 106: 171-182.

[30] Osherovich LZ, Weissman JS (2001) Multiple Gln/Asn-rich prion domains confer susceptibility to induction of the yeast [PSI(+)] prion. *Cell* 106: 183-194.

[31] Si K, Choi YB, White-Grindley E, Majumdar A, Kandel ER (2010) Aplysia CPEB can form prion-like multimers in sensory neurons that contribute to long-term facilitation. *Cell* 140: 421-435.

[32] Nader K, Schafe GE, Le Doux JE (2000) Fear memories require protein synthesis in the amygdala for reconsolidation after retrieval. *Nature* 406: 722-726.

[33] Sara SJ (2000) Retrieval and reconsolidation: Toward a neurobiology of remembering. *Learning & Memory* 7: 73-84.

[34] Lee SH, Kwak C, Shim J, Kim JE, Choi SL, et al. (2012) A cellular model of memory reconsolidation involves reactivation-induced destabilization and restabilization at the sensorimotor synapse in Aplysia. *Proc Natl Acad Sci USA* 109: 14200-14205.

[35] Cai D, Pearce K, Chen S, Glanzman DL (2012) Reconsolidation of long-term memory in Aplysia. *Curr Biol* 22: 1783-1788.

[36] Kruttner S, Stepien B, Noordermeer JN, Mommaas MA, Mechtler K, et al. (2012) Drosophila CPEB Orb2A mediates memory independent of Its RNA-binding domain. *Neuron* 76: 383-395.

[37] Pavlopoulos E, Trifilieff P, Chevaleyre V, Fioriti L, Zairis S, et al. (2011) Neuralized1 activates CPEB3: a function for nonproteolytic ubiquitin in synaptic plasticity and memory storage. *Cell* 147: 1369-1383.

[38] Fiumara F, Fioriti L, Kandel ER, Hendrickson WA (2010) Essential role of coiled coils for aggregation and activity of Q/N-rich prions and PolyQ proteins. *Cell* 143: 1121-1135.

[39] Raveendra BL, Siemer AB, Puthanveettil SV, Hendrickson WA, Kandel ER, et al. (2013) Characterization of prion-like conformational changes of the neuronal isoform of Aplysia CPEB. *Nat Struct Mol Biol* 20: 495-501.

[40] White-Grindley E, Li L, Mohammad Khan R, Ren F, Saraf A, et al. (2014) Contribution of Orb2A stability in regulated amyloid-like oligomerization of Drosophila Orb2. *PLoS Biol* 12: e1001786.

[41] Mastushita-Sakai T, White-Grindley E, Samuelson J, Seidel C, Si K (2010) Drosophila Orb2 targets genes involved in neuronal growth, synapse formation, and protein turnover. *Proc Natl Acad Sci USA* 107: 11987-11992.

[42] Bougie JK, Cai D, Hastings M, Farah CA, Chen S, et al. (2012) Serotonin-induced cleavage of the atypical protein kinase C Apl III in Aplysia. *J Neurosci* 32: 14630-14640.

[43] Sacktor TC (2011) How does PKMzeta maintain long-term memory? *Nature Reviews Neuroscience* 12: 9-15.

[44] Raveendra BL, Siemer AB, Puthanveettil SV, Hendrickson WA, Kandel ER, et al. (2013) Characterization of prion-like conformational changes of the neuronal isoform of Aplysia CPEB. *Nat Struct Mol Biol* 20: 495-501.

[45] Higgs HN, Pollard TD (2001) Regulation of actin filament network formation through ARP2/3 complex: activation by a diverse array of proteins. *Annu Rev Biochem* 70: 649-676.

[46] Weissmann C (2004) The state of the prion. *Nat Rev Microbiol* 2: 861-871.

[47] Meyer-Luehmann M, Coomaraswamy J, Bolmont T, Kaeser S, Schaefer C, et al. (2006) Exogenous induction of cerebral beta-amyloidogenesis is governed by agent and host. *Science* 313: 1781-1784.

[48] Osherovich LZ, Weissman JS (2002) The utility of prions. *Dev Cell* 2: 143-151.

[49] Shorter J, Lindquist S (2005) Prions as adaptive conduits of memory and inheritance. *Nat Rev Genet* 6: 435-450.

[50] Stephan JS, Fioriti L, Lamba N, Derkatch IL, and Kandel ER.2015. The CPEB3 protein important in memory persistence is a functional prion that interacts with the actin cytoskeleton. Cell Reports DOI: http://dx.doi.org/10.1016/j.celrep.2015.04.060

[51] Fioriti L, Myers C, Huang Y-Y, Li X, Stephan J, Trifilieff P, Kosmidis S, Drisaldi B, PavlopoulosE, Kandel ER. 2015. The Persistence of Memory and its Reconsolidation Require CPEB3-Mediated Protein Synthesis in the Hippocampus. *Neuron.* DOI: http://dx.doi.org/10.1016/j.neuron.2015.05.021

[52] Fiumara F, Rajasethupathy P, Antonov I, Kosmidis S, Sossin W, Kandel E. 2015. MicroRNA-22 gates long-term heterosynaptic plasticity in *Aplysia* through presynaptic regulation of CPEB and downstream targets. *Cell Reports.*

[53] White-Grindley E, Li L, Mohammad Khan R, Ren F, Saraf A, Florens L, Si K. Critical role of amyloid-like oligomers of *Drosophila* Orb2 in the persistence of memory. PLoS Biol. 2014 Feb 11;12(2):e1001786. doi: 10.1371/journal.pbio.1001786. eCollection 2014 Feb.

In: The Prion Phenomena in Neurodegenerative Diseases ISBN: 978-1-63483-399-8
Editors: Giuseppe Legname and Gabriele Giachin

Chapter 12

CONCLUDING REMARKS

Giuseppe Legname[1,*], Suzana Aulić[1] and Gabriele Giachin[1,2]
[1]Department of Neuroscience, Scuola Internazionale Superiore di Studi Avanzati (SISSA), Trieste, Italy
[2]Structural Biology Group, European Synchrotron Radiation Facility (ESRF), Grenoble, France

ABSTRACT

Prions are self-perpetuating proteinaceous infectious agent transmissible intra and inter species and are the primary causative agents of numerous human and animal neurological diseases, collectively denoted as transmissible spongiform encephalopathies or prion diseases. The physiological cellular form of the prion protein (PrP^C) undergoes a conformational transformation leading to aggregation into infectious prions. Prion-like protein aggregates spreading and transmission between cells have also been shown for other proteins associated with other neurological diseases such as Alzheimer's disease, Parkinson's disease and amyotrophic lateral sclerosis. This protein-only phenomenon may therefore have broader implications in neurodegenerative disorders. This final chapter recapitulates the recent advances in prion biology presented in this thematic book and highlights the unique roles of prions and prion-like proteins in neurodegenerative diseases.

Proteins are complex macromolecular systems playing crucial roles for cell and tissue functions in all living organisms. Finely regulated physiological processes depend on the correct assembly of protein architectures in key regulatory nodes of different pathways, such as signal transduction, DNA replication, RNA processing and translation. These functions can be jeopardized when proteins follow alternative folding conformations, by losing their biological function and being targeted for degradation. Although each living organism invests energy for the elimination of misfolded proteins, a possible inability of the cell to cope with this protein misfolding may result in a cascade of events leading to disease [1].

* Corresponding Author addresses: Email: legname@sissa.it and gabriele.giachin@esrf.fr

A traditional dogma in biology dictates that the protein native structure is entirely governed by its primary amino acid sequence, which is the final product of the DNA-to-RNA-to-protein cascade [2]. This notion started to be debated after that S.B. Prusiner coined the term prion in 1982 to describe a novel class of infectious agent solely composed of proteinaceous material and responsible for rare human and animal neurodegenerative disorders, collectively called transmissible spongiform encephalopathies (TSE) or prion diseases [3]. The revolutionary implications of this protein-only hypothesis lie in the existence of multiple stable conformations of a single protein in the absence of any post-translational modifications: the host encoded cellular isoform, PrP^{C}, and the misfolded and infectious isoform associated with prion diseases, PrP^{Sc} or prion. Unique from other bacterial or viral pathogens, prions can self-replicate *via* a conformational remodeling event whereby native α-helical folded PrP^{C} are converted into β-sheet enriched PrP^{Sc} in a template-directed fashion [4]. Furthermore, the existence of distinct PrP^{Sc} strains was seen as implausible without invoking mutations in the human DNA genome [5].

Nowadays, the protein-only hypothesis is widely accepted and proved by different groups with the demonstration that bacterially produced prion proteins can be *in vitro* refolded into infectious prions that cause prion diseases *in vivo* (termed also as "synthetic prions") [6].

In addition to constituting a unique biological paradigm, it has been recently suggested that the same pathological mechanisms observed for prion diseases may be found in much more common neurodegenerative diseases where other amyloidogenic proteins can become prion-like [7].

Several neurodegenerative disorders –e.g., Alzheimer disease (AD), Parkinson disease (PD) and amyotrophic lateral sclerosis (ALS)- are linked to an irreversible protein aggregation process whereby one or more proteins self-associate in oligomeric structures leading to cell-to-cell spreading, neurotoxicity, cell damage and dysfunction, and ultimately death. Similar to the pioneeristic studies employing bacterially expressed PrP to produce the first synthetic prions [8], different groups have succeeded in the production of synthetic amyloids made of amyloid-β (Aβ), α-synuclein, tau and SOD1 (Table 1).

There is considerable scientific and ethical debate over whether the term prion should be applied to other amyloidogenic proteins different from PrP^{Sc} [44]. Taking into account the original accepted sense of the term prion –i.e., natural, self-perpetuating proteinaceous infectious agent transmissible inter and intra species- there is no clear evidence that other neurodegenerative diseases are transmissible from person to person. However, nomenclature notwithstanding, a common consensus has emerged defining the amyloidogenic proteins responsible for these diseases as prion-like proteins due to their intrinsic ability to perform seeded aggregation, cell-to-cell spreading and *in vivo* neurotoxicity: properties reminiscent of prions [44].

In this book we have expanded the protein-only phenomenon responsible for TSE to the general prion phenomena in other neurodegenerative diseases. This thematic series consists in different contributions that cover this new paradigm at clinical, molecular, structural and functional levels. At first, the reader is introduced to a detailed description about human prion diseases and the current methods for *ante-mortem* diagnosis of TSE (Chapter 1).

Table 1. Synthetic amyloids involved in neurodegenerative disorders reported in literature

Protein	Structural features	Aggregation *in vitro*	Aggregation in cell culture	Aggregation *in vivo*	Intracellular transmission in cell culture	Transmission *in vivo* (serial passages)
PrP^{Sc}	β-folded MoPrP(89-143)	Yes [9]	n.d.	Yes [9]	n.d.	Yes [9]
	MoSP (MoPrP89-230)	Yes [8, 10, 11, 12, 13, 14, 15]	n.d.	Yes [8, 10, 11, 12, 13, 15]	n.d.	Yes [8, 10, 11, 12, 13, 15]
	$rPrP\text{-}res^{17kDa}$ $rPrP\text{-}res^{14kDa}$ MoPrP23-230	Yes [16, 17, 18] in presence of cofactors*	Yes [16]	Yes [17,18]	n.d.	Yes [17] only $rPrP\text{-}res^{17kDa}$
	SHa and Mo recPrP(23-230)	Yes [19, 20]	n.d.	Yes [20] No disease just deposits of PrP^{Sc}	n.d.	Yes [20]
	#4 and #28 recPrP amyloid forms (MoPrP 23-230)	Yes [6]	Yes [6]	n.d.	Yes [6]	n.d.
α-synuclein	Oligomers	Yes [21, 22]	Yes [21, 22]	n.d.	n.d.	n.d.
	Ribbons	Yes [23]	Yes [23]	n.d.	n.d.	n.d.
	Fibrils	Yes [23, 24, 25, 26, 27, 28,29]	Yes [23, 24, 25, 28, 29]	Yes [25, 26, 27]	Yes [24, 25]	n.d.
Aβ	Oligomers of Aβ40 and Aβ42	Yes [30, 31]	Yes [30,31]	n.d.	Yes [30, 31]	n.d.
	Fibrils of Aβ40 and Aβ42	Yes [32, 33]	n.d.	Yes [32, 33]	n.d.	n.d.
Tau	Fibrils	Yes [34, 35, 36, 37, 38]	Yes [34, 35, 36, 38]	Yes [37, 38]	Yes [37, 38]	Yes [38]
SOD1	Fibrils	Yes [39, 40]	Yes [40, 41]	Indirect evidence [42]	Yes [41, 43]	n.d.

n.d., not determined. *cofactors: polyanions, RNA, and lipids.

A complete comprehension of prion diseases is not possible without structural studies on PrP^{Sc}. Chapter 2 presents seminal work about the long-awaited structural architecture of different PrP^{Sc} strains investigated by X-ray fiber diffraction. Subsequently, Chapter 3 and Chapter 4 discuss the mechanisms of prion-induced neurotoxicity, the unfolded protein response and the role of glycosaminoglycans in prion and prion-like diseases.

The prion phenomena are explained to the heart of the matter with Chapter 5 and Chapter 6, which summarize the prion-like properties of α-synuclein, the protein responsible for PD. These chapters provide a lesson about the complexity of structures that α-synuclein may adopt when present in monomeric and aggregated states, and discusses the biological relevance of the observed α-synuclein assemblies. In the next chapter the reader is guided into an introduction of AD pathology, and then to a detailed description of the molecular processes underlying amyloid β (Aβ) and tau propagation and related pathologies. Particularly informative is the space that authors dedicated to the role of non-neuronal cells and other cellular cofactors in Aβ and tau spreading (Chapter 7). Like the seeded aggregation of Aβ, the pathogenesis of tauopathy appears in the prion paradigm, as discussed in Chapter 8.

Finally, the complex group of proteins associated with ALS pathology is presented in Chapter 9, which includes an introduction of the ALS topic, up-to-date contents about the prion-like features of SOD1, TDP-43 and other ALS-related proteins, and a discussion about prospective therapeutic targets in ALS.

Prion-like processes are not necessarily associated with accumulation of toxic aggregates that frequently accompany neurodegeneration, but may have a functional profit for the cell, particularly in lower organisms such as in yeasts. Chapter 10 provides an informative introduction about the criteria used to define yeast prions and the structural and molecular mechanisms responsible for yeast prion formation and interaction. As a conclusion to the book, the role of prions as functional epigenetic factors is discussed. Chapter 11 presents an exhaustive overview on seminal work that led to the discovery of *Aplysia californica* CPEB prions: the first class of prion-like proteins with functional activity in learning and memory processes.

In conclusion, the prion phenomena may extend from pathogenic proteins responsible for neurodegenerative disorders to functional protein aggregates involved in biological information transfer.

Aberrant protein folding underlies over 30 human diseases [45], therefore an exhaustive dissertation about all the proteins and the pathological mechanisms involved in protein misfolding diseases cannot be entirely covered in a book. For instance, recent findings extend the prion phenomena beyond the nervous system including aggregation-prone proteins –e.g., c-Abl and p53- involved in human cancer [46] or in type 2 diabetes where toxic aggregates of the islet amyloid polypeptide (IAPP) may contribute to β-cell dysfunction and disease onset [47]. Additionally, little is known about how toxic protein assemblies may spread from cell to cell contributing to rapid disease progression. Different groups are investigating the role of microvesicles, particularly exosomes, in shipping toxic α-synuclein, Aβ, tau and PrP^{Sc} aggregates from unhealthy neurons to their own neighboring cells [48, 49, 50, 51, 52, 53, 54, 55].

This comprehensive collection of chapters represents an up-to-date review of prion phenomena in different neurodegenerative diseases and serves as a useful introduction to those entering this new and exciting field of research.

ACKNOWLEDGMENTS

The authors wish to thank Kate E. Pischke for critical proofreading of the manuscript.

REFERENCES

[1] Knowles TP, Vendruscolo M, Dobson CM (2014) The amyloid state and its association with protein misfolding diseases. *Nat Rev Mol Cell Biol* 15: 384-396.

[2] Anfinsen CB (1973) Principles that govern the folding of protein chains. *Science* 181: 223-230.

[3] Prusiner SB (1982) Novel proteinaceous infectious particles cause scrapie. *Science* 216: 136-144.

[4] Colby DW, Prusiner SB (2011) Prions. *Cold Spring Harb Perspect Biol* 3: a006833.

[5] Aguzzi A, Heikenwalder M, Polymenidou M (2007) Insights into prion strains and neurotoxicity. *Nat Rev Mol Cell Biol* 8: 552-561.

[6] Le NT, Narkiewicz J, Aulic S, Salzano G, Tran HT, et al. (2014) Synthetic prions and other human neurodegenerative proteinopathies. *Virus Res.*

[7] Prusiner SB (2012) Cell biology. A unifying role for prions in neurodegenerative diseases. *Science* 336: 1511-1513.

[8] Legname G, Baskakov IV, Nguyen HO, Riesner D, Cohen FE, et al. (2004) Synthetic mammalian prions. *Science* 305: 673-676.

[9] Kaneko K, Ball HL, Wille H, Zhang H, Groth D, et al. (2000) A synthetic peptide initiates Gerstmann-Straussler-Scheinker (GSS) disease in transgenic mice. *J Mol Biol* 295: 997-1007.

[10] Colby DW, Giles K, Legname G, Wille H, Baskakov IV, et al. (2009) Design and construction of diverse mammalian prion strains. *Proc Natl Acad Sci USA* 106: 20417-20422.

[11] Legname G, Nguyen HO, Baskakov IV, Cohen FE, Dearmond SJ, et al. (2005) Strain-specified characteristics of mouse synthetic prions. *Proc Natl Acad Sci USA* 102: 2168-2173.

[12] Ghaemmaghami S, Colby DW, Nguyen HO, Hayashi S, Oehler A, et al. (2013) Convergent replication of mouse synthetic prion strains. *Am J Pathol* 182: 866-874.

[13] Legname G, Nguyen HO, Peretz D, Cohen FE, DeArmond SJ, et al. (2006) Continuum of prion protein structures enciphers a multitude of prion isolate-specified phenotypes. *Proc Natl Acad Sci USA* 103: 19105-19110.

[14] Colby DW, Zhang Q, Wang S, Groth D, Legname G, et al. (2007) Prion detection by an amyloid seeding assay. *Proc Natl Acad Sci USA* 104: 20914-20919.

[15] Colby DW, Wain R, Baskakov IV, Legname G, Palmer CG, et al. (2010) Protease-sensitive synthetic prions. *PLoS Pathog* 6: e1000736.

[16] Wang F, Wang X, Yuan CG, Ma J (2010) Generating a prion with bacterially expressed recombinant prion protein. *Science* 327: 1132-1135.

[17] Zhang Z, Zhang Y, Wang F, Wang X, Xu Y, et al. (2013) De novo generation of infectious prions with bacterially expressed recombinant prion protein. *FASEB J* 27: 4768-4775.

[18] Wang F, Wang X, Ma J (2011) Conversion of bacterially expressed recombinant prion protein. *Methods* 53: 208-213.

[19] Bocharova OV, Makarava N, Breydo L, Anderson M, Salnikov VV, et al. (2006) Annealing prion protein amyloid fibrils at high temperature results in extension of a proteinase K-resistant core. *J Biol Chem* 281: 2373-2379.

[20] Makarava N, Kovacs GG, Bocharova O, Savtchenko R, Alexeeva I, et al. (2010) Recombinant prion protein induces a new transmissible prion disease in wild-type animals. *Acta Neuropathol* 119: 177-187.

[21] Danzer KM, Krebs SK, Wolff M, Birk G, Hengerer B (2009) Seeding induced by alpha-synuclein oligomers provides evidence for spreading of alpha-synuclein pathology. *J Neurochem* 111: 192-203.

[22] Danzer KM, Haasen D, Karow AR, Moussaud S, Habeck M, et al. (2007) Different species of alpha-synuclein oligomers induce calcium influx and seeding. *J Neurosci* 27: 9220-9232.

[23] Bousset L, Pieri L, Ruiz-Arlandis G, Gath J, Jensen PH, et al. (2013) Structural and functional characterization of two alpha-synuclein strains. *Nat Commun* 4: 2575.

[24] Aulic S, Le TT, Moda F, Abounit S, Corvaglia S, et al. (2014) Defined alpha-synuclein prion-like molecular assemblies spreading in cell culture. *BMC Neurosci* 15: 69.

[25] Guo JL, Covell DJ, Daniels JP, Iba M, Stieber A, et al. (2013) Distinct alpha-synuclein strains differentially promote tau inclusions in neurons. *Cell* 154: 103-117.

[26] Masuda-Suzukake M, Nonaka T, Hosokawa M, Oikawa T, Arai T, et al. (2013) Prion-like spreading of pathological alpha-synuclein in brain. *Brain* 136: 1128-1138.

[27] Sacino AN, Brooks M, McGarvey NH, McKinney AB, Thomas MA, et al. (2013) Induction of CNS alpha-synuclein pathology by fibrillar and non-amyloidogenic recombinant alpha-synuclein. *Acta Neuropathol* Commun 1: 38.

[28] Volpicelli-Daley LA, Luk KC, Patel TP, Tanik SA, Riddle DM, et al. (2011) Exogenous alpha-synuclein fibrils induce Lewy body pathology leading to synaptic dysfunction and neuron death. *Neuron* 72: 57-71.

[29] Luk KC, Song C, O'Brien P, Stieber A, Branch JR, et al. (2009) Exogenous alpha-synuclein fibrils seed the formation of Lewy body-like intracellular inclusions in cultured cells. *Proc Natl Acad Sci USA* 106: 20051-20056.

[30] Domert J, Rao SB, Agholme L, Brorsson AC, Marcusson J, et al. (2014) Spreading of amyloid-beta peptides via neuritic cell-to-cell transfer is dependent on insufficient cellular clearance. *Neurobiol Dis* 65: 82-92.

[31] Nath S, Agholme L, Kurudenkandy FR, Granseth B, Marcusson J, et al. (2012) Spreading of neurodegenerative pathology via neuron-to-neuron transmission of beta-amyloid. *J Neurosci* 32: 8767-8777.

[32] Stohr J, Watts JC, Mensinger ZL, Oehler A, Grillo SK, et al. (2012) Purified and synthetic Alzheimer's amyloid beta (Abeta) prions. *Proc Natl Acad Sci USA* 109: 11025-11030.

[33] Stohr J, Condello C, Watts JC, Bloch L, Oehler A, et al. (2014) Distinct synthetic Abeta prion strains producing different amyloid deposits in bigenic mice. *Proc Natl Acad Sci USA*.

[34] Frost B, Jacks RL, Diamond MI (2009) Propagation of tau misfolding from the outside to the inside of a cell. *J Biol Chem* 284: 12845-12852.

[35] Guo JL, Lee VM (2011) Seeding of normal Tau by pathological Tau conformers drives pathogenesis of Alzheimer-like tangles. *J Biol Chem* 286: 15317-15331.

[36] Nonaka T, Watanabe ST, Iwatsubo T, Hasegawa M (2010) Seeded aggregation and toxicity of {alpha}-synuclein and tau: cellular models of neurodegenerative diseases. *J Biol Chem* 285: 34885-34898.

[37] Iba M, Guo JL, McBride JD, Zhang B, Trojanowski JQ, et al. (2013) Synthetic tau fibrils mediate transmission of neurofibrillary tangles in a transgenic mouse model of Alzheimer's-like tauopathy. *J Neurosci* 33: 1024-1037.

[38] Sanders DW, Kaufman SK, DeVos SL, Sharma AM, Mirbaha H, et al. (2014) Distinct tau prion strains propagate in cells and mice and define different tauopathies. *Neuron* 82: 1271-1288.

[39] Chia R, Tattum MH, Jones S, Collinge J, Fisher EM, et al. (2010) Superoxide dismutase 1 and tgSOD1 mouse spinal cord seed fibrils, suggesting a propagative cell death mechanism in amyotrophic lateral sclerosis. *PLoS One* 5: e10627.

[40] Grad LI, Guest WC, Yanai A, Pokrishevsky E, O'Neill MA, et al. (2011) Intermolecular transmission of superoxide dismutase 1 misfolding in living cells. *Proc Natl Acad Sci USA* 108: 16398-16403.

[41] Munch C, O'Brien J, Bertolotti A (2011) Prion-like propagation of mutant superoxide dismutase-1 misfolding in neuronal cells. Proc *Natl Acad Sci USA* 108: 3548-3553.

[42] Bruijn LI, Houseweart MK, Kato S, Anderson KL, Anderson SD, et al. (1998) Aggregation and motor neuron toxicity of an ALS-linked SOD1 mutant independent from wild-type SOD1. *Science* 281: 1851-1854.

[43] Grad LI, Yerbury JJ, Turner BJ, Guest WC, Pokrishevsky E, et al. (2014) Intercellular propagated misfolding of wild-type Cu/Zn superoxide dismutase occurs via exosome-dependent and -independent mechanisms. *Proc Natl Acad Sci USA* 111: 3620-3625.

[44] Walker LC, Jucker M (2015) Neurodegenerative Diseases: Expanding the Prion Concept. *Annu Rev Neurosci.*

[45] Chiti F, Dobson CM (2006) Protein misfolding, functional amyloid, and human disease. *Annu Rev Biochem* 75: 333-366.

[46] de Oliveira GA, Rangel LP, Costa DC, Silva JL (2015) Misfolding, Aggregation, and Disordered Segments in c-Abl and p53 in Human Cancer. *Front Oncol* 5: 97.

[47] Mukherjee A, Morales-Scheihing D, Butler PC, Soto C (2015) Type 2 diabetes as a protein misfolding disease. *Trends Mol Med.*

[48] Gotz J, Chen F, van Dorpe J, Nitsch RM (2001) Formation of neurofibrillary tangles in P301l tau transgenic mice induced by Abeta 42 fibrils. *Science* 293: 1491-1495.

[49] Fevrier B, Vilette D, Archer F, Loew D, Faigle W, et al. (2004) Cells release prions in association with exosomes. *Proc Natl Acad Sci USA* 101: 9683-9688.

[50] Bolmont T, Clavaguera F, Meyer-Luehmann M, Herzig MC, Radde R, et al. (2007) Induction of tau pathology by intracerebral infusion of amyloid-beta -containing brain extract and by amyloid-beta deposition in APP x Tau transgenic mice. *Am J Pathol* 171: 2012-2020.

[51] Vella LJ, Sharples RA, Lawson VA, Masters CL, Cappai R, et al. (2007) Packaging of prions into exosomes is associated with a novel pathway of PrP processing. *J Pathol* 211: 582-590.

[52] Coleman BM, Hanssen E, Lawson VA, Hill AF (2012) Prion-infected cells regulate the release of exosomes with distinct ultrastructural features. *FASEB J* 26: 4160-4173.

[53] Danzer KM, Kranich LR, Ruf WP, Cagsal-Getkin O, Winslow AR, et al. (2012) Exosomal cell-to-cell transmission of alpha synuclein oligomers. *Mol Neurodegener* 7: 42.

[54] Joshi P, Turola E, Ruiz A, Bergami A, Libera DD, et al. (2014) Microglia convert aggregated amyloid-beta into neurotoxic forms through the shedding of microvesicles. *Cell Death Differ* 21: 582-593.

[55] Victoria GS, Zurzolo C (2015) Trafficking and degradation pathways in pathogenic conversion of prions and prion-like proteins in neurodegenerative diseases. *Virus Res.*

INDEX

#

14-3-3 protein, 2, 5, 6, 8
2N4R human tau, 164

α

α-, β- and γ-secretases, 130
α-7nAChRs, 137
α-synuclein, v, 29, 33, 70, 71, 89, 90, 91, 92, 93, 94, 95, 96, 97, 98, 99, 102, 111, 112, 114, 115, 117, 120, 131, 137, 184, 187, 224, 256, 257, 258
α-synuclein (αsyn), 33, 34, 35, 36, 42, 45

β

β-solenoid, 17, 18, 19, 20, 21, 23, 24

A

AA amyloidosis (AA), 70, 77, 103
activating transcription factor 4 (ATF4), 41, 42, 43, 61
activating transcription factor 6 (ATF6), 40, 42, 43, 58
Adeno-associated virus (AAV), 194
Advanced Photon Source (APS), 18, 24
agyrophilic grain disease, 158, 159, 163, 164
akinetic mutism, 2
Alix [ALG-2 (apoptosis-linked gene 2)-interacting protein X], 133
ALZ17 mice, 135, 164
Alzheimer's disease (AD), vii, viii, 33, 34, 43, 47, 49, 59, 70, 77, 81, 84, 85, 129, 130, 131, 132, 133, 134, 135, 136, 137, 138, 139, 140, 141, 142, 143, 144, 158, 159, 160, 162, 163, 164, 174, 175, 204, 205, 206, 256, 258
Amantadine, 45, 63
AMPA receptor, 134
amyloid fibrils, 15, 16, 17, 24, 25, 26, 27, 33, 73, 81, 92, 96, 104, 105, 106, 111, 113, 119, 121, 123, 125, 153, 157, 181, 188, 213, 215, 217, 223, 260
Amyloid Lateral Sclerosis (ALS), vii, viii, 43, 47, 177, 178, 179, 180, 181, 182, 183, 184, 185, 186, 187, 188, 189, 190, 191, 192, 193, 194, 195, 196, 197, 198, 199, 200, 201, 202, 204, 205, 206, 207, 256, 258, 261
amyloid plaques, 3, 4, 7, 17, 35, 70, 80, 81, 130, 133, 151
amyloid precursor protein (APP), 33, 43, 46, 53, 130, 131, 132, 133, 142, 147, 150, 199, 261
amyloid-β (Aβ), v, 24, 33, 34, 35, 36, 43, 47, 70, 72, 74, 77, 96, 98, 129, 130, 131, 132, 133, 134, 136, 137, 138, 139, 140, 141, 142, 143, 144, 145, 146, 147, 148, 151, 152, 153, 154, 155, 164, 167, 256, 257, 258
anterior neocortical regions, 6
anti-apoptotic molecule Bcl-2, 37
apical dendrites, 7
Aplysia, vi, viii, 211, 237, 238, 239, 242, 243, 244, 245, 246, 247, 248, 250, 252, 253, 258
apolipoprotein E, 34, 53, 168
Argyrophilic Grain Disease (AGD), 135
astrocytes, 130, 135, 137, 138, 139, 148, 151, 152, 153, 196, 199, 202
Ataxia, 4
Aβ 3pyroglutamate-42, 132
Aβ*56, 34
Aβ11-42, 132
Aβ1-40, 132
Aβ1-42, 132
Aβ40, 94, 137, 257
Aβ40 peptide, 94
Aβ42, 134, 137, 139, 140, 143, 257

Aβ-derived diffusible ligand (ADDL), 142

B

BACE1, 43, 48, 60
Bim, 43
blood brain barrier (BBB), 44, 46, 48, 77
bovine spongiform encephalopathy (BSE), 16, 30

C

C57BL/6 mice, 136
C9ORF72, 178, 192, 196, 197, 206
central nervous system (CNS), 44, 45, 46, 48, 49, 199, 260
cerebellar cortex, 4, 5
cerebellum, 4, 5, 7, 8, 10, 130, 206
cerebral amyloid angiopathy (CAA), 130
cerebrospinal fluid (CSF), 2, 5, 8, 34, 49, 139, 164
chameleon, 102, 112, 122, 123, 124
chemokine IL-8, 138
Chinese hamster ovary (CHO) cells, 71
chondroitin sulfate (CS), 58, 65, 69, 74, 78, 105, 250
CHOP, 41, 42, 43
chronic traumatic encephalopathy, 157, 158, 159, 166
chronic wasting disease (CWD), 16, 19, 30
circular dichroism (CD) spectroscopy, 14, 16, 58, 66, 115, 116, 153, 199
ClpB, 215
Compound-B (cpd-B), 44
continuous wave (CW) spectrum, 59, 84, 102, 113, 123, 125, 174
copper, ix, 68, 71, 82, 105, 130, 180, 198, 200, 202
corticobasal degeneration, 150, 158, 159, 162, 163, 164, 168, 170, 173
corticobasal degeneration (CBD), 135, 162
Creutzfeldt-Jakob disease (CJD), 1, 2, 6, 7, 8, 9, 10, 11, 12, 13, 16, 30, 41, 56, 62, 63, 71, 73, 77, 86, 156, 178
cross-β diffraction, 21
^{ctm}PrP, 39, 40
cyclin-dependent kinase-5 (CDK5), 141
cytosolic PrP (cytPrP), 39, 40

D

D^2P^2 database, 90, 93
Dementia with Lewy Bodies (DLB), 34
dermatan sulfate (DS), 65, 69, 70, 80, 100, 122, 124, 146, 202
DJ-1, 35, 100
Doppel (Dpl), 37, 39
Doxycycline, 45, 63

E

EIF2AK3, 43
electroencephalogram (EEG), 2, 5, 6, 8, 63
electron crystallography, 16, 27
electron microscopy, 16, 23, 82, 95, 119, 162, 170, 213
electron paramagnetic resonance (EPR) spectroscopy, 95, 102, 111, 113, 116, 120
electron paramagnetic resonance (EPR) spectroscopy, 24
endoplasmic reticulum (ER), 39, 40, 42, 46, 58, 59, 60, 61, 64, 79, 84, 133, 137, 185, 190, 199, 202, 250, 252, 253
endothelial cells, 138, 140, 151
entorhinal cortex, 6, 129, 132, 142, 152, 164
equatorial diffraction, 15, 18, 19, 21, 22, 23
ER associated degradation (ERAD), 39, 40, 43
ER stress, 39, 40, 42, 46, 58, 59, 60, 61, 64, 185, 199
ESpritz, 90, 100
eukaryotic translation factor-2 (eIF2α), 40, 41, 42, 43, 46, 154
Ewing sarcoma breakpoint region 1 (EWSR1), 191, 197
exosomes, 48, 66, 133, 134, 135, 139, 143, 147, 148, 185, 189, 190, 193, 202, 258, 261
extrapyramidal signs, 2, 4

F

fatal familial insomnia (FFI), 2, 6, 30, 45
fibers, 16, 25, 70, 157, 163, 166
fibril conformation, 111, 120, 140, 162
fibrillation, 55, 84, 96, 101, 105, 106, 107, 108, 111, 112, 118, 119, 121, 126, 127
fibrils, 15, 16, 17, 18, 20, 24, 25, 26, 27, 33, 35, 49, 55, 72, 73, 74, 80, 81, 83, 92, 94, 95, 96, 97, 98, 99, 104, 105, 106, 108, 111, 113, 114, 117, 118, 119, 120, 121, 122, 123, 124, 125, 126, 127, 130, 132, 135, 137, 143, 147, 149, 150, 151, 153, 156, 157, 158, 159, 160, 161, 162, 163, 164, 165, 166, 170, 172, 173, 175, 178, 181, 183, 184, 188, 191, 192, 196, 205, 213, 215, 216, 217, 219, 223, 224, 257, 260, 261
flotillin-1, 133
Flupirtine, 45
Förster resonance transfer fluorescence (FRET), 106, 107, 111, 113

Fourier-transform infrared (FTIR) spectroscopy, 16, 115
frontotemporal dementia (FTD), 178, 206
fused in sarcoma/translocated in liposarcoma (FUS/TLS), 178, 197, 204, 205
FVB mice, 17
fyn kinase, 141

G

glia, 151, 202
gliosis, 2, 29, 40
glucuronic acid (GlcA), 69
glycogen synthase kinase 3β (GSK-3β), 43
glycogen synthase kinase-3beta (GSK3beta), 141
glycosaminoglycans (GAGs), 67, 68, 69, 70, 71, 72, 73, 74, 75, 76
glycosylphosphatidylinositol (GPI) anchor, 19, 30, 39, 68, 71, 79
GSK2606414, 41, 43, 46, 63

H

H/D exchange, 16, 96, 97
HEK cells, 121, 163
heparan sulfate (HS), 69, 70, 71, 72, 73, 74, 75, 198
heparin (Hep), 69, 70, 73, 74, 75, 78
HET-s prions, 16
hexosamine, 68, 69
hexuronic acid, 68, 69
hidden Markov Model algorithm, 187
hnRNPA2B1/A1, 179
Hsp104, 175, 212, 213, 215, 216, 218, 221, 222, 223
hub, 92, 101
human brain microvessel endothelial cells (hBMECs), 140
hyaluronic acid (HA), 27, 69, 107, 123, 144, 201, 203
hydroxypropyl cellulose (HPC), 98, 99

I

iduronic acid (IdoA), 69
IL-1β, 138, 140
IL-6, 138
inositol-requiring enzyme 1 (IRE1), 40, 42, 43
intrinsically disordered protein (IDP), 90
iron, 130
islet amyloid polypeptide (IAPP), 35, 70, 74, 258
ISRIB, 41, 46, 59
IUPred, 90, 93, 100

J

juxtanuclear quality control (JUNQ) pathway, 181

K

keratan sulfate (KS), 24, 61, 69, 86, 101, 154, 173, 196
kuru, 30, 68, 156

L

laminin receptor, 48, 65, 83
Lewy bodies (LB), 34, 90, 155, 170, 199, 207
long-term depression (LTD), 34
long-term potentiation (LTP), 34, 43, 155, 250
low density lipoprotein receptor-related protein 1 (LRP1)/APOE, 72, 83, 134
low-molecular-weight heparin (LMWHep), 67, 68, 73, 75, 76, 77, 78
LRRK2, 35, 65
Luminescent Conjugated Polymers (LCPs), 44
lymphoid organs,, 30

M

mad cow disease, 68
magic angle spinning (MAS), 113
magnetic resonance imaging (MRI), 2, 4, 5, 6, 8, 12, 65
Mahogunin (MGRN1), 40
Manganese, 42
MCP-1, 138
meridional diffraction, 15, 18, 19, 21, 22, 23
MES (mouse embryonic stem) cell line, 90
metabotropic glutamate-5 (mGlu5) receptor, 34
microchamber, 17
microglia, 130, 138, 139, 151, 153, 178, 202, 262
microspongiosis, 5
miRNA, 48, 49, 66, 248
miRNA-22, 248
MM2 cortical subtype, 13
MM2 thalamic subtype, 6
MoSP1, 23
MoSP2, 23
MoSP5, 23
MoSP6, 23
MoSP7, 23
mRNA, 32, 41, 42, 48, 66, 79, 135, 149, 160, 187, 204, 240, 241, 248, 251
multiple system atrophy (MSA), 34, 35

mutlivesicular bodies (MVB), 185
MV2 subtype, 13
MVU subtype, 7, 8
myoclonus, 2, 4, 6, 12

N

NAC region, 92, 118
N-acetylgalactosamine (GalNAc), 69
N-acetylglucosamine (GlcNAc), 69
nasal-brushing, 11
neurofibrillary tangles (NFT), 130, 135
neuronal loss, 2, 5, 6, 29, 34, 38, 42, 47, 49, 141, 164, 166, 173, 174, 187, 204
neurotoxicity, 29, 30, 31, 32, 33, 35, 37, 40, 41, 42, 44, 48, 49, 50, 54, 55, 57, 58, 73, 84, 127, 133, 140, 141, 142, 152, 153, 156, 175, 177, 196, 202, 205, 256, 258, 259
N-Methyl D-Aspartate (NMDA) receptor, 34, 52, 134, 148, 151, 175
NMR spectroscopy, 15, 16, 18, 19, 22, 25, 123
^{ntm}PrP, 39

O

olfactory epithelium, 11, 14
oligodendrocytes, 138
oligomers, vii, 32, 33, 34, 35, 36, 40, 45, 52, 53, 54, 55, 73, 74, 77, 83, 84, 92, 94, 95, 96, 97, 98, 103, 105, 106, 107, 108, 109, 115, 118, 119, 121, 122, 124, 126, 127, 132, 133, 134, 135, 136, 137, 139, 140, 141, 142, 143, 144, 146, 147, 148, 149, 150, 151, 153, 154, 155, 156, 173, 175, 184, 185, 190, 201, 202, 224, 227, 251, 253, 257, 260, 262
olivary nucleus, 6
Orb2, 229, 248, 251, 252, 253

P

P102L mutation, 10, 11, 14
P301S mice, 164, 166
p53, 71, 80, 83, 148, 258, 261
p75NTR (p75 neurotrophin receptor), 134
Parkin, 35
Parkinson's disease (PD), vii, viii, 33, 34, 35, 42, 43, 45, 47, 59, 70, 92, 95, 96, 172, 256, 258
pentosan polysulfate (PPS), 44, 45, 77
pericytes, 138
perivacuolar PrP^{Sc} deposits, 5
phosphorylated eIF2α (p-eIF2α), 40, 41, 42, 43
phosphorylated PERK (p-PERK), 41, 42, 43
phosphotungstate anions (PTA), 17, 18
PINK1, 35
PK-resistant PrP^{Sc}, 3, 32
POM2 antibody, 57
PONDR® VL3, 90
PONDR® VLXT, 90, 93
posttranslational modifications (PTMs), 90, 93
PrDOS, 90, 93, 100
pre-emptive quality control (pQC), 40
prion domain (PrD), 213, 215, 218, 220, 222, 223, 227, 228
prion protein gene (*PRNP*), 2, 11, 14, 26, 30, 32, 48, 56, 85
prion-like, 67, 68, 70, 80, 83, 89, 129, 131, 134, 135, 136, 137, 138, 139, 140, 144, 145, 150, 157, 159, 160, 161, 177, 178, 179, 181, 182, 183, 186, 187, 188, 189, 190, 191, 192, 193, 194, 197, 205, 206, 209, 210, 211, 212, 213, 217, 219, 222, 243, 244, 245, 247, 249, 250, 252, 255, 256, 258, 260, 262
pro-apoptotic stimuli Bax, 37
progressive supranuclear palsy, 60, 150, 158, 159, 163, 168
Progressive Supranuclear Palsy (PSP), 135, 152
Proteasome, 61, 153, 206
protein kinase RNA (PKR)-like ER kinase (PERK), 37, 40, 41, 42, 43, 46, 48, 59, 60, 63
protein-protein interaction networks (PPI), 92
proteoglycans (PGs), 68, 70, 73, 74, 77
protofibrils, 33, 34, 36, 55, 103, 118, 126, 171, 201
PrP 27-30, 10, 11, 15, 16, 17, 18, 19, 20, 23, 24, 71
PrP peptides, 21, 25
PrP^C, 16, 22, 29, 30, 31, 32, 33, 34, 35, 36, 37, 38, 39, 45, 46, 47, 48, 64, 67, 68, 70, 71, 72, 73, 74, 75, 82, 134, 142, 155, 178, 186, 255, 256
PrP^{Sc}, 1, 2, 3, 4, 5, 6, 7, 8, 9, 10, 11, 15, 16, 17, 18, 19, 20, 22, 23, 24, 25, 29, 30, 31, 32, 33, 34, 36, 37, 39, 40, 41, 44, 45, 46, 47, 48, 51, 52, 58, 64, 65, 68, 70, 71, 72, 73, 74, 75, 76, 82, 83, 129, 131, 178, 186, 189, 210, 211, 221, 249, 256, 257, 258
PrP^{Sc} glycotypes, 2, 3, 8, 9
PrP^{Sc} glycotyping, 2
PubMed, 74
PV2, 90, 93
pyramidal signs, 11

Q

Quinacrine, 44, 45, 61, 62

R

rabies virus glycoprotein (RVG), 48
Real-time quaking induced conversion (RT-QuIC), 11, 14, 73, 76
recombinant PrP, 19, 20, 22, 78
RNAi, 47, 48, 65
RONN, 90, 93, 100
ROS, 37, 137, 138

S

SALS, 178, 179, 180, 181, 185, 187, 192
SAXS, 118
scrapie, 19, 25, 49, 50, 64, 84
seed(s), 73, 75, 76, 83, 98, 103, 105, 118, 129, 131, 132, 133, 135, 137, 138, 139, 140, 142, 143, 144, 146, 147, 148, 152, 155, 162, 163, 164, 172, 183, 190, 191, 202, 205, 224
sensitivity, 11, 49, 182, 218, 220
serotonin, 237, 240, 248, 250
serum amyloid A (SAA), 70, 77
shRNA, 47, 48
SH-SY5Y cells, 134, 163
single chain Fv fragment, 37
siRNA, 47, 48, 66
skeletal muscle, 30
smooth muscle cells, 138, 148
SNCA gene, 112
solid-state NMR, 18, 19, 22, 25, 104, 105, 113, 116, 117, 119, 120, 121, 123, 126
spleen, 30, 62
spongiform changes, 1, 2, 5, 7, 8, 11
sporadic CJD (sCJD), 1, 2, 3, 4, 5, 6, 8, 9, 10, 11
sporadic fatal insomnia (sFI), 6
SSLOW, 23
Stanford Synchrotron Radiation Laboratory (SSRL), 18, 24
STRING (Search Tool for the Retrieval of Interacting Genes), 90
Sup35 amyloid fibrils, 16
superoxide dismutase (SOD1), 43, 60, 65, 178, 179, 180, 181, 182, 183, 184, 185, 186, 187, 188, 189, 190, 191, 192, 193, 194, 196, 197, 198, 199, 200, 201, 202, 204, 206, 256, 257, 258, 261
wynthetic prions, 259
synucleinopathies, 109
Syrian hamsters (SHa), 17, 19, 257

T

tangle-only dementia, 158, 159, 164, 168
TAR-DNA binding protein 43 (TDP-43), 43, 61, 94, 103, 178, 179, 187, 188, 189, 190, 191, 192, 193, 194, 196, 197, 203, 204, 205, 206, 207, 258
TATA-binding protein associated factor 15 (TAF15), 191, 197
tau, v, 8, 14, 26, 43, 53, 60, 70, 71, 81, 94, 96, 101, 103, 105, 109, 129, 130, 131, 132, 133, 134, 135, 136, 137, 138, 139, 140, 141, 142, 143, 144, 145, 148, 149, 150, 151, 152, 153, 154, 155, 156, 157, 158, 159, 160, 161, 162, 163, 164, 165, 166, 167, 168, 169, 170, 171, 172, 173, 174, 175, 176, 185, 187, 203, 256, 257, 258, 260, 261
tauopathies, 43, 60, 134, 136, 150, 152, 157, 158, 159, 160, 161, 163, 164, 167, 169, 170, 173, 176, 261
TDP-43, 43, 61, 94, 103, 178, 179, 187, 188, 189, 190, 191, 192, 193, 194, 196, 197, 203, 204, 205, 206, 207, 258
thioflavin T, 20, 210
TNF-α, 138
transmissible mink encephalopathy (TME), 18, 19
transmissible spongiform encephalopathies (TSEs), 1, 30, 68, 70, 71, 77, 143, 210
trimethylamine oxide (TMAO), 94
tunnelling nanotubes (TNTs), 133, 136, 137, 143
two-dimensional electrophoresis (2D-PAGE), 8, 9
type II diabete, 35, 70

U

ubiquitin/proteasome system (UPS), 36, 55
unfolded protein response (UPR), 40, 41, 42, 43, 44, 46, 141, 181

V

variant CJD (vCJD), 6, 30, 77
voltage-gated sodium channels, 134
VSL2, 90, 93
VV1 subtype, 8

W

withdrawal reflex, 238, 239, 247

X

X-ray crystallography, x, 15, 16, 92, 95
X-ray fiber diffraction, 15, 16, 17, 18, 19, 21, 22, 23, 24, 25, 258
X-ray scattering, 118

Y

Yeast, vi, 104, 188, 209, 210, 211, 213, 215, 217, 227, 230, 232, 234, 235, 236, 251
YFP reporter, 186